DOPPLER ECHOCARDIOGRAPHY

DOPPLER ECHOCARDIOGRAPHY

Stanley J. Goldberg M.D.

Professor of Pediatrics (Cardiology)

Hugh D. Allen M.D.

Professor of Pediatrics (Cardiology)

Gerald R. Marx M.D.

Associate Professor of Pediatrics (Cardiology)

Richard L. Donnerstein B.S.E.E., M.D.

Assistant Professor of Pediatrics (Cardiology)

Department of Pediatrics
University of Arizona
Health Sciences Center
Tucson, Arizona

Second Edition

LEA & FEBIGER   *Philadelphia*

1988

Lea & Febiger
600 Washington Square
Philadelphia, PA   19106-4198
U.S.A.
(215) 922-1330

First Edition, 1985

Library of Congress Cataloging-in-Publication Data

Doppler echocardiography.

1. Doppler echocardiography.   2. Heart—Diseases—
Diagnosis.   I. Goldberg, Stanley.   [DNLM: 1. Echo-
cardiography.   WG 141.5.E2 D6921]
RC683.5.U5D673   1988   616.1′207′543   87-22839
ISBN 0-8121-1106-0

PRINTED IN THE UNITED STATES OF AMERICA

Print number: 5   4   3   2   1

*To our families
who tolerated our many hours away from them
to write this book*

PREFACE

Doppler is now an accepted means of cardiac evaluation. Clinical acceptance, however, took over a decade. Our involvement occurred after we listened to a paper presented at the American College of Cardiology in 1973 by Dr. Johnson from the University of Washington. This paper was the first that we had heard regarding the use of Doppler interfaced with echocardiography. We thought that the potential for this type of evaluation was enormous. Until that time, the cardiologist had no direct noninvasive means for evaluating flow. We had a series of meetings, one on the back of a ferry boat departing Seattle, with Ralph Astengo, then President of Advanced Technology Laboratories. Mr. Astengo was developing a commercial instrument similar to the one Johnson had used. We were finally able to acquire that instrument two years later. Before leaving Seattle with our new instrument, we spent a productive and memorable day with Drs. Stevenson and Rubenstein, who taught us how to use the machine. We quickly became aware that many important contributions to Doppler knowledge had already been made, but only a few were in the American literature. Over the next several years, we conducted, presented, and published a number of investigations and through these had the opportunity to meet some of the true pioneers of Doppler, including Drs. Kalmanson, Peronneau, Light, Edler, and Mr. Baker, Mr. Brandestini, and Mr. Suskind.

The group of individuals performing clinical Doppler examinations and investigations remained relatively static and limited over the next few years. In 1978, our group and the group at Irvine acted as consultants to Honeywell for the construction of the first commercially available FFT analyzed pulsed Doppler system. Even though this machine became commercially available in 1979, the level of interest regarding Doppler in the United States still remained relatively low. At this time, in Norway, Drs. Hatle, Holen, Angelsen and their co-workers began publishing their remarkable observations regarding measurement of pressure drop by Doppler. Dr. Angelsen visited us and convinced us of the importance of pressure drop analysis. Clearly, Doppler was going to become important. By this time we had gathered enough clinical experience with Doppler echo to recognize its application and usefulness. With great trepidation, we decided to hold our first Doppler echo course in Los Angeles in 1982. Our goal was to attempt to increase the general clinical interest level in Doppler. We were surprised to see the large response; many interested cardiologists attended. The remainder of the story is relatively well known. Doppler became a major technique in cardiology, and now, at the end of 1987, this technique is used world-wide in most hospitals that treat cardiac patients. We have greatly appreciated the opportunity to participate in some of the development of Doppler echocardiography.

The first edition of this textbook was written in 1983 and was published in the summer of 1984. Our goal in the first edition was to provide the basic information necessary to incorporate Doppler cardiac examination with the echocardiographic examination for individuals who were already able to perform and interpret two-dimensional echocardiography. We attempted to provide the information in a readable form and decided to forego deep mathematical discussions of Doppler physics. In this second edition, we have attempted to considerably update the information in the first edition, to maintain readability and lucidity, and to catalog as much updated information as practical. Although we have attempted to be relatively inclusive in acknowledging the work of our colleagues, we recognize that we may have missed a favorite reference or even a publication authored by a reader. We apologize in advance for these omissions.

We would like to acknowledge the assistance we have received from so many different investigators, clinicians, and industrial representatives. Further we would like to acknowledge those individuals who have worked directly with us including Zoe Kececioglu-Draelos, Cleo Loeber, Susan Vasko, Jay Requarth, Heinz Hoeneke, Marcy Schwartz, Neil Wilson, David Dickinson, Olive Scott, Volkert deVilleneuve, Jose Areias, Ehud Grenadier, Teddy Hegesh, Halim Wahdan, Demetrio Kosturakis, Carlos Oliveira Lima, and Jesus Vargas Barron. Two individuals in the industrial world, Wayne Moore and James Gessert, have been of great assistance to us over the years. Finally, we would like to acknowledge the contributions made by our prior associates, Drs. Valdes-Cruz, Sahn and Flinn, and our present associates and co-authors, Drs. Gerald Marx and Richard Donnerstein. Although Drs. Marx and Donnerstein began their Doppler work a bit later, their backgrounds, research and capability in the field have provided us with immeasurable assistance.

Tucson, Arizona   Stanley J. Goldberg
                                                         Hugh D. Allen

CONTENTS

CHAPTER 1

HISTORY OF DOPPLER ECHOCARDIOGRAPHY

An Austrian professor of mathematics and geometry, Johann Christian Doppler (1803–1853), is generally credited with the initial description of what has come to be known as the "Doppler effect." His article, published in 1842,[1] established the relationship of frequency shift to velocity. Dr. Doppler applied the principle to shifts in red light from double stars (Fig. 1–1), but not directly to sound. Changes in light were used to track motion of celestial objects. This concept has since been used extensively in astronomy. Later in that same decade, Dr. Bays Ballot applied this principle to sound.

Following the Second World War, many scientific developments were put to peace-time use. Present cardiac applications of the Doppler principle could probably not have been realized as soon without the contributions of the many individuals who developed radar and sonar circuitry and concepts during the war. Early ultrasonic and Doppler machines were mainly adapted from military use.

Satomura first reported cardiac evaluation using the Doppler principle.[2] Accordingly, the first Doppler cardiac evaluation followed the initial imaging work by Edler[3] by only 2 years. During the next several years, the Doppler principle was utilized extensively for monitoring blood flow in animals using implanted Doppler transducers.[4–6] Although this initial work is far removed from present noninvasive Doppler application, much theoretical work and ordering of knowledge occurred in this early phase. The invasive techniques developed by Franklin,[6] Baker[7] and Rushmer[8] were eventually extended to humans.[9]

During the early phases of Doppler investigation a symbiotic relationship developed between industry and physicians. Although relationships exist in pharmaceutical, appliance and other medical electronic industries, this relationship in Doppler was perhaps closer and more interdependent than most others.

During the latter portion of the 1960s, Doppler was transformed into a noninvasive modality and was used by several investigative groups, including those led by Edler,[10] Kalmanson,[11,12] and Peronneau[13] but the invasive phase was reintroduced in 1972 by Benchimol and co-workers who utilized a catheter tip Doppler transducer to monitor velocities during the course of cardiac catheterization.[9] Doppler, however, could not become a major modality until a commercial instrument was available. Combined expertise of Donald Baker (University of Washington) and Ralph Astengo (president of a then fledgling Doppler

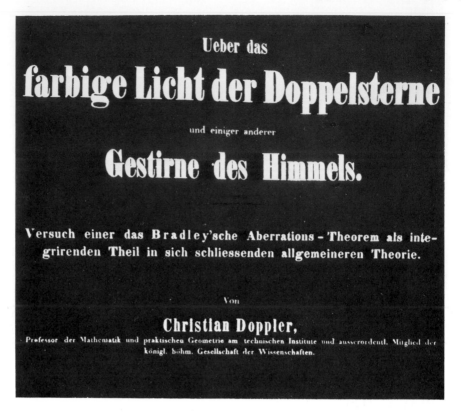

Ueber das

farbige Licht der Doppelsterne

und einiger anderer

Gestirne des Himmels.

Versuch einer das Bradley'sche Aberrations-Theorem als inte-
grirenden Theil in sich schliessenden allgemeineren Theorie.

Von

Christian Doppler,

Professor der Mathematik und praktischen Geometrie am technischen Institute und ausserordentl. Mitglied der
königl. böhm. Gesellschaft der Wissenschaften.

Fig. 1–1. Photographic reproduction of the cover page of Dr. Doppler's article published in 1842.

company, Advanced Technology Laboratories), resulted in the first commercial Doppler instrumentation in 1975–76. This instrument offered the first opportunity for the cardiologist who had no electronic development laboratory to experiment with pulsed Doppler. This instrument, however, had a serious problem: frequency shift was analyzed by a time interval histographic method which was an alinear analysis process. Although information could be gained regarding direction and, to some extent, flow disturbance, most signals could not be recorded accurately. For this reason the audio signal alone was utilized for most analyses. The prototype of this instrumentation was used by Johnson[14] at the University of Washington for an early clinical study which included "localization of cardiac murmurs" in the title. This title was unfortunate because many cardiologists confused Doppler with the then popular electronic stethoscope. Early cardiac Doppler investigators spent much time convincing audiences that Doppler and electronic stethoscopy were different.

Color Doppler had its origins at approximately the same time. Brandestini, working in Zurich, developed a multi-channel Doppler system which could be utilized to encode directional velocities onto an echocardiographic image by representing the velocities in a color code.[15] This aspect will be discussed separately later.

Although a few cardiac Doppler studies were published in the subsequent several years, further development had to wait until 1976–78, years which proved to be extremely important ones for Doppler. A remarkable observation by Holen and associates in 1976 laid the cornerstone for development of pressure drop measurement by continuous wave Doppler.[16] Hatle and co-workers developed the principles espoused by Holen et al. into an important clinical tool.[17–18] During these same years, Stevenson, from the University of Washington, published several important qualitative clinical papers regarding detection of congenital lesions including patent ductus,[19] mitral regurgitation,[20] and ventricular septal defects.[21] That group used the audio signal almost exclusively for analysis in each of these studies. At approximately the same time, Goldberg and co-workers published a series of papers demonstrating that analysis of the time interval histogram alone could be utilized to qualitatively assess the presence or absence of cardiac defects.[22–24]

In 1978, Gessert and Taylor, working for Honeywell, made a major technologic breakthrough by combining two-dimensional echocardiography with fast Fourier analysis of the pulsed Doppler signal. This combination provided linear signal analysis and a convenient method for pulsed Doppler sample volume placement by two-dimensional echocardiographic guidance. Although the time was ripe for development of clinical Doppler echocardiography, general clinical usage did not start until approximately 1982. Since that time Doppler has been incorporated into cardiac ultrasonic examinations on a regular basis in many noninvasive laboratories.

Several distinct subareas have now developed in Doppler and include estimation of cardiac output and pressure drop, and color velocity coding. Each of these areas have a separate history and each will be discussed individually.

CARDIAC OUTPUT

One early promise of Doppler was that cardiac output could be measured noninvasively and accurately. Theory suggested that flow could be computed by multiplying the mean velocity times the area through which that velocity passed. However, several factors clouded early development of accurate measurements of cardiac output. These factors included (1) linear Doppler signal analysis; (2) appropriate interrogation of the aorta prior to its branching; (3) development of a convenient methodology for determining mean velocity; and (4) accuracy in determination of the flow area.

Light and colleagues published a series of reports[25–26] demonstrating a method for interrogation of the aorta by continuous wave Doppler and computation of a velocity integral which was proportional to blood flow. They reported a reasonable correlation between cardiac output measured by Doppler and by electromagnetic flow catheters and indicator dilution and termed the Doppler method "transcutaneous aortovelography." Although this name never gained popularity, the general methodology was adopted by other investigators.[27–29] Their method, however, did not solve many of the problems of cardiac output measurement. Specifically, at that early date, vessel area was difficult to measure noninvasively, the aorta was not studied prior to branching, and a simple method for determination of mean velocity was not available.

The next important event occurred in 1978 when Griffith and Henry,[30] using pulsed Doppler with true spectral analysis and two-dimensional echocardiography, reported results from 20 human subjects. Although the form of spectral analysis was accurate, it provided information in a manner that was difficult to interpret and their output results were not compared to any standard cardiac output measurements. Later, Magnin et al.[31] studied pulsed Doppler cardiac outputs using a nonlinear zero crossing detector and compared results to Fick outputs. They demonstrated a favorable correlation, but the slope and intercept of the relationship were unfavorable, perhaps as the result of erroneous alinear processing of the frequency shift by the zero crossing detector. Shortly thereafter Goldberg and co-workers[32] reported results of simultaneous outputs derived by green dye indicator dilution and pulsed Doppler analyzed by fast Fourier transform. The result was a high correlation between invasive and Doppler output with a standard error of the estimate of about 500 ml. Standard error of the estimate is a descriptor of the measurement variability. Many subsequent studies have demonstrated similar correlations, slopes, intercepts, and standard errors of the estimate.

Since these early studies, newer methodologies have been used to measure aortic output. A most important early addition to the equipment of investigators of volumetric flow was development of an off-axis transducer (Honeywell 1981) which allows imaging down the axis of the ascending aorta. This transducer eliminated any appreciable intercept angle between flow and beam direction. Further, the transducer provided simultaneous imaging of the ascending aorta in the precise area of velocity measurement. Another important development was a simple microcomputer program for off line computation of mean velocity and cardiac output (Biodata Co., 1981). This program combined with a micro-computer of the Apple II series allowed an inexpensive method of computing mean velocity. More recently, non-imaging continuous wave Doppler directed from the suprasternal notch has been used to measure cardiac output, and reasonable correlations with invasive flows have been obtained.[33]

Flow has also been measured distal to other valves. Pulmonary diameter was difficult to measure by imaging echocardiography.[32] This problem was over-come by positioning the patient into a marked left decubitus position which allowed improved imaging of the pulmonary artery.[34] Pulmonary flow meas-urements by Doppler with this minor methodologic revision now also provides accurate measurements.

Mitral flow quantitation has continued to represent a significant problem for Doppler echocardiography. The mitral orifice is noncircular, and distal to the orifice leaflet separation changes during the diastolic phase. An early report by Fisher et al.[35] suggested a method to correct measured annulus size for diastolic leaflet separation that worked well in dogs, but human application gave less favorable results.[34] Lewis et al.[36] reported an improved relationship with invasive flows by utilizing a round orifice approximation. An elliptical orifice technique appeared to further improve results.[37]

The currently utilized tricuspid flow measurement technique was originally reported almost simultaneously by Loeber et al.[34] and Meijboom et al.[38] Both groups used a circular approximation for tricuspid valve orifice and achieved high correlations of flow measured by Doppler and by invasive techniques.

PRESSURE DROP MEASUREMENTS

The landmark investigation in pressure drop was presented in a paper by Holen and co-workers in 1976.[16] This initial but definitive work demonstrated that simultaneously measured pressure drops across the mitral valve by manometry and by Doppler ultrasound were highly correlated. Further, the investigators demonstrated an orderly time course of pressure drop by Doppler as compared to that measured by manometry. All later studies emanate from this single investigation. A followup study by the same group[39] demonstrated that the effective orifice area in mitral stenosis could be computed by adapting the Gorlin equation to Doppler. Subsequent studies demonstrated that Doppler could also compute the effective flow area of prosthetic valves.[40] Slightly after Holen et al. developed the method for estimating pressure drop by Doppler, Hatle et al.[41] published data regarding pressure drop in mitral stenosis. Careful analysis of this work shows that their results were generally similar to those of Holen, but perhaps because she published these results in a more widely read journal, or perhaps because these results confirmed previously published work, the Doppler method for pressure drop determinations became accepted in the cardiology community. Hatle and co-workers followed up their initial work on the mitral valve by demonstrating that gradients in aortic stenosis could also be measured by continuous wave Doppler.[42] Perhaps this paper had an even greater impact than the mitral valve publication because noninvasive assessment of aortic stenosis was more difficult than noninvasive assessment of mitral stenosis at that time. Hatle and co-workers later demonstrated that pulmonary artery pressure could be estimated by Doppler using the Burstin nomogram[43] and that mitral orifice areas could be approximated by a simpler application of the pressure half-time principle.[44] Most subsequent studies have been merely confirmation of the earlier work by Holen and Hatle and their co-workers. Perhaps the factor which most initiated increased awareness of the role of Doppler in pressure drop estimation was publication of the first clinical book in Doppler echocardiography by Hatle and Angelsen.[45]

COLOR-CODED VELOCITY MAPPING ON A TWO-DIMENSIONAL IMAGE

Most information regarding this qualitative technique has been published only in abstract form and is thus somewhat difficult to evaluate. The earliest paper[15] of which we are aware was published by Brandestini, who described a multi-channel digital Doppler system. Clearly, once additional channels were possible, velocity could be encoded by direction and magnitude. Such an instrument was built and was used initially by Stevenson.[46] This system permitted color velocity coding of an M-mode signal. Somewhat later Kitabatake[47] published results utilizing an expanded two-dimensional version of the instrument. Namekawa[48] published methodology for analyzing velocity by auto correlation. Much of the early work regarding color-coded velocity mapping was in the Japanese literature and frequently in abstract form. Perhaps the most important contribution which led to popularizing the technique was a book edited by Omoto which both detailed the theory and demonstrated the technique.[49] Since publication of the book, a considerable number of reports, again mainly in abstract form, began to become available. This technology, which is now almost 10 years old, is only now becoming more integrated into the general Doppler examination.

Doppler has already had a relatively long history, 30 years at the time of this summarization. Most major developments occurred prior to 1978, a time before Doppler was even recognized as a useful entity by most cardiologists. It seems obvious that additional noteworthy development will occur during the next few years and that Doppler will find its rightful place amongst other noninvasive modalities.

REFERENCES

1. Doppler, C.J.: Uber das farbige Licht der Doppelsterne. Abhandlungen der Koniglishen Bohmischen Gesellschaft der Wissenchaften. *11*:465, 1842.
2. Satomura, S.: A study on examining the heart with ultrasonics. I. Principles; II. Instrument. Jpn Circ J *20*:227, 1956.
3. Edler, I., Hertz, C.H.: Use of ultrasonic reflectoscope for continuous recording of movements of heart walls. Kung Fysiograf Sallsk Lund Fordhandl *24*:40, 1954.
4. Van Citters, R.L., Evonuk, E., Franklin, D.L.: Blood flow distribution in Alaska Sled dogs during extended exercise. Physiologist *9*:310, 1966.
5. Franklin, D.L., Van Citters, R.L., Watson, N.W.: Applications of telemetry to measurement of blood flow and pressure in unrestrained animals. Proceedings of the National Telemetry Conference 1965, pp. 233–234.
6. Franklin, D.L., Schlegal, W., Rushmer, R.F.: Blood flow measured by Doppler frequency shift of backscattered ultrasound. Science *134*:564, 1961.
7. Baker, D.W., Watkins, D.W.: A phase coherent pulsed Doppler system for cardiovascular measurement. Proc 20th ACEMB, *27*:2, 1967.
8. Rushmer, R.F., Baker, D.W., Johnson, W.L., Strandness, D.E.: Clinical applications of a transcutaneous ultrasonic flow detector. JAMA *199*:325, 1967.
9. Benchimol, A., Desser, K.B., Gartlan, J.: Bidirectional blood flow velocity in the cardiac chambers and great vessels studied with the Doppler ultrasonic flowmeter. Am J Med *52*:467, 1972.
10. Edler, I., Lindstrom, K.: Ultrasonic Doppler technique used in heart disease—I. An experimental study. Ultrasono Graphia Medica Separatum. 1st World Congress on Ultrasonic Diagnosis in Medicine and SIDUO III. Edited by Bock, J., Ossoinig, K. Vienna, Verlag der Wiener Medizinischen Akademia, 1969, p. 455.
11. Kalmanson, D., Toutain, G., Novikoff, N., Derai C., Chiche, P. Gabrol, C.: Le catheterisme velocimetrique du coeur et des gros vaisseaux pour sonde ultrasonique directionnelle a effet Doppler. Rapport Preliminaire. Ann Med Interne *120*:685, 1969.
12. Kalmanson, D., Veyrat C., Chiche, P.: Atrial versus ventricular contribution in determining systolic venous return. Cardiovasc Res *5*:293, 1971.
13. Peronneau, P., Hinglais, H., Pellet, M., Leger, F.: Velocimetre sanguin par effect Doppler a' emission ultras-sonore pulsee L'onde Electrique *59*:369, 1970.
14. Johnson, S.L., Baker, D.W., Lute, R.A., Dodge, H.T.: Doppler echocardiography. The localization of cardiac murmurs. Circulation *48*:810, 1973.
15. Brandestini, M.A., Eyer, M.K., Stevenson, J.G.: M/Q-mode echocardiography—the synthesis of conventional echo with digital multigate Doppler. *In* Echocardiology, edited by Lancee C. The Hague, Martinus Nijhoff, 1979, p. 441.
16. Holen, J., Aaslid, R., Landmark, K., Simonsen, S.: Determination of pressure gradient in mitral stenosis with a noninvasive ultrasound Doppler technique. Acta Med Scand *199*:455, 1976.
17. Hatle, L., Brubakk, A., Tromsdal, A., Angelsen, B.: Noninvasive assessment of pressure drop in mitral stenosis by Doppler ultrasond. Br Heart J *40*:131, 1978.
18. Hatle, L.: Noninvasive assessment and differentiation of left ventricular outflow obstruction by Doppler ultrasound. Circulation *64*:381, 1981.
19. Stevenson, J.G., Dooley, T.K., Kawabori, I.: Patent ductus arteriosus in a neonatal intensive care unit: Utility of pulsed Doppler echocardiography. Circulation *58*:110, 1978.
20. Stevenson, J.G., Kawabori, I., Guntheroth, W.G.: Differentiation of ventricular septal defect from mitral regurgitation by pulsed Doppler echocardiography. Circulation *56*:14, 1977.
21. Stevenson, J.G., Kawabori, I., Dooley, T., Guntheroth, W.G.: Diagnosis of ventricular septal defect by pulsed Doppler echocardiography. Sensitivity, specificity and limitations. Circulation *58*:322, 1979.
22. Areias, J.C., Goldberg, S.J., Spitaels, S.E., de Villeneuve, V.H.: An evaluation of range gated pulsed Doppler echocardiography for detecting pulmonary outflow tract obstruction in d-transposition of the great vessels. Am Heart J *96*:467, 1978.
23. Goldberg, S.J., Areias, J., Spitaels, S.E.C., de Villeneuve, V.H.: Use of time interval histographic output from echo Doppler to detect left-to-right atrial shunts. Circulation *58*:147, 1978.
24. Goldberg, S.J., Areias, J.C., Spitaels, S.E.C., de Villeneuve, V.H.: Echo Doppler detection of pulmonary stenosis by time-interval histogram analysis. J Clin Ultrasound *7*:183, 1979.
25. Light, H.: Transcutaneous aortovelography—a new window on the circulation? Br Heart J *38*:433, 1976.
26. Light, L.H., Closs, G., Hansen, P.L., Brotherhood, J. Hanson, G.C., Peisach, A.R., Sequeira, R.F.: *In* Clinical Blood Flow Measurement, edited by Woodcock, Bath, Pitman, 1974.

27. Colocousis, J.S., Huntsman, L.L., Curreri, P.W.: Estimation of stroke volume changes by ultrasonic Doppler. Circulation *56*:914, 1977.
28. Huntsman, L.L., Gams, E., Johnson, C.C., Fairbanks, E.: Transcutaneous determination of aortic blood flow velocities in man. Am Heart J, *89*:605, 1975.
29. Sequeira, R.F., Light, L.H., Cross, G, Raftery, E.B.: Transcutaneous aortovelography. A quantitative evaluation. Br Heart J *38*:443, 1976.
30. Griffith, J.M., Henry, W.L.: An ultrasound system for combined cardiac imaging and Doppler blood flow measurement in man. Circulation *57*:925, 1978.
31. Magnin, P.A., Stewart, J.A., Myers, S., von Ramm, O., Kisslo, J.A.: Combined Doppler and phased array echocardiographic estimation of cardiac output. Circulation *63*:388, 1981.
32. Goldberg, S.J., Sahn, D.J., Allen, H.D., Valdes-Cruz, L.M., Hoenecke, H., Carnahan, Y.: Evaluation of pulmonary and systemic blood flow by two-dimensional Doppler echocardiography using fast Fourier transform spectral analysis. Am J Cardiol *50*:1394, 1982.
33. Huntsman, L.L., Stewart, D.K., Barnes, S.R., Franklin, S.B., Colocousis, J.S., Hessel, E.A.: Noninvasive Doppler determination of cardiac output in man: Clinical validation. Circulation *67*:593, 1983.
34. Loeber, C.P., Goldberg, S.J., Allen, H.D.: Doppler echocardiographic comparison of flows distal to the four cardiac valves. J Am Coll Cardiol *4*:268, 1984.
35. Fisher, D.C., Sahn, D.J., Friedman, M.J., Larson, D., Valdes-Cruz, L.M., Horowitz, S., Goldberg, S.J., Allen, H.D.: The mitral valve orifice method for noninvasive two-dimensional echo Doppler determination of cardiac output. Circulation *67*:872, 1983.
36. Lewis, J., Kuo, L., Nelson, J. Limacher, M., Quinones, M.: Pulsed Doppler echocardiographic determination of stroke volume and cardiac output: Clinical validation of two new methods using the apical window. Circulation *70*:425, 1984.
37. Goldberg, S.J., Dickinson, D.F., Wilson, N., Scott, O.: Evaluation of an elliptical area technique for calculating mitral flow by Doppler echocardiography. Br Heart J *54*:68, 1985.
38. Meijboom, E.J., Horowitz, S., Valdes-Cruz, L.M., Sahn, D.J., Larson, D.F., Lima, C.O.: A Doppler echocardiographic method for calculating volume across the tricuspid valve: Correlative laboratory and clinical studies. Circulation *71*:551, 1985.
39. Holen, J., Aaslid, R., Landmark, K., Simonsen, S.: Determination of effective orifice area in mitral stenosis from noninvasive ultrasound Doppler data and mitral flow rate. Acta Med Scand *201*:83, 1977.
40. Holen, J., Nitter-Hauge, S.: Evaluation of obstructive characteristics of mitral disc valve implants with ultrasound Doppler techniques. Acta Med Scand *201*:429, 1977.
41. Hatle, L., Brubakk, A., Tromsdal, A., Angelsen, B.: Noninvasive assessment of pressure drop in mitral stenosis by Doppler ultrasound. Br Heart J *40*:131, 1978.
42. Hatle, L.: Noninvasive assessment and differentiation of left ventricular outflow obstruction by Doppler ultrasound. Circulation *64*:381, 1981.
43. Hatle, L., Angelsen, B.A.J., Tromsdal, A.: Noninvasive estimation of pulmonary artery systolic pressure with Doppler ultrasound. Br Heart J *45*:157, 1981.
44. Hatle, L., Angelsen, B., Tromsdal, A.: Noninvasive assessment of atrioventricular pressure half-time by Doppler ultrasound. Circulation *60*:1096, 1979.
45. Hatle, L., Angelsen, B.: Doppler Ultrasound in Cardiology. Physical Principles and Clinical Applications. 1st Ed. Philadelphia, Lea & Febiger, 1982; 2nd Ed., 1985.
46. Stevenson, J.G., Kawabori, I., Brandestini, M.A.: A twenty-month experience comparing conventional pulsed Doppler echocardiography and color coded digital multigate Doppler for detection of atrioventricular valve regurgitation and its severity. In: Rijsterborgh H Echocardiology. The Hague, Martinus Nijhoff, 1981.
47. Kitabatake, K., Inoue, M, Asao, M., et al.: Non-invasive visualization of intracardiac blood flow in human heart using computer-aided pulsed Doppler technique. Clinical Hemorheology, *1*:85, 1982.
48. Namekawa, K., Kasai, C., Tsukamoto, M., Koyano, A.: Imaging of blood flow using autocorrelation. Ultrasound Med Biol *8*:138, 1982.
49. Omoto, R.: Color Atlas of Real-Time Two-Dimensional Doppler Echocardiography. 1st Ed. Tokyo, Shindan-To-Chiryo, 1984; 2nd Ed., 1987.

CHAPTER 2

DOPPLER PHYSICS FOR PHYSICIANS AND TECHNOLOGISTS

Doppler echocardiography and imaging echocardiography share many physical properties, but certain differences also exist. When the echocardiographer looks at a diagnostic image, knowledge of the physics of how that image was obtained is, in most instances, of little importance. On the other hand, when an examiner looks at a velocity tracing, knowledge of the specific techniques utilized to obtain that tracing is important. Most cardiologists and technologists do not have an extensive background in physics. Accordingly, the purpose of this chapter is to present a nonmathematical approach to the essential physical concepts of Doppler. Readers who wish to delve more deeply into theoretical and mathematical considerations are referred to other publications.[1,2]

THE DOPPLER PRINCIPLE

The Doppler principle, as defined by J. Christian Doppler,[3] states that an apparent shift in transmitted frequency occurs as a result of motion of either the source or the target. Everyday examples of the Doppler principle are numerous. One example occurs when a stationary individual is approached by an automobile which is sounding its horn. As the automobile approaches the stationary individual, the pitch of the horn increases (higher frequency), and when the automobile moves away from the individual, the pitch of the horn decreases (lower frequency). This is only an apparent change in frequency, because the transmitted pitch of the horn remained constant. Nonetheless, the individual heard a change in pitch during passage of the automobile. The change in pitch (also called frequency) is directly proportional to velocity of the vehicle. This example differs somewhat from use of Doppler in cardiology, for in cardiology, the source, the transducer, remains stationary, and the target, blood cells, are in motion. Numerous other applications of the Doppler principle in astronomy, aviation, and burglar alarms are in common usage today.

FREQUENCY

Frequency defines the number of times an event occurs per unit time. For ultrasound purposes, the unit of frequency is cycles per second, and one cycle/second = 1 Hertz (Hz). Frequencies presently utilized in ultrasound range from 1 to 10 megahertz (1MHz = 1 million cycles/sec). These frequencies are far in excess of the audible range, which extends from 40 to approximately 15,000

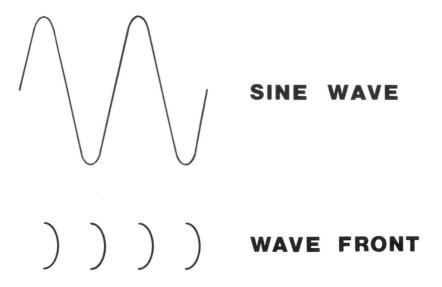

Fig. 2–1. Two cycles of a sine wave. For purposes of illustration, sine waves in the remaining figures will be represented as wavefronts.

Hertz. Doppler ultrasound frequency ranges are similar to those used for imaging echocardiography.

Figure 2–1 demonstrates a sinusoidal waveform. A sinusoidal waveform is one that constantly changes amplitude and periodically reverses direction. In order to simplify figures in this chapter, each peak and nadir will be presented by a simple curved line, as shown below the sine wave in Figure 2–1. As frequency increases, curved lines will be closer together, and as frequency decreases, the curved lines will be further apart.

TRANSDUCER

Ultrasonic transducers convert pressure into an electrical signal, or an electrical signal into pressure (Fig. 2–2). Transformation between the two states is accomplished with a piezoelectric crystal. The frequency at which a crystal oscillates is determined principally by its thickness and the material from which it was cut. Oscillation occurs when an electrical signal is imposed upon the crystal. If an oscillating crystal is placed upon a surface, oscillation of the crystal will cause alternating compressions and rarefactions of the molecules

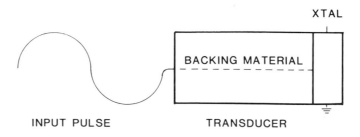

Fig. 2–2. Transducer. An input electrical sine wave is demonstrated. Most of the transducer casing is a backing material that is used to absorb the ultrasonic radiation passing toward the casing, and to concentrate most of the ultrasound energy to the face of the crystal.

of the surface (Fig. 2–3). Each compression and rarefaction represents one cycle. Thus, the electrical signal has been changed into a pressure wavefront which passes through the material on which the crystal was placed. The reverse process is equally important. Pressure wavefronts may be reflected, under certain conditions, from the material, and passed back to the transducer. If the transducer is not transmitting when the reflection returns, it will be in a receiving mode. When these pressure wavefronts arrive, the crystal will begin to oscillate, creating an electrical signal. Thus, the transducer can both send and receive pressure wavefronts. Although sophisticated techniques and crystals have been developed to use in ultrasonics, the basic principle governing the transducer is similar for all crystals.

Thus far, a transducer has been considered to consist of one crystal, but, under certain circumstances, a somewhat similar beam can also be formed by firing a number of crystals which have the appropriate physical relationship. This is an application of the Huygen principle which suggests that a single large wavefront may be equivalent to a group of smaller summed wavefronts (Fig. 2–4). This principle forms the basis for the phased array, which has become a common transducer for ultrasonic imaging. If all crystals are fired simultaneously, a beam will be propagated perpendicular to the face of the

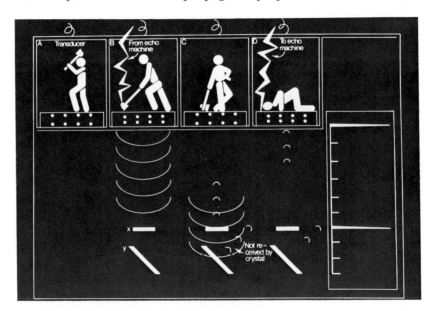

Fig. 2–3. A pictorial representation of the general properties of a transducer (panels *A* through *D*). When an electrical signal, usually a pulse, is imposed upon the crystal, the molecules alternately are pushed more closely together, and during the opposite portion of the cycle, are located farther apart. The latter is not demonstrated pictorially. This compression and rarefaction causes a wavefront to be emitted. If the wavefront strikes a stationary target (panel *C*), some of the wavefront will be reflected back toward the crystal, and some will pass through the material. A stationary target causes the reflected wavefronts to be of the same frequency as the transmitted wavefront. Panel *D* demonstrates that the returning wavefront can strike the crystal and again set up cycles of compression and rarefaction that will induce an electrical current. An A-mode display is demonstrated at the far right, which indicates that the timing from the transmission of the pulse until the reception will permit computation of the distance of the reflecting site. This figure also demonstrates that if the wavefront strikes an angled plate, reflections occur that may not be sensed by the transducer. (From Goldberg, S.J., Allen, H.D., and Sahn, D.J.: Pediatric and Adolescent Echocardiography: A Handbook. 2nd Ed. Chicago, Year Book Medical Publishers, 1980.)

HUYGEN PRINCIPLE

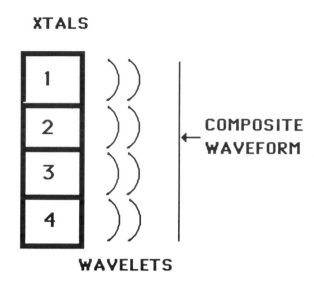

XTALS

WAVELETS

Fig. 2–4. Demonstration of the Huygen principle. The wavelets produced by each crystal are additive to form the composite waveform.

array, a situation which has little advantage over the waveform transmitted from a single crystal. On the other hand, firing all crystals simultaneously is not necessary. Figure 2–5 shows the effect of firing each subsequent crystal slightly later than the preceding one. In this situation the emitted wavefront may be transmitted at an angle to the face of the array, a capability not available for the single crystal. By altering the firing sequence, the angle between the beam and the face of the array can be adjusted. For imaging, the beam can be progressively stepped through an arc so that an entire sector of information is available (Fig. 2–6A). In a similar manner, a Doppler beam may be steered to any desired area of the sector. Unfortunately, no system is ideal. As the beam is swept laterally, the effective aperture (transducer face area) is progressively reduced (Fig. 2–6B). Reduced aperture alters focal depth. Single crystals, while unable to participate in beam steerage other than by mechanical movement, are somewhat more sensitive and have less "refractory" period between firings than do phased arrays. Manufacturers and eventually users must make many choices and compromises, and this is one of them.

TRANSMITTERS AND RECEIVERS

Equipment for ultrasonic investigation has become quite elaborate. However, a transmitter and a receiver underlie all of the expensive circuitry (Fig. 2–7). The transmitter sends an electrical signal to the crystal each time that an oscillation is required. In a pulsed system, the transmitter is turned off after sending the pulse to the crystal and the receiver is then turned on. The receiver waits for pressure wavefronts to return to the crystal and amplifies those returning wavefronts to allow further processing. The transmitter and receiver usually have one basic control each, transmit power and receiver gain. Transmit power controls how much power is transferred from the crystal into the tissue.

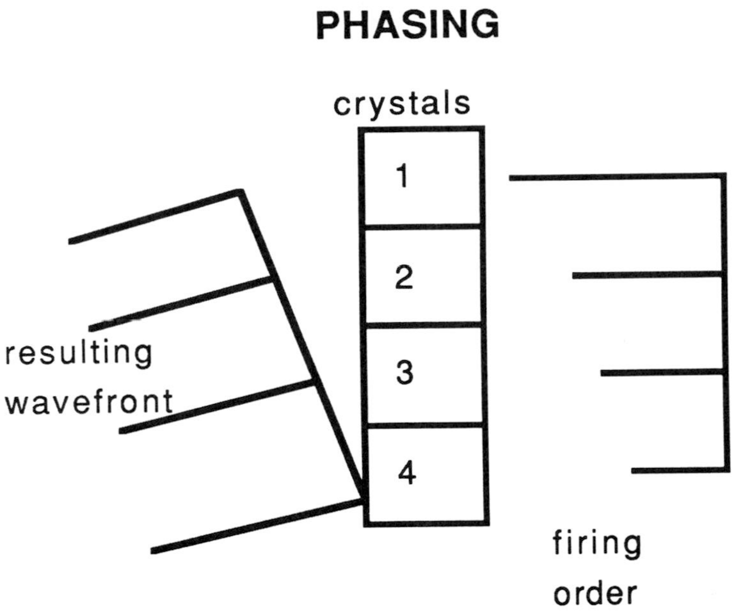

PHASING

crystals

Fig. 2–5. Phasing. The firing order is sequentially delayed for each crystal. This causes the resulting waveform to be directed at an angle to the transducer face rather than perpendicular to the transducer face.

In some instruments the upper available power level may exceed the recommended power for imaging ultrasound without warning. The greater the transmitted power, the stronger will be each reflection. However, if too much power is transmitted, tissue damage could occur. The exact safe limit is uncertain. Receiver gain control amplifies the level of reflected wavefronts which strike the crystal during the listening phase. Increasing receiver gain, in contrast to increasing transmitted power, has no tissue effect. For strong signals, increasing receiver gain performs a function similar to that of increasing transmit power. However, for weak signals, both signal and noise are amplified and little or no actual improvement occurs. Some instruments further simplify control by fixing either transmitter power or receiver gain. Thus, for these instruments only one major control is available to the operator.

TARGETS

An ultrasonic target is a surface that causes reflection of ultrasound, and reflection of ultrasound occurs when the wavefront encounters an interface between two different materials. To have an ultrasonic interface, the two materials must have a different density or pass ultrasound wavefronts at a different velocity, or both. These two properties, density and speed of ultrasound through the material, are the components of acoustical impedance. Thus, reflection occurs when ultrasound strikes an interface of two tissues or two materials which have different acoustical impedances. Two general types of reflectors are recognized, specular and diffuse. Specular reflectors are relatively large with respect to the incident wavelength and reflect wavefronts in a direction easily predicted by their position within the beam. Diffuse reflectors, on the

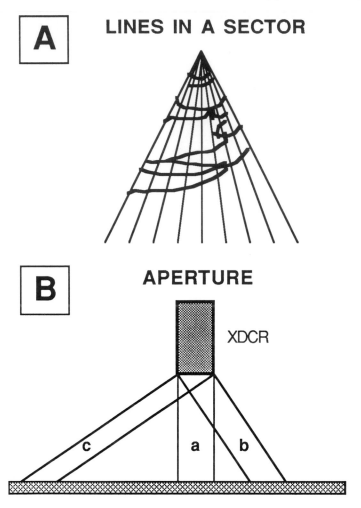

Fig. 2–6. Panel A: A sector is composed of numerous lines of information each created by one crystal firing. Panel B. Aperture refers to the effective crystal area. Note that the aperture decreases as the sector deviates from firing directly perpendicular to the crystal. The aperture is widest in a, and least wide in c.

other hand, are small with respect to the incident wavelength and reflect waveforms in multiple directions. Accordingly, if a specular reflector is angled rather than perpendicular within the beam it is unlikely that any reflections will return to the transducer. Diffuse reflectors, irrespective of their position within the beam, will return some reflections, mainly very weak ones, to the transducer. Specular targets in imaging echocardiography include valves, endocardial surfaces, pericardial surfaces, and, unfortunately, other structures which interfere with ultrasonic studies such as ribs and lung. Each tissue has a different acoustical impedance than blood, and thus, blood and tissue form an interface from which sound waves are reflected. In fact, the difference in acoustical impedance between blood and tissue is usually sufficient to cause a relatively high intensity reflection.

For Doppler, targets are blood cells. Most reflections occur from red cells because of their size and number in the blood, but Doppler signals can also be

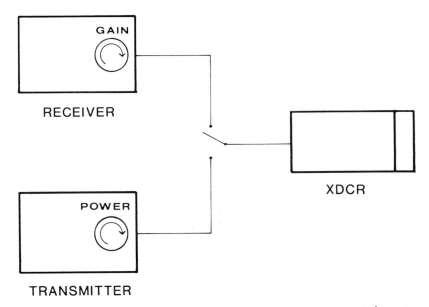

Fig. 2–7. Basic Doppler systems can be a receiver and a transmitter connected to a transducer through a switch. First, the transmitter is connected to the crystal and a wave-form is transmitted into tissue, then the switch is thrown so that the transducer is connected to the receiver. The transmitter and receiver may contain a control that increases power or gain, respectively.

detected from white cells and platelets. Since the acoustical impedance difference between blood cells and plasma is very small, reflected signal strength is very low. Therefore, for most imaging echocardiography, reflections from blood cells are too low in magnitude to be detected. Signal strength for cellular reflection approaches the noise level of the receiver, and these signals are usually rejected during imaging echocardiography. Occasionally, with some instruments, reflections from red cells in low flow areas can be seen during standard imaging echocardiography, but these weak signals are usually ignored or suppressed by the examiner. In contrast, Doppler echocardiography is based exclusively on studying reflections from moving red blood cells. Thus, the Doppler receiver differs from a standard imaging echocardiographic receiver primarily by being able to process very low amplitude signals arising from reflections from moving blood cell elements.

FREQUENCY ANALYSIS

Thus far, the shift in frequency between transmitted and received wavefronts has been indicated as increasing or decreasing, depending upon motion of the target toward or away from the source. However, for Doppler echocardiography, precise quantitation of frequency shift is required. Fundamentally, this means that at each instant in time, the received frequency or frequencies must be compared to the transmitted frequency. Since the difference in frequency falls within the audio range, the ear can be used as a frequency analyzer. Unfortunately, the ear is not a quantitative instrument. The situation is even further complicated by the fact that red cells within the sample volume may be moving at different velocities. Accordingly, several frequency shifts may occur within the sample volume simultaneously. A quantitative frequency analyzer must determine rapidly all frequencies within the sample volume.

Prior to 1979, most cardiologic Doppler spatial analyses were performed by zero crossing detectors. The zero crossing detector simply determined the time interval between zero crossings of the sine wave. Time interval is related to frequency as shown in Figure 2–8A and the output is displayed as a time interval histogram (TIH). Although this frequency analyzer provided accurate information for a single sine wave, it was ill-suited for Doppler echocardiography because simultaneous analysis of several sine waves is usually required. The zero crossing detector permits analysis of only a single frequency at any time interval. For time interval histography, multiple simultaneous signals arriving back to the transducer could cause an error in frequency analysis as shown in Figure 2–8B. Inability to simultaneously analyze more than one sine wave at a time demonstrates that the zero crossing detector is a nonlinear detector. A linear detector is defined, in part, as one which allows simultaneous analysis of numerous sine waves within the sample volume.

A most important breakthrough for Doppler echocardiography, which allowed development of commercial instrumentation, was the incorporation in Doppler instrumentation of linear frequency analysis devices. The most commonly employed linear method for performing frequency analysis is fast Fourier transform (FFT). This digital method permits simultaneous analysis of various frequency components within the sample volume by converting received data from the time and amplitude domain to the frequency domain. Another method, Chirp Z analysis, provides approximately similar information with analog techniques. Another method of frequency analysis requires direct solution of the Fourier equation and this method is usually referred to as discrete Fourier analysis. The latter requires considerable computer power. These several related techniques have supplanted the zero crossing detector for analysis of the Doppler shift frequency.

Recently, development of color-coded Doppler has required a much more rapid method of analysis of frequency shift than is provided by any technique discussed thus far. An autocorrelation method was developed to meet this need and will be discussed in more detail later in this chapter.

VELOCITY DETERMINED BY DOPPLER

Doppler can provide direct determination of blood cell velocities. The formula for conversion of frequency shift to velocity is:

$$V = (c) \, \Delta F / \, 2 \, f_0 \, (\cos \Theta)$$

where V = velocity of blood cells, c = the speed of ultrasound in the medium, ΔF = the frequency shift in kHz, f_0 = transmitted frequency, and $\cos \Theta$ = the cosine of the intercept angle. Most Doppler machines contain microprocessors which can directly compute velocity from frequency shift.

CONVENTIONAL DOPPLER TECHNIQUES

Study of reflections from blood cell elements may be accomplished with several types of ultrasonic transmission and processing techniques, including pulsed, continuous wave and high pulse repetition frequency (PRF) Doppler.

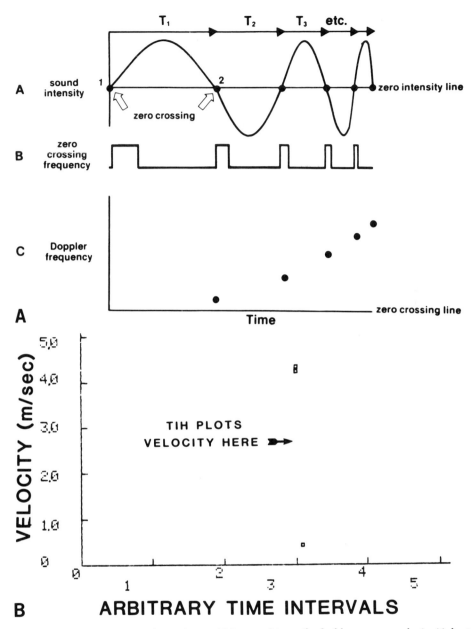

Fig. 2–8. *A,* Demonstration of time-interval histographic method of frequency analysis. (Adapted from Baker, D.W., et al.: Pulsed Doppler Echocardiography. *In* Echocardiology. Edited by N. Bom. The Hague, Martinus Nijhoff Medical Division, 1977, p. 207.) *B,* Comparison of time interval histography (TIH) and fast Fourier transform (FFT). At a given instant in time, three separate frequencies were found by FFT, one at 4 m/sec, another at 4.1 m/sec, and a third at 0.4 m/sec. FFT would provide an output for each of the frequencies. A time interval histogram would take an average of the frequencies and plot a single point. The time interval histogram would probably plot a frequency that never existed in the original signal.

In the remainder of the book, these modalities will be called conventional Doppler. Further, one variant of pulsed Doppler permits color coded velocities to be superimposed on a two-dimensional image. The following sections will be concerned with the several types of Doppler.

Pulsed Doppler

Pulsed Doppler bears many similarities to imaging echocardiography. Figure 2–9 demonstrates the principle of pulsed Doppler. An electrical signal is sent to a piezoelectric crystal which creates a short oscillation; the crystal then ceases oscillation and "listens" for reflected signals. Figure 2–9, panel A demonstrates that if a transmitted wavefront encounters a stationary or perpendicularly moving target, the reflected frequency will be equal to the transmitted frequency. On the other hand, if the transmitted wavefront strikes a moving target which is not moving perpendicularly to the transducer (Panels B and C), a difference in frequency will be detected between the transmitted frequency and the received frequency. If the target is moving toward the transducer, the returned frequency will be increased (Panel B). If the target is moving away from the transducer (Panel C), the returned frequency will be decreased. Accordingly, analysis of the Doppler reflected frequency indicates whether the target is moving toward the transducer or away from it. Although it is possible to provide directional information simultaneously for all tissue depths along the transmitted beam, pulsed Doppler also offers the opportunity to interrogate only a small area at a time.

Range Gating. Interrogation of one small area along the beam is known as

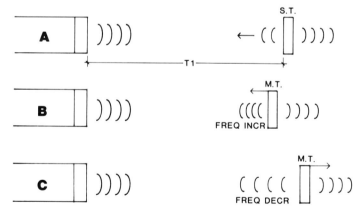

Fig. 2–9. Doppler principle in the pulsed system. In panels *A*, *B*, and *C*, the transducer remains in a constant position and transmits a wavefront of the same frequency and amplitude. In panel *A*, the wavefront strikes a stationary target (ST). Some of the wavefront passes through the stationary target and some of the decreased amplitude is reflected back toward the transducer. Note that the distance between wavefronts of the transmitted and reflected signal is exactly identical. In panel *B*, the target is moving toward the transducer. Again, some of the incident wavefront passes through the target and is attenuated, as demonstrated by a decrease in the amplitude of the wavefronts. Some of the wavefront is reflected, and the distance between reflected wavefronts is smaller than that for the transmitted signal, which means that the frequency of the reflected signal has increased by comparison to the incident frequency as a result of motion of the target (MT) toward the transducer. In panel C, motion of the target is away from the transducer, and space between the reflected wavefronts is increased. Thus, the frequency of the incident and reflected waves are similar if the source and target are motionless, increased if the target moves toward the source, or decreased if the target moves away from the source.

"range gating" (Fig. 2–10). Range gating is possible because the speed of ultrasound through tissue is constant at 1540 meters/sec. Accordingly, it is possible to measure the time required for information from a chosen depth to return to the crystal. Since the velocity and time are known, it becomes simple to solve for the depth of reflection. Analysis of the reflected signal for change in frequency exclusively at a given depth is accomplished by analyzing only for that time interval and totally disregarding reflections from all other depths. Although a point in space as small as the pulse length could be sampled, the range gate in practical terms is variable in length usually from 1 to 20 mm. The area encompassed within the range gating is called the "sample volume." The advantages of a variable sample volume length are that its length can be tailored to the anatomy under consideration and longer sample volumes usually improve the signal to noise ratio over smaller ones. This is particularly important for study of small hearts. Sample volume length, in most instruments, can be operator adjusted, whereas in others, sample volume length is fixed. Further, in most instruments the length of the sample volume is shown on the image. In a few instruments the length is not shown on the image. Sample volume width is always equal to beam width at the sample volume site. Since beam width expands in the far field, sample volume width also expands in this area. Beam width is a function of transducer frequency, aperture size, and sample volume depth

All pulsed Doppler instruments allow the operator to set the sample volume at various depths along a cursor line within the heart. This is usually accomplished by demonstrating simultaneously the sample volume location and a two-dimensional image of the heart. Thus, the operator can set the sample volume within a chamber or great vessel of interest, and then lengthen or shorten the sample volume so that its length fits into the area of interest throughout the entire cardiac cycle. Further, most mechanical and phased array instruments allow the cursor line to be moved right or left within the image. A

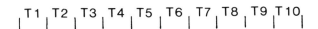

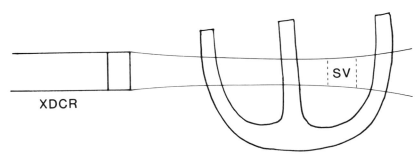

Fig. 2–10. Range gating. The transducer (XDCR) emits an ultrasonic beam that changes width as it passes distally. Above the pictorial heart is a group of time zones. The operator may select any zone for Doppler interrogation of cellular velocities. In this example, the operator selected time zone 8 and information reflecting from all other zones is disregarded. Zone 8 was selected for analysis on the basis of the time required for the beam to go from the transducer to zone 8 and return. Zone 8 has a length, width, and shape. See text for details.

few have a fixed position cursor, which means that the cardiac image must be moved around the fixed cursor. The latter is difficult to perform.

Pulsed Doppler has limited high velocity measurement capability. The limitation occurs because pulsed Doppler permits only a single pulse to be within the examining range at any one time. This pulse may either be traveling toward or reflecting from the target. Since ultrasound travels through tissue at a fixed speed, two factors will determine whether more than one pulse will be in the body at one time, (1) the pulse repetition frequency (PRF) (i.e. a determination of the time interval between pulses) and (2) the distance (called "range" by engineers) that the pulse must travel to the farthest target. The user deals with this situation by moving the sample volume to an area of interest. Instruments are programmed to determine depth of the sample volume and for this depth to transmit the maximum possible PRF. The higher the PRF, the greater the velocity that can be recorded. Accordingly, all velocities within the sample volume will be assessed, however, only a certain range of velocities can be determined accurately without ambiguity.

Continuous Wave Doppler

Continuous wave (CW) Doppler uses two crystals, one of which continuously sends and the other continuously receives ultrasound (Fig. 2–11 top). As a result of frequency, crystal size, and inherent characteristics, CW beams are usually wider than those of pulsed Doppler. Since transmission is continuous, reception is also continuous. Accordingly, information from the full length of the beam is continuously present, a situation which eliminates any possibility of determining the depth from which any given waveform originated. Inability to determine the depth of origin of a waveform is referred to as "range ambiguity." A major advantage of CW over pulsed Doppler is that CW can measure

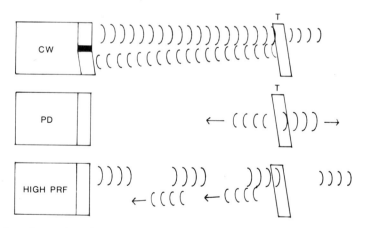

Fig. 2–11. Doppler modes. The top panel demonstrates a continuous wave (CW) Doppler system. One crystal continuously transmits wavefronts, and a second, independent crystal, continuously receives reflections from the target (T). Usually, the second crystal is at a slight angle to the first. Pulsed Doppler system (PD) is demonstrated in the middle panel. In this mode, a single pulse is transmitted and the receiver listens. No second pulse is transmitted until the wavefronts from the first have been received from the maximal depth. Therefore, all received wavefronts are the result of one single transmitted pulse. The third panel demonstrates a high pulse repetition frequency (PRF) system. In this mode, pulses are transmitted so frequently that multiple pulses are within the system at any time. Accordingly, reflections may occur, but there is no way to determine whether a given reflection resulted from one pulse or another.

very high velocities because the PRF is very high (continuous). CW can be obtained from two crystals within a phased array, and the beam may be phased (moved to a desired portion of the sector). Further, for a phased array, the image and Doppler may be presented in a manner that seems simultaneous.

High PRF

An intermediate modality, high pulse repetition frequency (high PRF) Doppler, which is a cross between continuous and pulsed Doppler, has been developed. High PRF uses single crystal technology and thus conventional transducers can be used. The major difference between high PRF Doppler and standard pulsed Doppler is that the listening period for high PRF Doppler is too short to allow reflections to return to the crystal from deep structures. In conventional pulsed Doppler, only one pulse is considered to be in the body at any time. In CW Doppler a continuous waveform is transmitted. In high PRF Doppler, several pulses are in the body simultaneously (Fig. 2–11 bottom). This factor makes high PRF an intermediate form between pulsed and CW Doppler. Each pulse can be considered to form one sample volume. Instead of using one sample volume, as is customary in standard pulsed Doppler, two or more pulses are within the heart simultaneously at different depths. The logic for this approach is that high velocity resolution is a function of the PRF. Thus, increasing PRF allows resolution of higher velocities, but the depth from which the velocity was reflected is unknown (range ambiguity) because more than one pulse was in the body simultaneously. Velocity measured by high PRF is accurate.

A fundamental reason that high PRF Doppler evolved is that it requires only a single crystal and conventional pulsed Doppler circuitry. For applications in which CW might be preferable, high PRF Doppler, in many ways, simulates CW Doppler without the necessity or expense for the manufacturer of developing dual crystal technology and continuous wave electronics. Further, the interrogation line can be visualized on the two dimensional image, and this is a distinct advantage over non-imaging CW but less desirable than imaging combined with CW. High PRF Doppler, however, uses a narrow beam which makes jet detection more difficult than with CW Doppler. Further, the system may not be as sensitive as conventional pulsed Doppler. After initial enthusiasm, high PRF Doppler seems to have diminishing clinical usage.

MAJOR DIFFERENCES BETWEEN CONVENTIONAL DOPPLER MODES

Although all three modes provide generally similar information, at least two important differences exist. Standard single sample volume pulsed Doppler is the only mode that permits velocity to be sampled *exclusively* from the area of interest, the sample volume. However, the very same principle that permits exclusive interrogation of the sample volume also limits the maximal velocity that can be recorded within that sample volume. CW and high PRF Doppler permit much higher velocities to be sampled, but the point along the line of interrogation from which the velocity was recorded is unknown. This tradeoff is a major one and the reasons for it and methods for maximizing the yield from any system must be understood in depth by anyone who uses Doppler. The advantage of locating with precision the site from which a velocity is sampled is obvious, but the advantage of detecting high velocities needs additional explanation.

The need to measure high velocities arises from the clinical reality that velocities as high as 8 m/sec occur in certain abnormal circulations. Pulsed Doppler techniques, even under almost ideal conditions, are limited to velocities less than the maximal that occurs in the circulation. Under common but less than ideal circumstances, pulsed Doppler can detect only velocities that are far lower than those encountered in most patients with cardiac disease. Worse yet, if pulsed Doppler encounters a velocity in excess of its ability to plot magnitude properly, the analysis system causes the velocity to depart from the zero velocity baseline, progress to the maximal velocity limit and then wrap around the velocity scale beginning again at the bottom until the complete velocity is inscribed (Fig. 2–12). Accordingly, the signal wraps through the velocity domain one or more times, and the precise magnitude of this wrapped velocity may become completely obscured. The magnitude of the velocity is ambiguous. This process is called "aliasing."

ALIASING

Aliasing occurs when the sampling rate is too slow to appreciate events that occurred between samples. One common non-Doppler example, with which most individuals are familiar, occurs in western movies. As the wagon wheel of the stage-coach begins to roll, the appropriate forward direction of wheel motion appears on the screen. As the wagon wheel spins faster, it suddenly appears to reverse direction; this occurs because the camera which is photographing the wagon wheel has a frame rate which is too slow to correctly interpret the true direction of the turning motion. A high speed camera would record the correct direction of rotation.

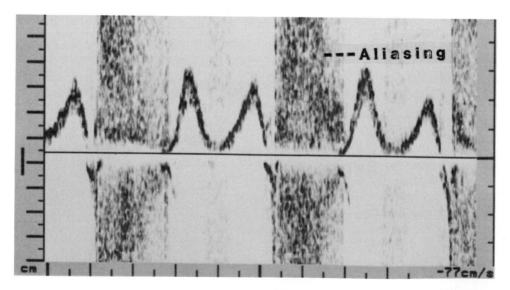

Fig. 2–12. Aliasing. Calibrated velocity amplitude is plotted on the vertical axis and time is plotted on the horizontal axis. Two distinct patterns are shown on this record, an M-shaped complex and a band of aliasing. In the aliasing band, no distinct velocity pattern is obvious.

ALIASING

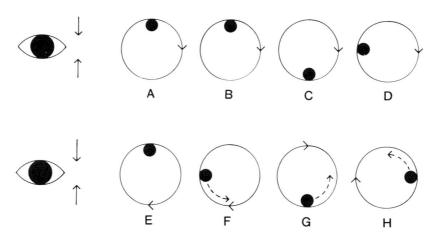

Fig. 2–13. A graphic explanation of aliasing. See text for details.

Figure 2–13 illustrates aliasing. On the left portion of the figure is an eye viewing motion of a ball placed within a circular track. Assume that an opaque window is closed except at times we choose to open it. In this context the device behaves much like the shutter of a camera. The objective is to predict the motion of the ball throughout its entire travel within the circular track. However, the eye is restricted in viewing the ball because the shutter only opens at certain times. If the circle is turning at precisely one or more complete revolutions per shutter opening, the eye will always see the ball in the same position. This could indicate that no motion has transpired, or that the ball had moved once, twice, or some other complete multiple between shutter openings. On the other hand, if more opportunities to view the ball were available, it could be seen in other positions such as the 12, 3, 6, 9 o'clock and again at the 12 o'clock positions. Under these conditions it would be possible to conclude that the ball had made a single revolution and that it had been tracked precisely. In fact, if the ball were visualized in two positions during each cycle, the rate and direction of travel of the ball could be predicted with accuracy. In Doppler, sampling twice per revolution is known as the Nyquist frequency limit. Nyquist indicated that if at least two samples could be obtained within each cycle, frequency could be determined without ambiguity.

Next, the lower panel will be examined to determine the apparent patterns which occur when sampling rate is too slow. In this instance, the assumption is made that the ball is traveling faster than the rate at which the shutter opens to permit viewing. If the first shutter opening (E) finds the ball at 12 o'clock, and if the ball is making more than one revolution between each viewing opportunity, the next time that the shutter opens, the ball will be viewed at the second position (F). It has not yet completed the second revolution, but has completed more than one revolution. The shutter then opens again to visualize the ball at the third position (G), and even though the ball is moving clockwise, as the eye views the ball, the ball appears to be moving counterclockwise because the sampling rate is too slow to determine forward progress. This is the principle of aliasing. For a Doppler frequency analyzer, the result is that the velocity appears to be going in the wrong direction, exactly as it did for the ball in the example, and, therefore, velocity may be plotted as away from the transducer, when, in fact, targets are moving toward the transducer at a velocity too rapid to be analyzed by the system. The Nyquist limit principle indicates that at least two points on each sine wave are required to accurately plot velocity direction. Thus, the maximal velocity that can be determined without ambiguity is related to the number of transmitted pulses/unit time. The higher the pulsing rate of the system, the greater the capability to measure high velocities. However, the time required for a pulse to reach the reflecting interface and return limits the number of pulses/unit time. If too many pulses are issued/unit time, not enough time is left for reflecting pulses from deep structures.

METHODS TO MAXIMIZE VELOCITY LIMITS FOR PULSED DOPPLER

Baseline Shift. If the operator does not have continuous wave or high PRF Doppler, and if the velocity determined by standard pulsed Doppler is too high to record without aliasing, several techniques are available to increase velocity measurement capability of the equipment. The first and simplest technique is to set zero velocity at either the top or the bottom of the recording paper. This technique allocates all of the velocity range to either positive or negative velocities rather than assigning half the range to positive and the other half to negative velocities. This method works best if velocity is unidirectional. Some Doppler machines do not allow movement of the zero line; therefore the top of the velocity tracing, which moves into the "wrong" directional area, must be added to the portion that was in the correct area, but the result is accurate.

Transducer Frequency. Another method for increasing the velocity limit is to use a lower frequency transducer. Increased velocity resolution is a direct function of reducing transducer frequency. Thus if a 3 MHz transducer permits measurement of x cm/sec, a 1.5 MHz transducer increases the maximal velocity to 2x. The effect of frequency change on maximal velocity is shown in Figure 2–14.

Reduction of the Distance to the Target to Increase PRF. A major method for increasing the velocity limit is increasing pulse repetition frequency. This is a practical solution since the maximal recordable velocity is a direct function of the PRF. Unfortunately, a major tradeoff occurs with an increased PRF because only one pulse may be in the area of interest at any one time. If two or more pulses were in the area of interest simultaneously, uncertainty exists as to which reflection belonged to which pulse. Accordingly, the only way to increase PRF is to reduce the distance between the transducer and target so that pulse travel time (at a constant 1540 m/s) is shorter. In fact, a constant relationship exists for each frequency transducer between the maximal velocity that can be recorded and the range between transducer and target. This relationship, shown in Figure 2–14, is called the range velocity product. This figure makes an assumption that is not valid for any commercial machine. The assumption is that the instrument has continuous compensation in PRF for every change in depth. For actual instrumentation, only 3 to perhaps 8 different PRFs

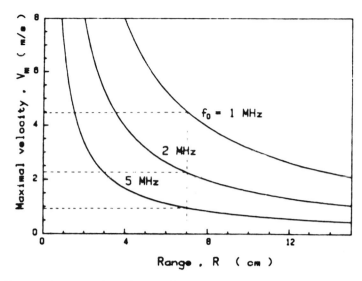

Fig. 2–14. Range velocity product. See text for details. (From Hatle, L., Angelsen, B.: Doppler Ultrasound in Cardiology. 2nd Ed., Philadelphia, Lea & Febiger, 1985.)

are available. Accordingly, if the operator reduced range by, for example, 1 cm, PRF would change only if that range change caused the instrument to enter a different range band. One instrument that we use has the same PRF for the entire range between 6 and 10 cm. Accordingly, a reduction in range from 8 to 7 cm for this machine would not change PRF, whereas a change from 9.5 to 10.5 would reduce PRF since range alteration beyond 10 cm crossed a band programmed by the manufacturer. Most often, the optimal PRF is not achieved because of these bands. Clearly, the shortest path to the area of interest is the best because the maximal velocity recordable will be the highest and the signal to noise ratio will probably be better than at farther range. As a practical issue, reduction of distance from transducer to target to improve PRF is, at times, possible but at other times it is not.

BEAM FLOW INTERCEPT ANGLE

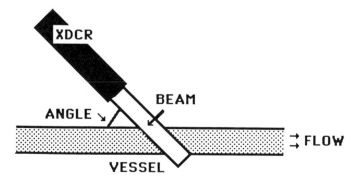

Fig. 2–15. Beam-flow intercept angle. A beam is emitted from the transducer (XDCR) which intercepts flow in the vessel at an angle. Under ideal conditions the beam would be parallel to flow. Any intercept angle reduces the amplitude of the Doppler signal by the cosine of the beam-flow intercept angle.

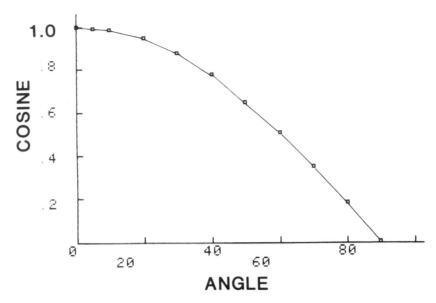

Fig. 2–16. Relationship of the value of the cosine (vertical axis) and the angle in degrees (horizontal axis). Note that if the angle is zero, the value of the cosine is +1. If the angle is 20°, the value of the cosine is still 94%. As the angle increases beyond 20°, however, the value of the cosine drops rapidly. Negative cosines are not shown.

Beam-Flow Intercept Angle. The angle between the interrogating beam and the blood flow path is another determinant of the recorded velocity amplitude. In order to record the full magnitude of velocity, the interrogating Doppler beam must be perfectly parallel to the direction of blood flow. If the beam is not aligned with flow an intercept angle occurs (Fig. 2–15), and recorded velocity will be less than true velocity. The relationship between true and measured velocity is the cosine of the intercept angle. Figure 2–16 shows the cosine function and the magnitude by which velocity will be reduced. Note that a 20° intercept angle causes a velocity reduction of only 6%. Intercept angles beyond 20°, however, cause considerable reduction in displayed amplitude. Further, the angle required is the spatial angle, not the angle in the two visualized dimensions. The interaction of velocity magnitude and beam-flow intercept angle suggests one more method to extend the velocity range of pulsed Doppler: increasing the beam-flow intercept angle. If velocity aliases, the angle between the transducer and flow could be increased until the velocity falls within the range-velocity product. The intercept angle could be measured and total velocity could then be computed by correcting according to the cosine function. This method works and provides accurate results if the precise spatial angle is known. In clinical situations the intercept angle may be measured in two dimensions, but no method exists to measure the angle simultaneously in the unseen third dimension (also called elevational or azimuthal dimension). As a result, the increased angle method to reduce aliasing is seldom if ever used.

DIRECTION OF VELOCITY

Thus far only the magnitude of velocity has been discussed in detail. One additional feature that Doppler offers is determination of the direction of flow.

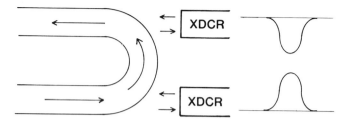

Fig. 2–17. Relationship of beam and flow. Flow occurs in a counterclockwise direction. Two transducers evaluate the flow. The top transducer evaluates velocity moving away from the transducer, and the reflected signal moves toward the transducer Accordingly, flow and the reflected signal are moving in the opposite direction, so velocity is plotted as a negative deflection. In the other instance, both flow and the reflected signal move toward the transducer; therefore, flow is shown as an upright signal. Doppler frequency shift magnitude is a function of intercept angle. See text for details.

Direction of velocity is determined by a quadrature detector, the details of which are beyond the scope of this chapter other than to indicate that this is a reliable, rapid, and well-documented methodology. The basic concept for directional information can be deduced from the beam-flow intercept angle principle. Doppler waveform polarity (direction) is always inscribed with respect to the transducer. Figure 2–17 provides a pictorial way to think about this concept. A zero degree intercept means that flow and beam direction are parallel and flow is going away from the transducer. The only problem relates to deciding the direction of the beam. Two possibilities exist. Beam direction could refer to the transmitted or the received beam. The first Doppler displays were made with reference to the received beam and not the transmitted beam. All manufacturers now use this convention. Accordingly, if the reflected beam and blood flow travel in the opposite direction the intercept angle is 180°, the cosine is − 1, and the waveform will be displayed below baseline (upper panel, Fig. 2–17). If the reflected beam and direction of blood flow are in the same direction, the intercept angle is 0° (360° is the same angle), the cosine is + 1, and the waveform will be printed above the baseline (lower panel, Fig. 2–17).

An Application Example

The magnitude of velocity is a function of the cosine of the intercept angle between beam direction and the path of blood cell elements. The combination of angles, velocity amplitudes, and directional information is explained by study of Figure 2–18. In this figure, pulsed Doppler is used to determine velocity in the root of the aorta. The root of the aorta may be studied from subcostal, precordial and suprasternal positions. Since the cosine of 180° is − 1 and 0° is + 1, signal amplitude will be greatest if the Doppler beam is parallel to flow at either 180° or 0°. If the reflected beam and blood flow path are related to one another at any other angle, recorded velocity will be diminished by the cosine of the angle. If the root of the aorta is studied from the subcostal position (position I), flow and reflected wavefront will proceed away from one another (180°), and therefore, the magnitude of the velocity signal will be the true magnitude. However, since the direction of cell elements is opposite to the reflected path of the beam (cosine = − 1), the direction will be registered as

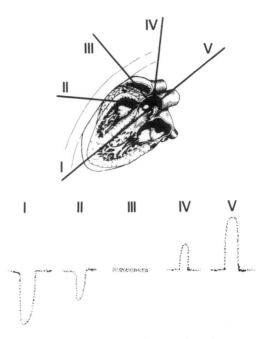

Fig. 2–18. Doppler directivity. Various locations for sampling the aortic root and corresponding velocity diagrams. See text for details.

negative. Precisely the same magnitude of velocity can be recorded from the suprasternal position V where the intercept angle is 0 or 360° (cosine = +1). The direction of cell elements is similar to the path of the reflected beam and therefore the velocity pattern will be demonstrated above baseline. Velocity patterns recorded from subcostal and from the suprasternal notch represent precisely the same magnitude of flow, but the directional component is opposite because of the different location of the transducer. Velocity directional registration is always plotted with respect to the cosine of the intercept angle as determined by the direction of the reflected wavefront.

The transducer can also be placed on the precordium to record velocity in the root of the aorta. For example, the transducer can be placed at position III, which represents an intercept angle of 90° to flow. The cosine of 90° is 0, and therefore no velocity will be recorded even though the sample volume is placed within the root of the aorta. However, if the transducer is moved to positions II or IV, the intercept angle is no longer 0°, and therefore velocity can be recorded. However, the magnitude of velocity is less than true velocity and the reduction is the result of the intercept angle. The exact magnitude is the product of true velocity and cosine of the intercept angle. Direction is again dependent on transducer location. Fortunately, within 20° of either 180° or 0°, the magnitude of velocity will be reduced only by a maximum of 6% (Fig. 2–16). At greater angles the magnitude of the recorded velocity drops rapidly. Methods for proper alignment will be covered in later chapters.

GRAY SCALE DEPICTION OF DOPPLER VELOCITIES

Cells within the Doppler sample volume often move at different velocities and, at times, in different directions. In laminar flow, velocities will probably be normally distributed. Some cells will move a bit faster, some a bit slower and many will move at nearly the same velocity (modal velocity) (Fig. 2–19). In theory, each cell should return a reflection. In practice every one of the millions of cells within the sample volume may not return a reflection, but multiple reflections will be received from blood particles.

These multiple velocities, on a printed or viewed Doppler record, should be depicted in a manner that will allow the operator to interpret the velocity pattern in a meaningful manner. Ordinarily, this is accomplished by depicting the strength of reflected echos as shades of gray. The strength of a reflected Doppler signal, if aligned with flow direction, is, in major part, determined by the number of cells traveling at that velocity. Accordingly, if a few cells travel at maximal velocity, their velocity should be depicted (encoded) as a light shade of gray. The velocity at which most cells travel, the modal velocity, should be encoded as black (Fig. 2–20). The modal velocity is usually represented as a dark envelope but a few cells move faster and a few move slower. The velocity for other groups of cell should be encoded in intermediate gray scale shades as a function of the number of cells moving at that velocity.

The gray scale capability of an instrument is usually stated in specifications by the number of bits. Each bit has two states, on and off. A one bit gray scale device would have two possible shades of gray, just black and white. The general principle is that the number of shades is equal to 2^n, where the "n" refers to the number of bits. A four bit gray scale machine would have 2^4, or 16 shades of gray. An example of the range of shades of gray in a 4 bit display is shown in Figure 2–21. The object is to attempt to provide enough gray scale to blur the transition between one shade and the next in order to avoid step changes. Probably 512 or more shades does this best, but the expense of having this capability outweighs its advantages. Manufacturers must compromise and not too much is lost by decreasing to 128 or 256 shades. The reason that not too much is lost is that little interpolation is necessary between the 128 or 256 steps. Another way of thinking about the situation is that 128 or 256 possible shades approach an analog display. Unfortunately, 8, 16, or 64 shades are probably on the inadequate side of the expense:effect ratio.

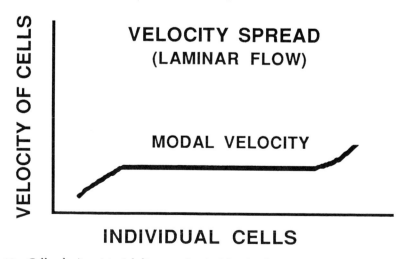

Fig. 2–19. Cell velocity pictorial diagram. See text for details.

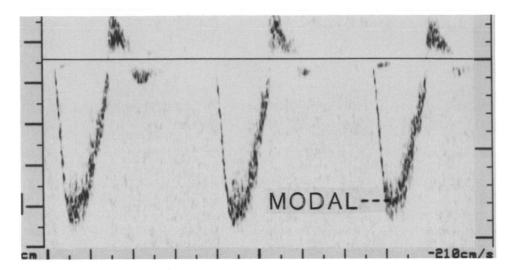

Fig. 2–20. A Doppler echocardiogram showing cells moving at different velocities. The velocity at which most cells move is marked "modal." Note, however, that some cells are moving at greater or lesser velocities than the modal and are depicted in less intense shades of gray.

One way to think of the number of gray levels available is as a third dimension. The first two dimensions consist of the number of pixels in the vertical and horizontal directions, for example an array of 512 by 256. Each pixel, however, can have many possible shades (but only one at any given time); for example, the range of possible shades might be 256. Accordingly, an engineer would refer to this as a 512 by 256 by 256 array.

Two general methods (shown pictorially in Fig. 2–22) are currently used to control gray scale for Doppler signals. The first is to assign gray scale in fixed steps of reflected signal strength, a so-called fixed gain method. Implementation of this method is quite simple. The design engineer decides how many millivolts of signal will be required to inscribe black and then divides that value by the number of shades of gray to set the millivolt range for each gray shade. This simple system is used by most manufacturers. The other system uses an adaptation of automatic gain control (AGC). In this system, the strongest signal, irrespective of its millivolt amplitude, is encoded as black, and lower level signals are encoded proportionately. A fixed gain encoder works well in a strong signal environment, but in Doppler we frequently work in low signal environments. The latter situation causes signals to be encoded only in gray tones (or tone) or, in some low signal cases, not to be encoded at all. In the latter case the signal is heard but never reaches the millivolt level to be encoded as the first shade of gray. It is invisible on the monitor. The AGC encoder works well in a lower level signal environment.

COLOR-CODED VELOCITIES—AN ADAPTATION OF PULSED DOPPLER

The concept of a conventional single sample volume has been discussed. Both velocity direction and magnitude within the sample volume can be determined by analysis of the Doppler shift. Simultaneous analysis of Doppler

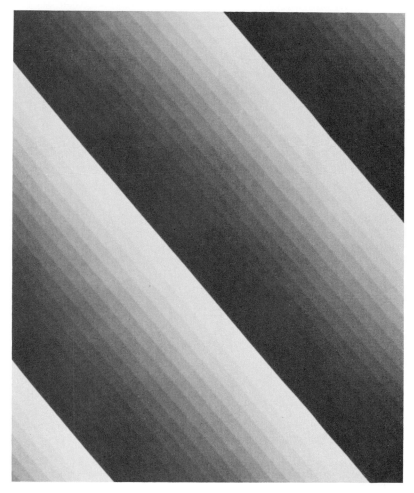

Fig. 2–21. An example of 16 shades of gray scale. Note the significant steps in gray scale between adjacent bars.

shifts in multiple sample volumes would be convenient. Two major problems (and innumerable technical problems) had to be faced before such an instrument could be built. First, FFT provides an output every few milliseconds. In fact, the FFT must receive a significant duration of waveforms before it can perform a spectral analysis. Thus the number of analyses that would be desirable for multiple sample volumes would far exceed the capability of a single or even several FFTs. The second problem regards how to display the information. Velocities from a single sample volume can be viewed using a conventional strip chart display. Such a display might even work for two or three sample volumes, but a truly effective display of many sample volumes would

GRAY LEVEL ALLOCATION

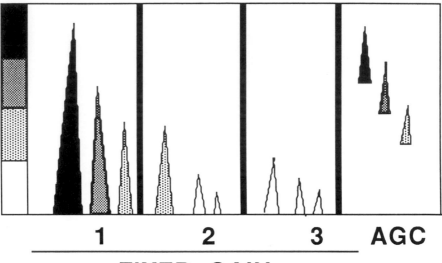

FIXED GAIN

Fig. 2–22. Gray scale allocation, a pictorial diagram. On the far left is a 2 bit gray scale representation extending from black to white. The first three panels show simultaneously detected fixed gain signals of different amplitudes. Panel #1 shows signals of optimal amplitude. The highest amplitude signal reaches the encoding threshold for black, the second reaches the gray level below black, and the third reaches the gray level two steps below black. However a weaker set of signals is shown in panel #2; only the strongest signal reaches the threshold for minimal gray encoding. The other two frequencies are heard but not seen because their signal levels fall in the white encoded range. In panel #2 no signal reaches threshold for encoding as other than white. Accordingly, all are heard and none are seen on the record. For automatic gain control, AGC, signals are approximately the same amplitude as in panel #3, but in AGC the highest amplitude signal is always encoded black, and lower level signals are encoded proportionately. Accordingly, in a weak signal environment, AGC still uses full gray scale, whereas fixed gain does not.

probably require a different strategy. Brandestini[4] was the first to build a machine which addressed some of these issues. His instrument analyzed velocity direction only (not magnitude) in multiple sample volumes distributed along a single line of interrogation. Directional information was displayed on an M-mode echocardiogram by encoding velocity direction as a color. Although only a single prototype unit was built, decisions made for design of this instrument affected future instrumentation.

Readers wishing a mathematical explanation of color coded Doppler are referred to the first three chapters of Omoto's book[5] in which these issues are covered in a clear manner. The purpose here will be to provide a conceptual explanation.

The objective of color-coded Doppler is to display directional and magnitude information for velocity on a two-dimensional echocardiographic image. Further, to aid maximally in diagnosis and physiologic interpretation, data should be acquired often enough to permit information to appear as though it were obtained in real time.

In order to obtain adequate utility from color-coded Doppler, numerous sample volumes must be present. Most commercial instruments today scan convert the television display to a digital display. This means that every portion of the

PIXELS WITHIN AN IMAGE

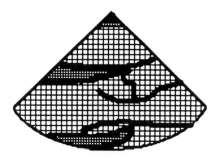

Fig. 2–23. Pictorial of pixels within an image. The oscilloscopic screen is subdivided into a large number of equal sized pixels. Each pixel can be displayed a shade of gray or color. The pixel size in this pictorial diagram, for display purposes, is enlarged many times over actual pixel size.

screen can be controlled by a computer. Each controllable portion is called a picture element, which is usually referred to as a pixel. Figure 2–23 shows a diagrammatic representation of pixels which make up an imaging sector. In an actual sector many more pixels are present. The total number of pixels in a display is usually referenced by the number in the vertical direction and the number in the horizontal direction. For example, a 512 by 512 matrix would contain 262,144 pixels. Obviously, numerous pixels lie outside the image sector, and computer control of these is less important than for those within the sector. The area outside the sector usually contains information useful to the operator such as instructions, values, or patient identification. A pixel can display only a shade of gray or a shade of color. The computer, on the other hand, can maintain much more information regarding each pixel than just its shade of gray or color. For each frame the computer can alter the information in each pixel independently, and such an alteration will change the appearance of the composite picture.

The first task in creating a color-coded Doppler image is to obtain a cardiac image on which to superimpose color coded velocities. This can be done in a manner similar to that used to create any conventional two-dimensional image. The next step, however, requires determining the flow direction and magnitude for each pixel within the sector image. It is most instructive to think of each pixel as a small sample volume. Accordingly, many thousands of pixels are present and each requires an analysis for each frame. Ordinarily, 15 to 30 frames per second are required to provide the sense of "real time motion." Clearly, many hundreds of thousands of frequency and directional analyses are needed each second. Determination of flow direction can be performed rapidly by a quadrature detector to meet this requirement. However, an FFT, the conventional spectral analyzer which is used to determine velocity magnitude, is capable of only hundreds of analyses, at maximum, each second. An autocorrelation method for velocity analysis was developed[6] which permitted the number of analyses required. This method provides true calibrated velocities. Other algorithms have also been developed which can also measure velocities rapidly, but details of these have not been released by their developers.

The easiest method for viewing this massive amount of Doppler information appears to be to convert it to color and to overlay this color information on the image. Both directional and velocity magnitude information need to be encoded into a single color. One further obvious problem regards separating structural and blood cell reflections. Structures, however, usually move more slowly and reflections are much stronger than those originating from blood cells. Accordingly, a "filter" is used which recognizes signals by strength and velocity. This process is called "pixel prioritization." Effectively, color is omitted from any pixel whch is defined as an image pixel. Although the pixel prioritization process can be misled into classifying rapidly moving, low amplitude tissue signals as blood cell signals, the method usually works fairly well.

Brandestini assigned color only for direction. Red and blue were used to depict whether blood was flowing toward or away from the transducer; however, in his first prototype, velocity magnitude was not encoded in addition to the primary color. Most current instruments encode flow toward the transducer as red and flow away from the transducer as blue. Some instruments reverse this color scheme and others allow the user to assign the color scheme. Further, most current instruments vary the shade of blue or red to depict the magnitude of velocity. Accordingly, the brighter the color, the higher the velocity.

Some color-coded Doppler displays also include a function termed variance. Variance, usually color coded as green, is thought to detect turbulent flow although no convincing evidence has been advanced to support the contention that green coded velocities are recorded from turbulent flow and that red and blue coded flows are recorded only from laminar flow. One variant is that green can be mixed with red or blue to create a mosaic pattern.

In order to understand variance, a more detailed look at color coded signal processing is required. To construct a conventional image only a single transmit

PIXELS WITHIN A LINE

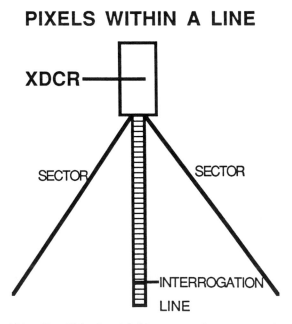

Fig. 2–24. Pixels within a line. This pictorial shows a transducer transmitting down a single line. The line is subdivided into a number of pixels. Multiple transmissions are sent down this single line in order to determine velocity by the autocorrelation method.

pulse is fired. After reflections are returned, the next transmit pulse is aimed down the next adjacent line. This process is repeated until all lines in a frame are complete. For color Doppler, and particularly for systems that use auto-correlation, a number of pulse transmissions and receptions are aimed down the same line before moving to the next line. Obviously, many pixels lie along a single line (Fig. 2–24), but it is most instructive to consider events that occur for only one pixel. Reflections from the first pulse go to a quadrature detector where velocity direction with respect to the transducer is determined (Fig. 2–25). This result determines primary color, red or blue. The code for primary color is then stored in the portion of computer memory that controls information for the given pixel. However, the process is not completed because the shade of the primary color which depicts velocity information remains to be determined. All subsequent pulses transmitted down the same line are used to determine velocity (Fig. 2–25). When the first pulse is transmitted down a line, no prior information is available for comparison. To overcome this transient problem, the first pulse is autocorrelated with an arbitrary fixed reference voltage and a velocity is computed. This velocity will be in significant error because it was compared to a fixed reference voltage rather than to a true velocity. The resultant velocity and all subsequent velocities determined from subsequent pulses are stored in a memory that may look like that in Figure 2–25. As each subsequent set of reflections is autocorrelated to the prior one, the influence of the fixed reference voltage is gradually diminished until it has trivial influence (Fig. 2–26, left). After a number of pulses are transmitted down the same line and each computed velocity is stored in memory for the concerned pixel, a "velocity history" for that pixel is available. Figure 2–26 shows in a pictorial manner the way this velocity history might look. The computer can then determine the average of the most representative velocity for that set of

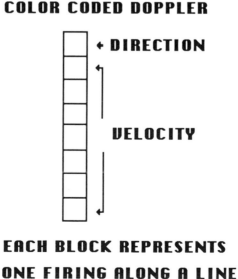

COLOR CODED DOPPLER

← DIRECTION

VELOCITY

EACH BLOCK REPRESENTS
ONE FIRING ALONG A LINE

Fig. 2–25. Time history of a single pixel during eight firings down the line in which that pixel resides. The first firing determines direction and encodes the pixel red or blue. All subsequent firings are used for quantitative pixel velocity.

VELOCITY "QUALITY"

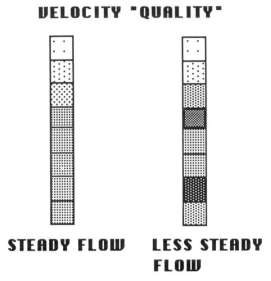

STEADY FLOW   LESS STEADY FLOW

Fig. 2–26. Velocity quality. This pictorial diagram depicts two possible states in a pixel velocity history. On the left, the top pixel contains directional information which will not be the point of this figure, but considered toward the transducer (red). The second pixel from the top contains velocity information left from the past frame, which is the starting place for velocity computation for this new pixel. The second firing is autocorrelated with information from the prior frame and determines that the velocity is now higher than in the last frame and encodes this data (more dots in the pictorial). In this left example, velocity remains the same during each firing. After the third autocorrelation (box 4) a constant velocity is found. The resultant velocity for this pixel will be encoded as a shade of red, the exact shade determined by the velocity found in the bottom box. On the right the same process takes place, but the velocity is varying during the 8 firings down the line. Accordingly, no stable velocity is found and this pixel is encoded green to show the velocity variance.

firings and code the resultant velocity as a shade onto the previously determined primary color. Thus, both direction and velocity magnitude are encoded in one pixel.

This process has several possible outcomes. If all velocities are similar (Fig. 2–26 left), no problem is encountered. On the other hand, velocities determined by each firing could be slightly to significantly different (Fig. 2–26 right). The method in which this variability is displayed is dealt with differently by each manufacturer. Some ignore the problem and simply encode the average or modal velocity. Others determine when velocity variability exceeds some limit determined by the manufacturer and when that variability is found, the pixel will be encoded as green, a color intended to suggest turbulence. The user should be aware that the method for making this decision is arbitrary and does not prove (1) that non-green encoding ensures laminar flow or (2) that green encoding ensures turbulent flow.

This chapter has covered an everchanging field of knowledge. Newer solutions (and newer problems) may occur before or after this book is published. Our purpose has been to provide a non-engineering viewpoint. Simplifications were an effort to translate a complex topic into terms and concepts that were more familiar to physicians and technologists. A reader who understands the aspects presented will be better prepared to perform examinations and to speak to representatives of industry.

REFERENCES

1. Hatle, L. Angelsen, B.: Doppler Ultrasound in Cardiology. 2nd Ed. Lea & Febiger, Philadelphia, 1985.
2. Baker, D.W., Forrester, F.K., Daigle, R.E.: Doppler Principles and Techniques. *In* Fry, F.G. (Ed.) Methods and Phenomena 3. Ultrasound—Its Applications in Medicine and Biology, New York, Elsevier, 1978, Ch. 3.
3. Doppler, C.J.: Uber das farbige licht der doppelsterne. Abhandlungen der Koniglishen Bohmischen Gesellschaft der Wissenchaften. *11*:465, 1842.
4. Brandestini, M. A., Eyer, M. K., Stevenson, J. G.: M/Q-mode echocardiography—the synthesis of conventional echo with digital multigate Doppler. *In* Echocardiology, edited by Lancee, C. The Hague, Martinus Nijhoff, 1979, p. 441.
5. Omoto, R.: Color Atlas of Real-Time Two-Dimensional Doppler Echocardiography. 2nd Ed., Tokyo, Shindan-To-Chiryo Co, Ltd, 1987.
6. Namekawa K., Kasai, C., Tsukamoto, M., Koyano A.: Imaging of blood flow using auto-correlation. Ultrasound Med Biol *8*:138, 1982.

CHAPTER 3

PERFORMANCE OF A NORMAL EXAMINATION AND NORMAL FINDINGS

Understanding and performing the normal Doppler examination are essential for differentiating normal from pathologic states (Chapters 4 and 6), and for measuring flow by Doppler (Chapter 5). Goals of this chapter are to: (1) detail techniques used to obtain normal Doppler tracings, (2) describe normal Doppler tracings, and (3) present normal Doppler values. Since many excellent texts on conventional imaging are available,[1-4] imaging will not be emphasized.

Performance of a complete examination requires an echocardiographic system capable of good imaging, pulsed and continuous wave Doppler. Since all three modalities are essential, one should not be sacrificed for the other. Color-coded Doppler is a newer technology which increases the rapidity of acquisition of certain information by displaying Doppler information as an overlay on the two dimensional image. However, color-coded Doppler has not supplanted standard pulsed and continuous wave Doppler because of velocity and recording limitations. Color-coded Doppler should, nonetheless, be included in an optimal system.

This chapter will detail a systematic Doppler echocardiographic examination. Each echocardiographer may prefer his own sequence, but an organized approach should be used for all examinations to prevent diagnostic errors.

PATIENT

Patients must be quiet, relaxed and comfortable in order to accomplish a complete and accurate imaging and Doppler echocardiographic examination. Sedation is often required to accomplish these objectives for infants and small children. Chloral hydrate appears to be safe and reliable. In fact, we schedule almost all patients between ages 2 months and 3 years for sedation prior to examination.

Optimal Doppler tracings require alignment of the Doppler beam parallel with flow. Alignment can be significantly aided by appropriately positioning the patient during the examination. Pillows or foam wedges may be used to maintain patient position and aid patient comfort during the examination.

We allow 1 hour for performance, interpretation and dictation of the imaging and Doppler examination. A technician initially performs a standard examination. The cardiologist then reviews the study while the patient remains on the table so that the cardiologist can repeat any questionable portion of the examination. We believe that Doppler and imaging examinations should be taken as seriously as catheterizations, and all efforts are made to obtain a complete study before the patient leaves the laboratory.

NORMAL DOPPLER TRACINGS

Optimal Doppler waveforms are obtained when flow is laminar, and the Doppler sample volume or cursor is aligned parallel to flow. Most normal flow is laminar, although specific examples may be cited to the contrary. Laminar flow is considered to be present when the majority of red blood cells are moving in the same direction, and have approximately the same velocity (Chapter 4). Non-laminar flow is frequently found in patients with anatomic defects and is characterized by red blood cells moving in different directions or at significantly different velocities.

Laminar flow usually indicates absence of disease. However, jets resulting from discrete anatomic stenoses may also have laminar flow. This "jet region" can usually be differentiated from normal flow because jet velocities are much higher than normal, a parajet is present, and the jet terminates in a lower velocity postjet flow disturbance (Chapter 4). Jets, representing reversed flow through normal valves, may be found in many individuals, and this occurrence will be discussed later in this chapter.

Doppler waveforms should reach their highest velocities and contain the least velocity spread when the Doppler sample volume or cursor is aligned parallel to laminar flow. Velocity spread refers to the vertical width of the Doppler velocity signal at any instant in time (Fig. 3–1A). "Acceptable" velocity spread is usually achieved when the vertical width of the Doppler velocity signal is less than 30% of the maximum height of the Doppler velocity envelope (Fig. 3–1B). Alignment with flow is aided significantly by listening for the highest, "pure" audio signal. Non-laminar, or disturbed flow sounds much rougher and contains numerous simultaneous tones (frequencies). A book format, unfortunately, does not allow demonstration of the audio separation of laminar and disturbed flow.

GENERAL GUIDELINES FOR OBTAINING OPTIMAL TRACINGS

Several guidelines may assist in acquiring optimal Doppler tracings. First, multiple transducer locations should be used to interrogate velocities for each cardiac chamber and vessel. For example, aortic velocities can be obtained from a suprasternal notch (Fig. 3–2A), apical (Fig. 3–2B), or subcostal (Fig. 3–2C) plane. Further, transducer shapes and types sometimes define the best locations for interrogation. For example, ascending aortic velocities are generally best obtained with an off-axis transducer placed in the suprasternal notch (Fig. 3–3).

Doppler alignment with flow is usually possible and, therefore, correction for beam-flow intercept angles not only is unnecessary, but should be avoided (Chapters 4 and 5). In most instances, as shown by color-coded Doppler, flow in great vessels aligns with vessel walls (Plate 1). At ventricular inlets, inflow generally aligns with the septum in the right ventricle or the wall in the left ventricle (Plate 2). Initially, the sample volume is placed parallel to these structures or in the direction of flow as indicated by color-coded Doppler.

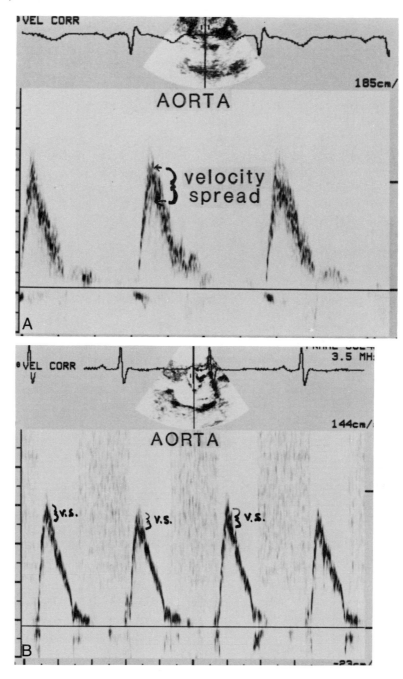

Fig. 3–1. *A.* Pulsed wave ascending aortic tracings showing excessive velocity spread. *B.* Pulsed wave ascending aortic tracings showing minimal velocity spread (v.s.) on three consecutive beats.

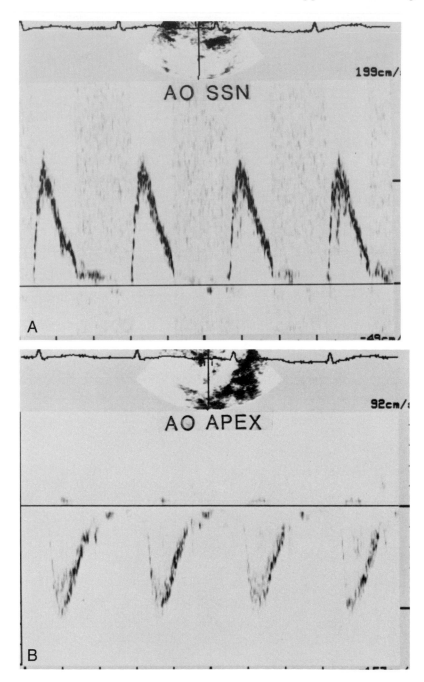

Fig. 3–2. Ascending aortic velocity tracings obtained in the same individual from the suprasternal notch (a), apex five chamber (b), and subcostal views (c). In this patient the highest velocities with the least velocity spread were obtained from the suprasternal notch.

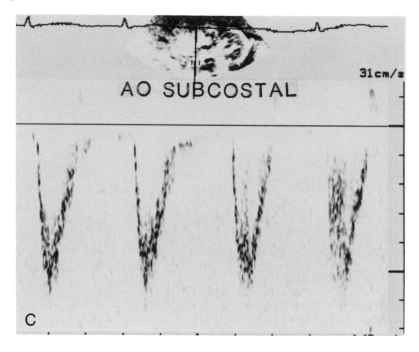

AO SUBCOSTAL

31cm/s

C

Fig. 3–2 (continued).

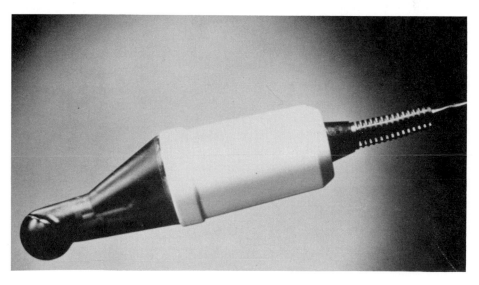

Fig. 3–3. Off-axis transducer used for imaging and velocity interrogation from the suprasternal notch.

This maneuver, however, approximates alignment with flow only in the two visualized dimensions and spatial alignment is required in three dimensions. Transducer direction is then altered concurrently in both the visualized and non-visualized planes until recordings with highest velocity and least velocity spread are obtained. Velocities, thus recorded, are assumed to be spatially aligned.

Abnormally high velocities can occur distal to cardiac valves in the absence of a discrete stenosis. These high velocities have been attributed to increased flow. Goldberg and co-workers reported that the velocity gradient across anatomically normal valves does not usually exceed 20 to 30 cm/sec even in high flow states.[5] In order to apply this criterion, interrogation proximal and distal to the valve should occur in a location where flow area remains constant. This is accomplished by moving the sample volume just proximal and just distal to the leaflet coaptation site within the ring area while recording velocity.

SYSTEMATIC EXAMINATION

We start the examination from the precordial planes, progressing to the subcostal and suprasternal notch planes. This sequence is followed regardless of patient age, or suspected diagnosis. Many subjects find the suprasternal notch examination uncomfortable and, therefore, this part of the examination is performed last.

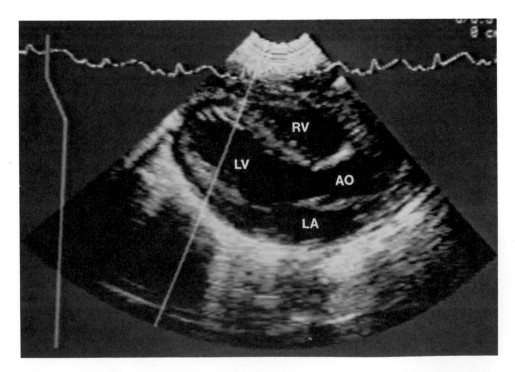

Fig. 3–4. Long axis parasternal view of the left ventricle (LV), aorta (AO), left atrium (LA), and right ventricle (RV).

Precordial Plane

LONG-AXIS PARASTERNAL PLANE

The long axis parasternal plane provides initial anatomic orientation (Fig. 3–4). Although abnormal flow associated with a ventricular septal defect or valve regurgitation or stenosis may be detected, this plane provides little information for quantitative analysis of normal Doppler velocities since alignment of the transducer parallel to flow across the mitral or aortic valve is not possible. The parasternal long axis plane also allows measurement of the left ventricular outflow tract diameter for subsequent calculation of Doppler cardiac outputs from that area.[6] Ascending aortic diameters can also be measured in this plane. However, the diameter measured here may be at the sinuses of Valsalva which will lead to an overestimation of aortic flow.[7]

Color-coded Doppler permits excellent evaluation of the left ventricular inflow and outflow regions in this plane.[8] Transducer position can be adjusted to obtain a large beam-flow intercept angle that will reduce aliasing in the aortic and mitral region. Reduced aliasing occurs because the large beam-flow intercept angle reduces the velocity by the cosine of the intercept angle until it fits within the non-aliasing limit. When imaging from a low long axis parasternal plane, diastolic flow traversing the mitral valve will be directed toward the transducer and will be encoded red (Plate 3). Systolic flow through the left ventricular outflow tract and aorta will be directed away from the transducer and will be encoded blue (Plate 4). Imaging from the high parasternal area brings the left ventricular outflow tract and aorta closer to the transducer. This location will usually result in mitral flow passing away from the transducer (blue) and aortic flow being directed toward the transducer (red) (Plate 5). Care should be taken to assure that flows in the areas of interest are not perpendicular to the imaging plane, since this position will result in velocities too low for adequate analysis and visualization. Therefore, to obtain satisfactory signals without aliasing, several transducer positions should be used to thoroughly investigate flow through the various regions of the left ventricle.

SHORT AXIS PARASTERNAL PLANE

The parasternal short axis is the preferred plane for interrogation of pulmonary velocities. Right ventricular outflow tract velocities can also be interrogated with minor variations from this same plane. However, for infants and young children the subcostal short axis plane may be preferable for interrogation of right ventricular outflow tract velocities. Tricuspid velocities can also be recorded from short axis parasternal planes but alignment with flow across the tricuspid valve is usually best accomplished from the apical four chamber plane.

Highest pulmonary velocities with least velocity spread are often best achieved by placing the patient in an exaggerated left lateral decubitus position. This position places the pulmonary artery more anteriorly, and displaces overlying lung laterally. It may be necessary to place the patient at an angle with respect to the examining table of greater than 90° in order to obtain adequate velocities from patients with lung disease. Sometimes the transducer must be aligned off the true short axis plane in order to obtain the best pulmonary artery Doppler signals. Pulmonary velocities recorded in these short axis parasternal

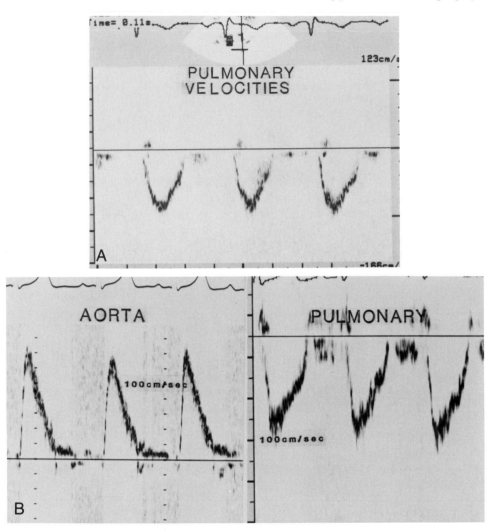

Fig. 3–5. (A) Pulmonary velocities from a short axis parasternal view. (B) Ascending aortic and pulmonary artery velocity tracings from the same individual. Note difference in amplitude.

planes are directed away (negative) from the transducer (Fig. 3–5A) and have a slower upstroke, lower maximal velocity, and later occurring peak than is found for aortic velocities (Fig. 3–5B). The lower pulmonary velocity can be explained, in part, by the difference in vessel areas. Aortic flow equals pulmonary flow in the absence of intracardiac shunting or semi-lunar valve insufficiency. Since the area of the pulmonary artery is usually larger than that of the aorta, pulmonary velocities are lower than aortic velocities.

In normal pulmonary velocity tracings a low amplitude negative diastolic waveform coincident with rapid ventricular filling through the tricuspid valve may be recorded.[9] A second low, negative, late diastolic peak ("A" wave) immediately precedes the systolic upstroke in patients with normal pulmonary artery pressure (Fig. 3–5) and is thought to be related to right atrial contraction. These diastolic waveforms are also shown in Fig. 3–7. Both diastolic waveforms probably represent minimal diastolic flow through the pulmonary valve. If the transducer is placed laterally in the main pulmonary artery near the wall, pulmonary velocity decreases in amplitude in late systole and reverses direction in early diastole. It is, therefore, preferable to record pulmonary velocity in the central portion of the vessel. Narrow high velocity spikes of pulmonary valve opening and closure can be seen when the sample volume is near the leaflets (Fig. 3–6). (These velocity patterns, which are called valve clicks, can be found for all four valves).

Adequate velocity tracings should allow measurement of peak pulmonary velocity, and time to peak velocity (acceleration time) (Fig. 3–7). Peak velocity is measured at the midpoint of the modal velocity. Acceleration time is defined as the interval from onset of the systolic velocity tracing as it leaves baseline, to attainment of peak systolic velocity. Additional measurements include pre-ejection period and ejection time (Fig. 3–7). Table 3–1 summarizes reported values for normal individuals. In normal subjects ranging in age from 14 days to 35 years, Wilson et al.[10] noted a slight decrease in the pulmonary artery peak velocity and a significant increase in the acceleration time with age. These changes are probably related to a decrease in pulmonary artery pressure and increase in vessel area in young subjects. Gardin et al. found no significant changes in these parameters in an older population.[11]

Serwer et al. noted a strong negative correlation in children between pulmonary acceleration time and cardiac rate,[12] but Isobe and associates found no similar correlation in adults.[13] The latter study substituted velocities in the right ventricular outflow tract for pulmonary artery velocities. Whether acceleration time should be adjusted for heart rate remains controversial.

Right ventricular outflow tract velocities in this plane are best measured by placing the transducer inferiorly and laterally on the chest wall, (fourth to fifth intercostal space along the mid clavicular line), and directing the beam superiorly (Fig. 3–8). This maneuver elongates the right ventricular outflow tract and main pulmonary artery and allows the Doppler sample volume to be placed parallel to the walls. Velocity waveforms in the outflow tract are similar in configuration to those in the pulmonary artery but are of lower amplitude and have more velocity spread because the outflow tract has more area than the pulmonary artery.

Positive, early diastolic velocities in both the pulmonary artery and right ventricular outflow tract may be found in most normals (Fig. 3–9). This velocity profile probably represents diastolic retrograde blood flow from the pulmonary artery into the right ventricular outflow tract, suggesting that "pulmonary regurgitation" commonly occurs. Since the term pulmonary regurgitation has a connotation of disease, we use the term "pulmonary backflow" for this condition to separate it from pathologic pulmonary regurgitation. However, pulmonary backflow may be difficult to differentiate from mild pulmonary regurgitation in individuals with normal pulmonary artery pressure. Right ventricular dilatation and pulmonary hypertension are often associated with significant pulmonary regurgitation. Chapter 5 details the procedure for quantitation of pulmonary regurgitant fraction, which is useful for assessing the magnitude of regurgitation.

Parasternal short axis imaging with color-coded Doppler permits recording right ventricular outflow tract and pulmonary artery velocities. Systolic pulmonary artery velocities are encoded blue since flow is away from the transducer. Since normal pulmonary artery velocities frequently exceed the Nyquist limit for color-coded Doppler, aliasing is commonly found (Plate 6). Flow

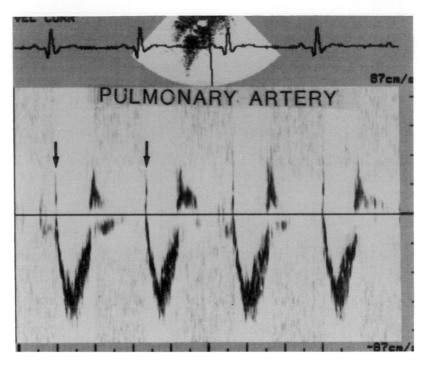

Fig. 3–6. Pulmonary artery velocities obtained with the sample volume placed near the pulmonary valve. High velocity spikes (arrows) associated with valve motion can be seen.

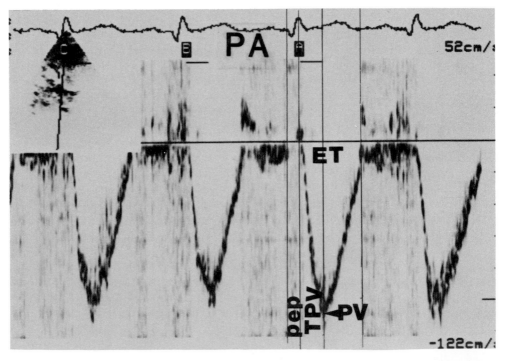

Fig. 3–7. Pulmonary artery (PA) velocity tracings demonstrating measurement of peak velocity and various time intervals; ejection time (ET); pre-ejection period (PEP); time to peak velocity or acceleration time (TPV); and peak velocity (PV).

Table 3–1. Normal Pulmonary Velocity Findings (Short Axis Precordial Plane)

PEAK VELOCITY

Site	Ref	N	Ages	Range (CM-SEC)	Mean ± SD (CM/SEC)
MPA	25	11	0d–3d	53–90	71 ± 9
MPA	26	18	0d–5d	33–100	63 ± 11
MPA	27	97	3d–22y	50–105	76 ± 13
MPA	10	108	14d–35y	52–131	81 ± 17
MPA	28	20	21y–46y	44–78	63 ± 9
MPA	22	30	1y–16y	70–110	90
MPA	22	40	18y–72y	60–90	75

TIME TO PEAK VELOCITY

Site	Ref	N	Ages	Range (MSEC)	Mean ± SD (MSEC)
MPA	26	12	<6h	35–72	51 ± 13
MPA	26	13	6h–24h	43–84	69 ± 14
MPA	26	17	1d–5d	52–101	78 ± 13
MPA	10	108	14d–35y	60–180	121 ± 27
MPA	29	15	4y–22y	105–182	151 ± 25
MPA	28	20	21y–46y	130–185	159 ± 18
RVOT	30	16	46y±15y		137 ± 24
RVOT	13	32	47y±16y	112–198	157 ± 25

PRE-EJECTION PERIOD

Site	Ref	N	Ages	Range (MSEC)	Mean ± SD (MSEC)
MPA	29	15	4y–22y	71–104	88 ± 3
RVOT	13	32	47y–16y		91 ± 21

EJECTION TIME

Site	Ref	N	Ages	Range (MSEC)	Mean ± SD (MSEC)
MPA	29	15	4y–22y		317 ± 33
MPA	28	20	21y–46y	280–380	331 ± 23
RVOT	30	16	46y–15y		304 ± 38
RVOT	13	32	47y–16y		317 ± 33
MPA	11	18	21y–30y		330
MPA	11	20	61y–70y		320

MPA = main pulmonary artery; RVOT = right ventricular outflow tract

reversal (positive or red) is often seen in the right ventricular outflow tract during early diastole (Plate 7). As described above, this small amount of "pulmonary backflow" should be considered a normal finding.

In the right pulmonary artery, Doppler interrogation parallel to flow can be difficult since this vessel lies perpendicular to the imaging plane. The left pulmonary artery, on the other hand, lies mainly parallel to the beam, thus permitting Doppler alignment with flow. Peripheral pulmonary artery Doppler tracings are similar to those in the main pulmonary artery except that they may have a higher amplitude, absence of the "A" wave, and absence of a reversal of flow pattern. We have serially followed branch pulmonary artery velocities in some infants and found that the increased branch artery velocities regress

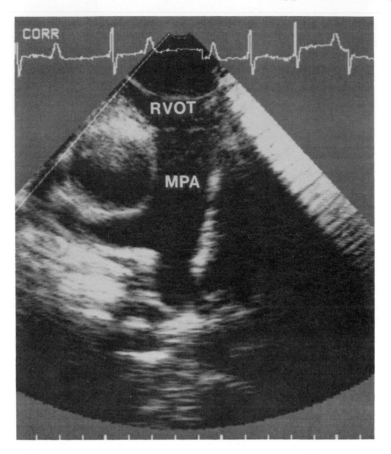

Fig. 3–8. Right ventricular outflow tract and main pulmonary artery from a precordial short axis plane with the transducer placed in the fourth to fifth intercostal space in the mid-clavicular line.

over time. The etiology for this change is unclear, but may relate to alterations in the ratio of main and branch pulmonary artery areas.

APICAL FOUR CHAMBER PLANE

The apical four chamber plane is preferred for interrogation of velocities across the mitral and tricuspid valves. In this plane velocities are "mapped" anteriorly from the pulmonary veins, through the left atrium and across the mitral valve. Similarly, velocities are mapped anteriorly through the right atrium and across the tricuspid valve. Superior and inferior vena caval inflow enter the right atrium nearly perpendicular to the apical four chamber imaging plane and are not studied in this plane.

Pulmonary venous velocities in children are of low amplitude and continuous throughout the cardiac cycle. We and others[14] usually find two or three pulmonary venous velocity peaks (Fig. 3–10) in infants and children which seem to depend upon the interaction of left atrial and pulmonary hemodynamics. The first peak occurs in early diastole with opening of the mitral valve. There is frequently reversal of flow into the pulmonary veins during atrial systole with a second forward peak occurring with atrial relaxation. A third peak occurs later in ventricular systole. Investigators[15] have reported two peaks

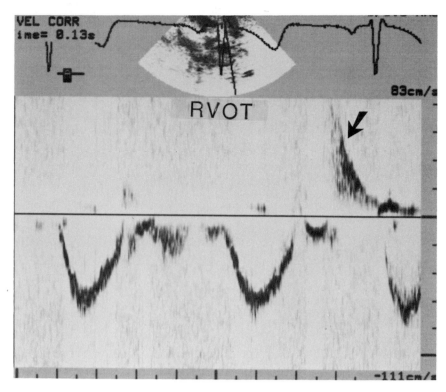

Fig. 3–9. Pulsed wave velocities from the right ventricular outflow tract showing positive, early diastolic velocities associated with "pulmonary backflow."

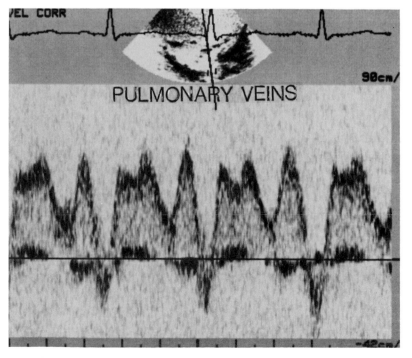

Fig. 3–10. Pulmonary venous inflow velocities from an apex four chamber view demonstrating three distinct peaks.

in adult subjects. The first peak was attributed to pulmonary venous inflow with mitral valve opening, and the second to atrial relaxation following atrial systole.

Left atrial velocities are dependent upon pulmonary venous and mitral flow, and their amplitude varies with sample volume location. Velocities proximal to the mitral valve are similar to biphasic transmitral velocities but are of lower amplitude, the magnitude of which is commensurate with area changes within the atrium. Velocity spread tends to be wide (Fig. 3–11).

Mitral velocities are obtained by placement of the Doppler sample volume within the valve leaflets just distal to the annulus. The sample volume is aligned parallel to the interventricular septum and then adjusted in the non-visualized plane until optimal waveforms are found. Mitral velocities (Fig. 3–12), are characterized by an early diastolic "E" wave associated with the rapid left ventricular filling phase followed by an "A" wave associated with atrial contraction. Table 3–2 lists normal mitral velocities. The absolute height, ratio of height, and area under these two time velocity waveforms have been associated with diastolic properties of the left ventricle. These relationships are discussed in detail in Chapter 6. However, characteristics and amplitude of both the "E" and "A" waveforms may change with slight alterations of the Doppler beam in any plane and with sampling site. Velocities within the annulus area just proximal to the mitral valve are similar to those just distal to the valve. Drinkovic et al.[16] demonstrated that the velocities at the tips of the mitral valve leaflets were significantly higher than those at the annulus due to the smaller flow area at the leaflet tips. The early diastolic "E" wave has been shown to decrease with age while the "A" wave and A/E ratio increase.[17,18] This finding has been attributed to changes in ventricular distensibility. The A wave amplitude has also been shown to increase with heart rate secondary to shortening of the total diastolic filling period.[19] In tachycardic individuals separate "E" and "A" waves may be difficult to differentiate because of the shortened diastolic period.

Increased negative systolic velocities of aortic outflow can be simultaneously recorded with mitral velocities when the sample volume is placed medially in the region of the left ventricular outflow tract (Fig. 3–13). Low amplitude negative diastolic velocities can also be seen (Fig. 3–14). These velocities are attributed to flow reversing direction at the apex during diastole.

Right atrial velocities are dependent upon systemic venous and tricuspid flow, and hence their amplitude also varies with sample volume location. The velocity waveform is similar to the biphasic tricuspid velocity waveform but is of lower magnitude and has more velocity spread. Right atrial velocity amplitude is affected by the respiratory cycle, and increases during inspiration.

Miyatake and associates[20] have provided insight into normal right atrial velocity patterns observed with color-coded Doppler. They found that flow passes toward the tricuspid valve near the region of the atrial septum in mid to late systole, and reverses near the tricuspid valve in late systole. Positive (red) flow streams along the atrial septum into the right ventricle in early diastole (Plate 8) and again during atrial systole.

Tricuspid velocities are obtained by placing the Doppler sample volume within the valve leaflets distal to the annulus. The sample volume is aligned parallel to the interventricular septum and then adjusted in the non-visualized

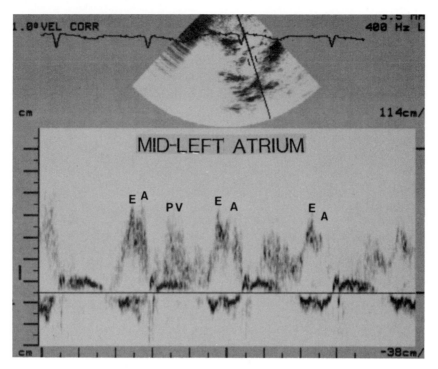

Fig. 3–11. Mid left atrial velocities from an apex four chamber view. Note the marked spectral width, and low amplitude "E" and "A" waves. Pulmonary venous velocities (PV) can be seen during systole.

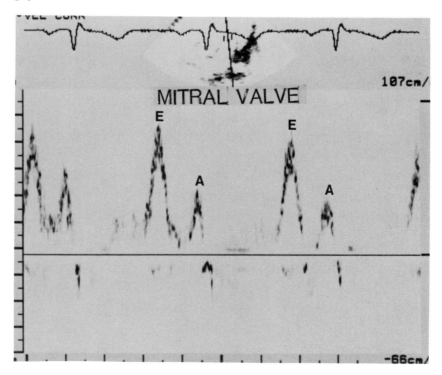

Fig. 3–12. Transmitral velocities from an apex four chamber view demonstrating "E" and "A" waves.

Table 3–2.   Normal Mitral Valve Velocity Findings—Apical Plane

PEAK VELOCITY

Ref	N	Ages	Range (CM/SEC)	Mean ± SD (CM/SEC)
25	11	0d–3d	41–70	53 ± 8
27	48	3d–22y	61–120	78 ± 13
10	110	14d–35y	44–128	77 ± 16
22	30	1y–16y	80–130	100
22	40	18y–72y	60–130	90

PEAK E WAVE VELOCITY

Ref	N	Ages	Range (CM/SEC)	Mean ± SD (CM/SEC)
26	18	0d–5d	28–70	50 ± 10
31	18	18y–64y		61 ± 7
32	52	21y–78y		54 ± 12
17	69	22y–69y	34–94	62
33	19	54y ± 15y		53 ± 10
18	8	21y–30y		66 ± 11
18	18	61y–70y		45 ± 10

PEAK A WAVE VELOCITY

Ref	N	Ages	Range (CM/SEC)	Mean ± SD (CM/SEC)
26	18	0d–5d	27–72	45 ± 11
31	18	18y–64y		40 ± 11
32	52	21y–78y		47 ± 11
17	69	22y–69y	28–69	48
33	19	54y ± 15y		47 ± 12
18	8	21y–30y		41 ± 7
18	18	61y–70y		55 ± 11

A/E RATIO

Ref	N	Ages	Range (CM/SEC)	Mean ± SD (CM/SEC)
26	18	0d–5d	0.56–1.42	0.91 ± 0.17
31	18	18y–64y		0.64 ± 0.18
32	52	21y–78y		0.94 ± 0.4
21	10	52y ± 7y		0.44 ± 0.14
33	19	54y ± 15y		1.0 ± 0.4
18	8	21y–30y		0.6 ± 0.1
18	18	61y–70y		1.2 ± 0.3

plane until optimal waveforms are found. Tricuspid velocities are similar in configuration to mitral velocities but are generally of lower amplitude. There is an early diastolic "E" wave associated with the rapid right ventricular filling phase followed by an "A" wave related to right atrial contraction (Fig. 3–15). The A/E ratio has been associated with diastolic properties of the right ventricle.[21] As diastole shortens, the "E" and "A" waves tend to occur close together and in tachycardic individuals separate peaks may be difficult to differentiate. Tricuspid velocities vary significantly with the respiratory cycle, whereas mi-

COLOR PLATES

Plate 1. Color-coded Doppler pulmonary velocities from precordial short-axis view of the pulmonary outflow tract. Blue color (double arrows) represents systolic pulmonary flow, away from the transducer, aligned within the walls of the pulmonary artery.

Plate 2. Color-coded Doppler mitral and tricuspid inflow velocities from an apex four-chamber plane. Red-orange color represents diastolic inflow velocities toward the transducer. Right ventricular inflow parallels the ventricular septum (A), while flow into the left ventricle tends to align with the lateral wall (B).

Plate 3. Color-coded Doppler velocities from a low long axis parasternal view. Diastolic velocities across the mitral valve are directed toward the transducer and are encoded as red-orange.

Plate 4. Color-coded Doppler velocities from a low long axis parasternal view. Systolic velocities through the left ventricular outflow tract and aortic valve are directed away from the transducer and are encoded as blue.

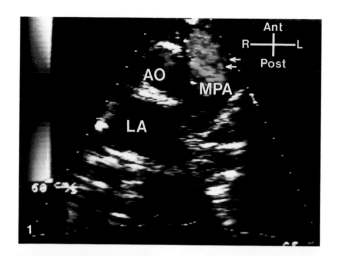

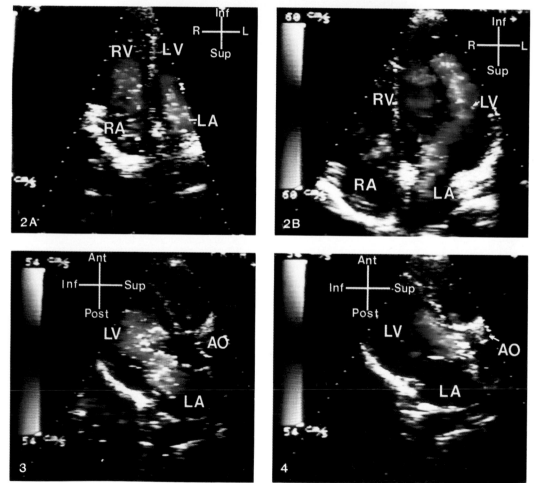

Plate 5.   Color-coded Doppler velocities from a high long axis parasternal view. Systolic velocities through the left ventricular outflow tract and aortic valve are directed toward the transducer and are encoded as red-orange.

Plate 6.   Color-coded Doppler pulmonary velocities from a short axis parasternal view. Velocities are coded as blue (away from the transducer). Red-orange velocities within the pulmonary artery indicate aliasing since these velocities exceed the Nyquist limit.

Plate 7.   Color-coded Doppler pulmonary velocities in the right ventricular outflow tract (RVOT) and pulmonary artery in a normal individual demonstrate "pulmonary backflow." Red-orange color in the right ventricular outflow tract represents diastolic flow toward the transducer.

Plate 8.   Color-coded Doppler velocities from an apex four chamber view. Diastolic flow into the right ventricle streams along the right atrial surface of the atrial septum.

Plate 9.   Color-coded Doppler velocities from an apex four chamber view demonstrate "tricuspid backflow." The narrow blue area (double arrows) in the right atrium represents early systolic retrograde flow from the right ventricle.

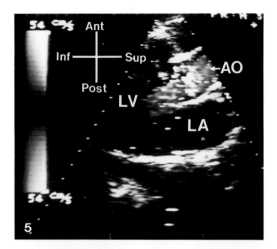

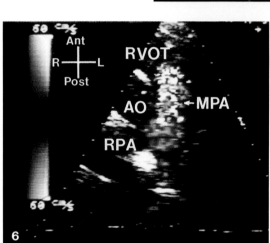

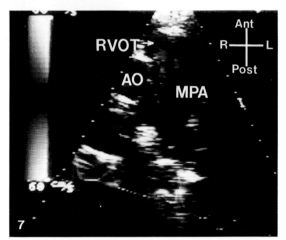

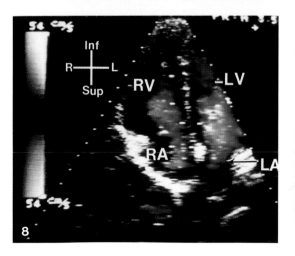

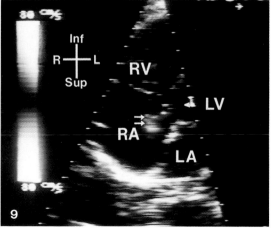

Plate 10. Color-coded Doppler velocities from an apex four chamber view demonstrate diastolic flow into the right ventricle. Velocities are toward the transducer and are encoded as red-orange. Flow in the right ventricle aligns with the ventricular septum.

Plate 11. Color-coded Doppler velocities from an apical five chamber view demonstrate systolic flow in the left ventricular outflow tract (LVOT) and ascending aorta. Flow is away from the transducer and is encoded as blue.

Plate 12. Color-coded Doppler velocities from the suprasternal notch demonstrate superior vena caval and ascending aortic flow. The superior vena caval flow is away from the transducer and is encoded as blue. Ascending aortic flow is toward the transducer and is encoded as red-orange. Descending aortic flow is shown as blue.

Plate 13. Color-coded Doppler velocities from the subcostal plane showing superior vena caval flow (arrow) entering the right atrium. Flow is toward the transducer and is encoded as red-orange.

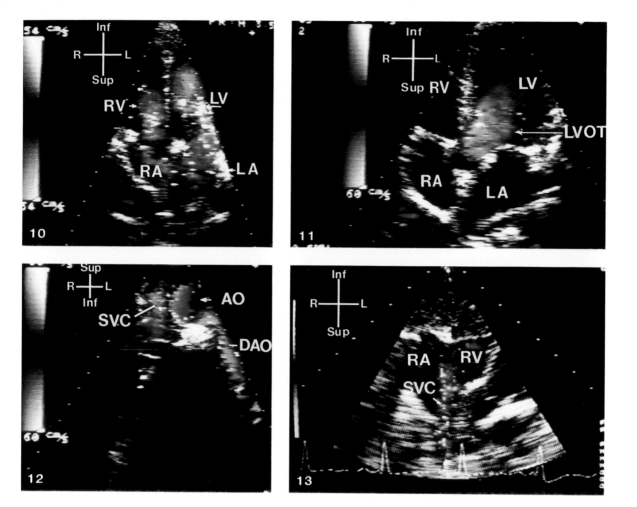

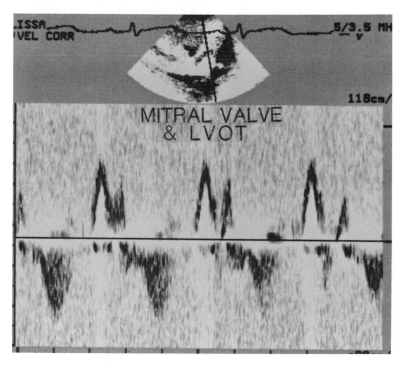

Fig. 3–13. Simultaneous left ventricular outflow and mitral inflow velocities obtained from an apical five chamber view.

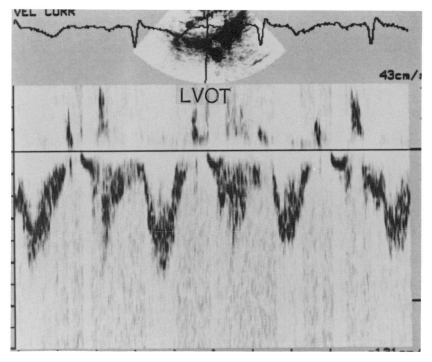

Fig. 3–14. Velocities with the sample volume placed medial to the mitral valve near the aortic outflow tract. Systolic negative velocities of aortic outflow can be seen with negative diastolic velocities of mitral inflow traversing around into the outflow tract.

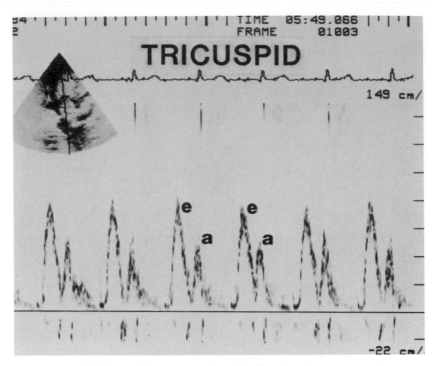

Fig. 3–15. Tricuspid velocities from an apex four chamber plane demonstrating the "E" wave of ventricular filling, and "A" wave associated with atrial contraction.

Table 3–3.   Normal Tricuspid Valve Velocity Findings— 4 Chamber Apex Plane

		PEAK VELOCITY			
Site	Ref	N	Ages	Range (CM/SEC)	Mean ± SD (CM/SEC)
RV	25	11	0d–3d	37–76	47 ± 11
RA	27	22	3d–22y	38–74	48 ± 9
RV	27	43	3d–22y	41–84	62 ± 12
RV	10	110	14d–35y	33–81	51 ± 12
	22	30	1y–16y	50–80	60
	22	40	18y–72y	30–70	50

	PEAK E WAVE VELOCITY			
Ref	N	Ages	Range (CM/SEC)	Mean ± SD (CM/SEC)
26	18	0d–5d	22–61	36 ± 9

	PEAK A WAVE VELOCITY			
Ref	N	Ages	Range (CM/SEC)	Mean ± SD (CM/SEC)
26	18	0d–5d	30–76	48 ± 12

	A/E RATIO			
Ref	N	Ages	Range (CM/SEC)	Mean ± SD (CM/SEC)
26	18	0d–5d	0.65–2.06	1.35 ± 0.30
21	10	52y ± 7y		0.51 ± 0.10

tral velocities are influenced minimally. Normal tricuspid valve velocity values are listed in Table 3–3. Peak tricuspid velocities decrease with age,[10] probably related to the increase in tricuspid valve annulus area with age and changes in right ventricular distensibility.

A negative right atrial systolic waveform can be seen in normals when the Doppler sample volume is directed medially along the atrial septum near the septal leaflet of the tricuspid valve (Fig. 3–16). On color-coded Doppler this is seen as a narrow blue area (Plate 9). This velocity pattern represents systolic retrograde flow from the right ventricle, and suggests that tricuspid backflow exists in normals. These negative systolic waveforms, as opposed to "pathologic" tricuspid regurgitation, occupy only a small area in the right atrium close to the valve. Similar waveforms may be found in the left atrium in a few normal subjects. Both may have significant duration.

Color-coded Doppler shows rapid positive (red) tricuspid velocities in early diastole, and these velocities are occasionally aliased (Plate 10). The initial filling phase is followed by positive velocities associated with atrial contraction.

APICAL FIVE CHAMBER PLANE

Optimal alignment with flow in the aortic outflow tract is probably best accomplished from the apical five chamber plane, although in infants and young children, alignment may also be achieved in a subcostal or suprasternal plane. Velocities in the proximal ascending aorta may also be interrogated from the apical five chamber plane (Fig. 3–17). However, velocities are generally of

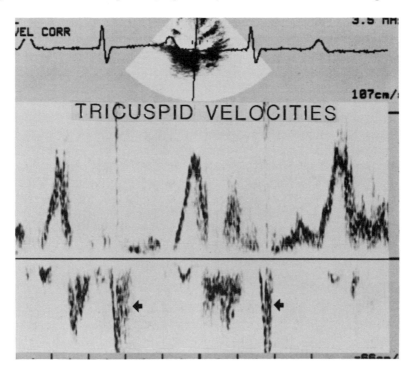

Fig. 3–16. Tricuspid velocities from an apex four chamber plane in a normal individual. The arrows demonstrate early systolic negative velocities of "tricuspid backflow."

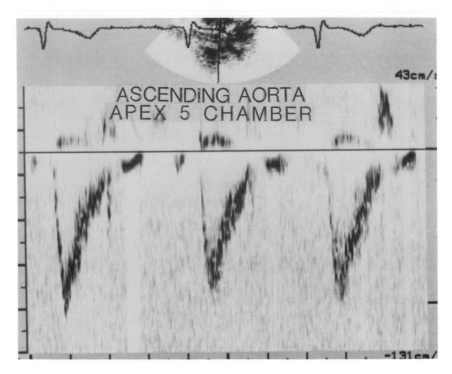

Fig. 3–17. Ascending aortic velocities from an apex five chamber view.

lower peak amplitude, and have greater velocity spread than ascending aortic velocities recorded from the suprasternal notch or right upper sternal border. This implies that optimal alignment with flow is better achieved from a more superior plane in most individuals.

The left ventricular outflow velocity waveform (Fig. 3–18), which is negative in polarity, is similar to that obtained in the ascending aorta. The systolic upstroke is rapid, and velocity dispersion is encountered. As mentioned above, low amplitude negative diastolic velocities may be seen (Fig. 3–14). These represent mitral inflow coursing around the anterior leaflet of the mitral valve and into the aortic outflow tract. Positive diastolic velocities of mitral inflow can occur simultaneously with negative systolic velocities of aortic outflow when the sample volume is placed laterally (Fig. 3–13).

Color-coded Doppler in the apical five chamber plane shows systolic aortic flow away from the transducer (blue) (Plate 11). Aliasing is frequently present since normal aortic velocities exceed the Nyquist limit. Mitral flow patterns are similar to those seen in the apical four chamber plane.

Suprasternal Notch Plane

The suprasternal notch is the preferred plane for interrogation of ascending, transverse and descending aortic velocities. In some patients, improved alignment with flow in the ascending aorta can be obtained by placement of the transducer in the right supraclavicular area. However, ascending aorta velocities may be better obtained from the right upper parasternal region or apical five chamber plane in some larger or older subjects. Therefore, other areas

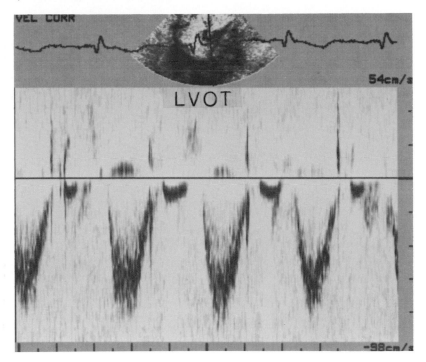

Fig. 3–18. Pulsed Doppler velocities from the left ventricular outflow tract obtained from the apical five chamber view.

should be interrogated and results compared to those obtained from the suprasternal notch.

We use an off-axis transducer designed for imaging and Doppler interrogation from the suprasternal notch (Fig. 3–3). The distal end of the transducer is dome shaped, which allows easier adjustment in all planes. This transducer images the ascending aorta in the center of the sector (Fig. 3–19). The subvalvar left ventricular outflow tract is imaged as a direct continuation of the ascending aorta allowing the sample volume to be moved along the axis of the left ventricular outflow tract and ascending aorta.

Ascending aortic velocities are positive, with a rapid systolic upstroke which exhibits minimal velocity spread (Fig. 3–20). Velocity spread routinely occurs at peak velocity and may persist through some or all of the deceleration phase. A brief negative velocity is frequently seen at the end of systole which is most likely due to a reversal of blood flow associated with closure of the aortic valve.[22] Poorly defined fluctuations around the baseline may be found throughout diastole.

Interrogation of ascending aortic velocities is obtained by placement of the sample volume superior to the sinuses of Valsalva and parallel to the walls of the aorta. The sample volume site rarely needs to be higher than the level where the right pulmonary artery traverses behind the ascending aorta. Above this level the aorta begins to curve in a posterior-leftward direction. Doppler aortic tracings in the curvature area are of lower velocity, and have significant velocity spread as a result of poor beam flow alignment.

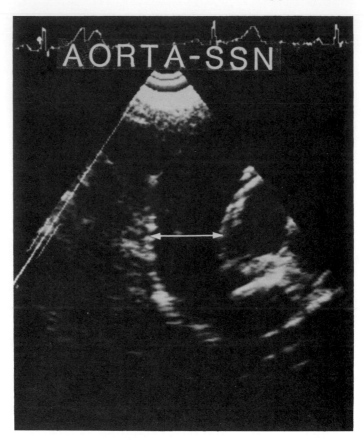

Fig. 3–19.   Suprasternal notch image of the ascending aorta. Arrows show the aortic diameter from middle of one wall to the other. Reprinted with permission from American Heart Journal.[7]

Hegesh et al. reported that subjects with aortic diameters greater than 25 mm have increased velocity spread both during peak velocity and the deceleration phase.[23] The wall influences the central core of velocities considerably less in larger vessels. These central core velocities may move at considerably higher velocities than those found in smaller vessels, accounting for the greater velocity spread.

Several problems may prevent adequate Doppler examinations from the suprasternal notch in some individuals. These factors include hypertrophied neck muscles, insertion of the sternocleidomastoid muscle on the contralateral side of the suprasternal notch, and patient discomfort due to tracheal compression.

Optimal ascending aortic tracings should allow accurate measurement of peak velocity, acceleration time, pre-ejection period, and ejection time (Fig. 3–21). Table 3–4 summarizes values for these measurements in normal individuals. Aortic peak velocities decrease with age probably, in part, due to an age related increase in aortic diameter.[11] Peak velocities at age 70 are approximately 60% of those found at age 20.[11,24] Acceleration time, or time to peak velocity, is the time interval from the onset of the systolic velocity tracing as it leaves baseline to attainment of peak systolic velocity. Aortic acceleration time has been used as an indicator of ventricular performance and is discussed

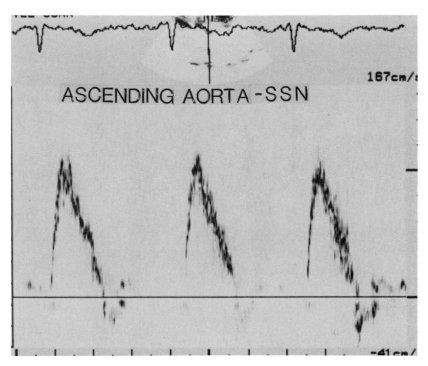

Fig. 3–20. Pulsed wave ascending aortic velocities from the suprasternal notch. Note the minimal velocity spread on the upstroke, and increased velocity spread during the deceleration phase.

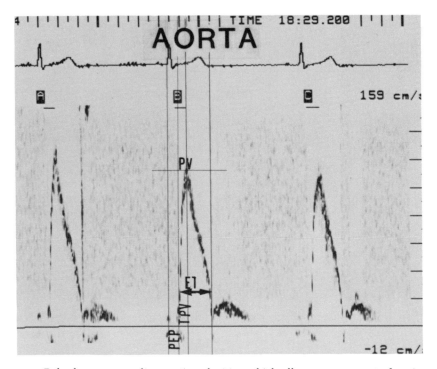

Fig. 3–21. Pulsed wave ascending aortic velocities which allow measurement of various time intervals including; pre-ejection period (PEP); ejection time (ET); time to peak velocity or acceleration time (TPV). Abbreviation: PV = peak velocity.

Table 3–4. Normal Ascending Aortic Velocity Findings

PEAK VELOCITY				
Ref	N	Ages	Range (CM/SEC)	Mean ± SD (CM/SEC)
25	11	0d–3d	61–103	85 ± 11
26	15	0d–5d	60–114	77 ± 11
27	23	3d–22y	60–116	89 ± 15
10	107	14d–35y	76–115	104 ± 19
28	20	21y–46y	72–120	92 ± 11
22	30	1y–16y	120–180	150
22	40	18y–72y	100–170	135
24	140	15y–80y		102 ± 25
34	12	62y–80y		100 ± 15
11	18	21y–30y		93 ± 11
11	20	61y–70y		65 ± 12

TIME TO PEAK VELOCITY				
Ref	N	Ages	Range (MSEC)	Mean ± SD (MSEC)
10	107	14d–35y	50–150	92 ± 23
28	20	21y–46y	83–118	98 ± 10
34	12	62y–80y		85 ± 9
11	18	21y–30y		100 ± 10
11	20	61y–70y		103 ± 32

EJECTION TIME				
Ref	N	Ages	Range (MSEC)	Mean ± SD (MSEC)
28	20	21y–46y	265–325	294 ± 19
34	12	62y–80y		233 ± 28
11	18	21y–30y		297 ± 19
11	20	61y–70y		296 ± 43

Table 3–5. Normal Descending Aortic Velocity Findings

PEAK VELOCITY				
Ref	N	Ages	Range (CM/SEC)	Mean ± SD (CM/SEC)
25	11	0d–3d	81–140	107 ± 14
27	20	3d–22y	51–104	88 ± 13
10	105	14d–35y	70–160	101 ± 17

TIME TO PEAK VELOCITY				
Ref	N	Ages	Range (MSEC)	Mean ± SD (MSEC)
10	107	14d–35y	50–190	107 ± 28

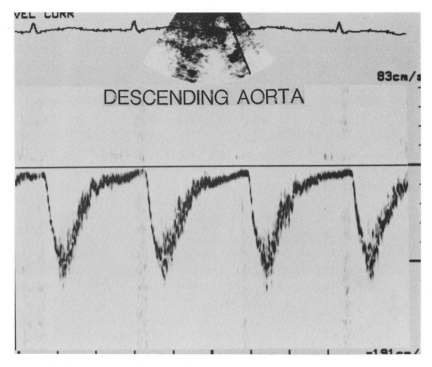

Fig. 3–22. Pulsed wave descending aortic velocities from the suprasternal notch.

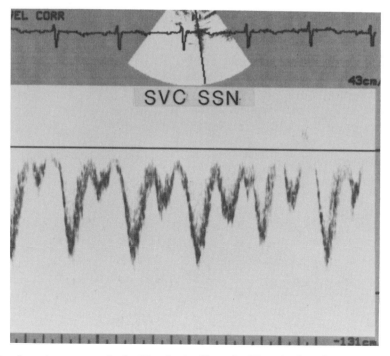

Fig. 3–23. Superior vena caval velocities obtained by pulsed Doppler from the suprasternal notch.

in detail in Chapter 6. As is true for pulmonary acceleration time, heart rate adjustment remains controversial and needs additional study.

Alignment with flow in the descending aorta is also best obtained from the suprasternal notch. The Doppler waveform in the descending aorta is similar to that in the ascending aorta except for negative polarity and increased velocity spread (Fig. 3–22). Increased velocity spread probably occurs because: (1) the best alignment occurs at the junction of the transverse and descending aorta where flow is changing direction, (2) flow has passed far from the aortic inlet and is becoming more parabolic and (3) centripetal forces may create a non-laminar flow pattern as the aorta curves posteriorly and inferiorly. In many neonates, velocities in the proximal descending aorta may be increased secondary to mild narrowing in the region of the aortic isthmus. This finding is rarely seen after the neonatal period. Normal values for descending aortic velocities are shown in Table 3–5.

Superior vena caval velocities are usually obtained from the suprasternal notch. In young subjects these velocities can also be obtained from the subcostal plane. The waveform is predominantly biphasic, with a larger negative peak during early systole, and a smaller negative peak during early to mid diastole (Fig. 3–23). Peak velocities in the superior vena cava increase during inspiration. Although not well studied in older adults, Wilson et al. found, in a group ranging up to 35 years, a significant decrease in the peak velocities with both age and body surface area.[10] This change was related, in part, to increasing vessel diameter with age.

In the suprasternal notch plane, color-coded Doppler will easily differentiate the negative (blue) flow found in the SVC from the positive (red) flow of the ascending aorta (Plate 12). Velocities found in normal individuals may frequently cause signal aliasing when imaging the ascending aorta in this plane. Further, in-line transducers used with color-coded Doppler may not image the ascending aorta parallel to flow. This is both an advantage (apparent lower velocities) and a disadvantage (inability to see left ventricular outflow tract and ascending aorta as a continuous structure). Since most aortic velocities are aliased, we have not found the suprasternal notch or right upper sternal border examination as rewarding as other planes of examination for color-coded Doppler.

Subcostal Plane

LONG AXIS

The preferred plane for Doppler interrogation of the atrial and ventricular septum is the subcostal long axis plane. The Doppler sample volume can be placed nearly perpendicular to both of these structures from this location (Fig. 3–24). Doppler interrogation of an intact atrial or ventricular septum shows continuous, positive, low amplitude velocities (Fig. 3–25), probably related to wall motion or red blood cell motion impacting the septa. Normal velocity tracings are clearly delineated from those in which a defect exists (Chapter 6).

Superior vena caval inflow velocities at the entrance to the right atrium can be interrogated from the long axis plane (Fig. 3–26). Except for waveform

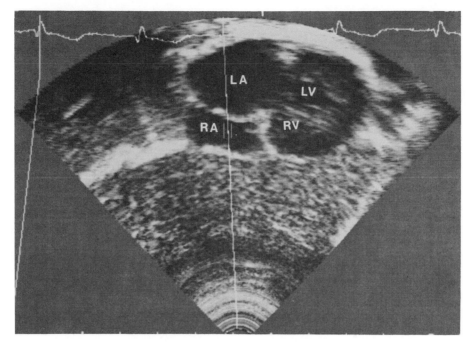

Fig. 3–24. Subcostal long axis image showing the atrial septum.

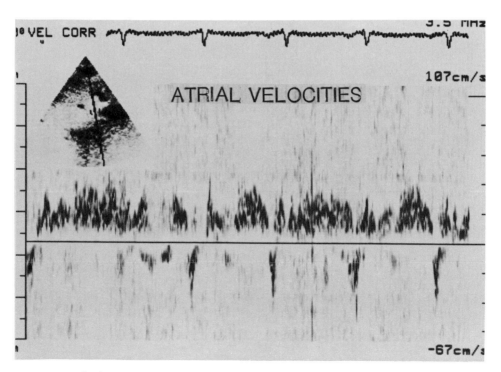

Fig. 3–25. Pulsed wave Doppler velocities with the sample volume placed nearly perpendicular to the right atrial septal surface from a subcostal short axis plane.

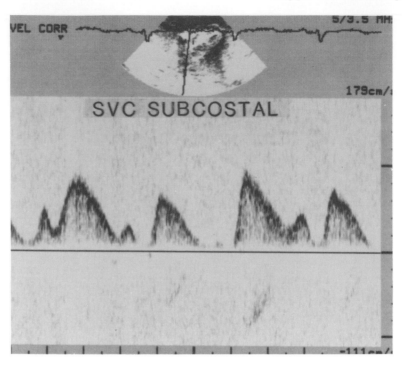

Fig. 3—26. Pulsed wave Doppler velocities at the entrance of the superior vena cava to right atrium from the subcostal view.

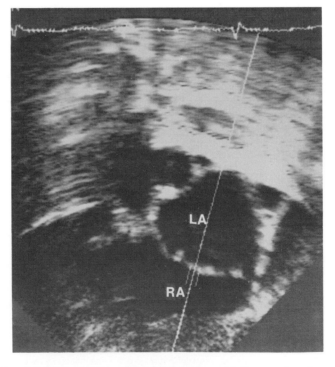

Fig. 3—27. Subcostal short axis view of the atrial septum with the sample volume aligned nearly perpendicular.

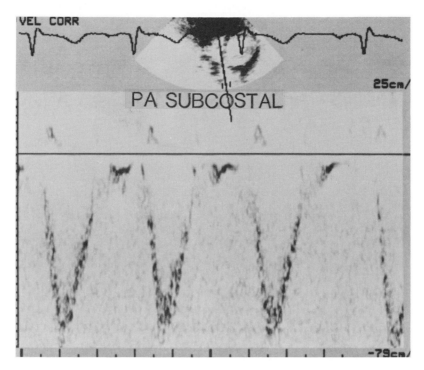

Fig. 3–28. Pulsed wave Doppler pulmonary waveforms from a subcostal plane.

polarity, these tracings are similar to the biphasic pattern seen in the suprasternal notch (Fig. 3–23).

Superior and clockwise transducer rotation allows interrogation of ascending aortic velocities. However, the preferred plane for ascending aortic velocities is the suprasternal notch where aortic velocities are usually of higher amplitude and contain less velocity spread.

Color-coded Doppler imaging in this plane can be used to investigate flow in the superior vena cava, ascending aorta, and the four cardiac chambers. As an example, Plate 13 shows superior vena caval flow entering the right atrium. In this plane superior vena caval flow is toward the transducer, and therefore is encoded as red. Velocities across the atrioventricular valves are unlikely to show aliasing from the subcostal plane due to the large beam flow intercept angle.

SHORT AXIS PLANE

Interrogation of atrial septal velocities can also be performed in a short axis plane. Perpendicular alignment with the atrial septum can be more easily performed in this plane (Fig. 3–27).

Optimal alignment with flow in the right ventricular outflow tract is best accomplished in the subcostal plane in infants, small children, and some adults. The Doppler pulmonary velocity waveform is similar to that obtained from a short axis parasternal plane (Fig. 3–28). In the adult, the distance from the subcostal approach is excessive and abdominal musculature is frequently too tense to permit adequate alignment. Accordingly, velocities in the right ventricular outlow tract in the adult are usually obtained from the parasternal short axis plane.

REFERENCES

1. Goldberg, S.J., Allen, H.D., Sahn, D.J.: Pediatric and Adolescent Echocardiography, 2nd Ed. Chicago, Year Book Medical Publishers, Inc., 1980.
2. Feigenbaum, H.: Echocardiography, 4th Ed. Philadelphia, Lea & Febiger, 1986.
3. Williams, R.G., Bierman, F.Z., Sanders, S.P.: Echocardiographic Diagnosis of Cardiac Malformations. Boston, Little, Brown & Co., 1986.
4. Silverman, N.H., Snider, A.R.: Two-dimensional Echocardiography in Congenital Heart Disease. Norwalk, CT, Appleton-Century-Crofts, 1982.
5. Goldberg, S.J., Wilson, N., Dickinson, D.F.: Increased blood velocities in the heart and great vessels of patients with congenital heart disease: An assessment of their significance in the absence of valvar stenosis. Br Heart J *53*:640, 1985.
6. Huntsman, L.L., Stewart, D.K., Barnes, S.R., Franklin, S.B., Colocousis, J.S., Hessel, E.A.: Noninvasive Doppler determination of cardiac output in man. Circulation *67*:593, 1983.
7. Marx, G.R., Goldberg, S.J., Allen, H.D.: Two methods for measurement of ascending aortic diameter by 2D echocardiography as compared with cineangiography. Am Heart J *112*:172, 1986.
8. Miyatake, K., Okamoto, M., Kinoshita, N., Izumi, S., Owa, M., Takao, S., Sakakibara, H., Nimura, Y.: Clinical applications of a new type of real-time two-dimensional Doppler flow imaging system. Am J Cardiol *54*:857, 1984.
9. Gibbs, J.L., Wilson, N., Witsenburg, M., Williams, G.J., Goldberg, S.J.: Diastolic forward blood flow in the pulmonary artery detected by Doppler echocardiography. J Am Coll Cardiol *6*:1322, 1985.
10. Wilson, N., Goldberg, S.J., Dickinson, D.F., Scott, O.: Normal intracardiac and great artery blood velocity measurements by pulsed Doppler echocardiography. Br Heart J *53*:451, 1985.
11. Gardin, J.M., Davidson, D.M., Rohan, M.K., Butman, S., Knoll, M., Garcia, R., Dubria, S., Gardin S.K., Henry, W.L.: Relationship between age, body size, gender, and blood pressure and Doppler flow measurements in the aorta and pulmonary artery. Am Heart J *113*:101, 1987.
12. Serwer, G.A., Cougle, A.G., Eckerd, J.M., Armstrong, B.E.: Factors affecting use of the Doppler-determined time from flow onset to maximal pulmonary artery velocity for measurement of pulmonary artery pressure in children. Am J Cardiol *58*:352, 1986.
13. Isobe, M., Yazaki, Y., Takaku, F., Koizumi, K., Hara, K., Tsuneyoshi, H., Yamaguchi, T., Machii, K.: Prediction of pulmonary arterial pressure in adults by pulsed Doppler echocardiography. Am J Cardiol *57*:316, 1986.
14. Smallhorn, J.F., Freedom, R.M., Olley, P.M.: Pulsed Doppler echocardiographic assessment of extraparenchymal pulmonary vein flow. J Am Coll Cardiol *9*:573, 1987.
15. Keren, G., Bier, A., Sherez, J., Miura, D., Keefe, D., LeJemtel, T.: Atrial contraction is an important determinant of pulmonary venous flow. J Am Coll Cardiol *7*:693, 1986.
16. Drinkovic, N., Smith, M.D., Wisenbaugh, T., Friedman, B., Kwan, O.L., DeMaria, A.N.: Influence of sampling site upon the ratio of atrial to early diastolic transmitral flow velocities by Doppler. (Abstr.) J Am Coll Cardiol *9*:16A, 1987.
17. Miyatake, K., Okamoto, M., Kinoshita, N., Owa, M., Nakasone, I., Sakakibara, H., Nimura, Y.: Augmentation of atrial contribution to left ventricular inflow with aging as assessed by intracardiac Doppler flowmetry. Am J Cardiol *53*:586, 1984.
18. Gardin, J.M., Rohan, M.K., Davidson, D.M., Dabestani, A., Sklansky, M., Garcia, R., Knoll, M.L., White, D.B., Gardin, S.K., Henry, W.L.: Doppler transmitral flow velocity parameters: Relationship between age, body surface area, blood pressure and gender in normal subjects. Am J Noninvas Cardiol *1*:3, 1987.
19. Herzog, C.A., Elsperger, K.J., Manoles, M., Murakami, M., Asinger, R.: Effect of atrial pacing on left ventricular diastolic filling measured by pulsed Doppler echocardiography. J Am Coll Cardiol *9*:197A, 1987.
20. Miyatake, K., Izumi, S., Shimizu, A., Kinoshita, N., Okamoto, M., Sakakibara, H., Nimura, Y.: Right atrial flow topography in healthy subjects studied with real-time two-dimensional Doppler flow imaging technique. J Am Coll Cardiol *7*:425, 1986.
21. Fujii, J., Yazaki, Y., Sawada, H., Aizawa, T., Watanabe, H., Kato, K.: Noninvasive assessment of left and right ventricular filling in myocardial infarction with a two-dimensional Doppler echocardiographic method. J Am Coll Cardiol *5*:1155, 1985.
22. Hatle, L., Angelsen, B.: Doppler Ultrasound in Cardiology. Physical Principles and Clinical Applications, 2nd Ed., Philadelphia, Lea & Febiger, 1985.
23. Hegesh, J.T., Goldberg, S.J., Schwartz, M.L.: Analysis of causes of velocity spread during initial deceleration in the ascending aorta in children and young adults. Am J Cardiol *59*:967, 1987.
24. Mowat, D.H.R., Haites, N.E., Rawles, J.M.: Aortic blood velocity measurement in healthy adults using a simple ultrasound technique. Cardiovasc Res *17*:75, 1983.
25. Mahoney, L.T., Coryell, K.G., Lauer, R.M.: The newborn transitional circulation: A two-dimensional Doppler echocardiographic study. J Am Coll Cardiol *6*:623, 1985.

26. Wilson, N., Reed, K., Allen, H.D., Marx, H.D., Goldberg, S.J.: Doppler echocardiographic observations of pulmonary and transvalvular velocity changes after birth and during the early neonatal period. Am Heart J *113*:750, 1987.

27. Grenadier, E., Lima, C.O., Allen, H.D., Sahn, D.J., Barron, J.V., Valdes-Cruz, L.M., Goldberg, S.J.: Normal intracardiac and great vessel Doppler flow velocities in infants and children. J Am Coll Cardiol *4*:34, 1984.

28. Gardin, J.M., Burn, C.S., Childs, W.J., Henry, W.L.: Evaluation of blood flow velocity in the ascending aorta and main pulmonary artery of normal subjects by Doppler echocardiography. Am Heart J *107*:310, 1984.

29. Kosturakis, D., Goldberg, S.J., Allen, H.D., Loeber C.: Doppler echocardiographic prediction of pulmonary arterial hypertension in congenital heart disease. Am J Cardiol 53:1110, 1984.

30. Kitabatake, A., Inoue, M., Asao, M., Masuyama, T., Tanouchi, J., Morita, T., Mishima, M., Uematsu, M., Shimazu, T., Hori, A., Abe, H.: Noninvasive evaluation of pulmonary hypertension by a pulsed Doppler technique. Circulation *68*:302, 1983.

31. Kitabatake, A., Inoue, M., Asao, M., Tanouchi, J., Masuyama, T., Abe, H., Morita, H., Senda, S., Matsuo, H.: Transmitral blood flow reflecting diastolic behavior of the left ventricle in health and disease—a study by pulsed Doppler technique. Jpn Circ J *46*:92, 1982.

32. Gardin, J.M., Dabestani, A., Takenaka, K., Rohan, M.K., Knoll, M., Russell, D., Henry, W.L.: Effect of imaging view and sample volume location on evaluation of mitral flow velocity by pulsed Doppler echocardiography. Am J Cardiol *57*:1335, 1986.

33. Takenaka, K., Dabestani, A., Gardin, J.M., Russell D., Clark, S., Allfie A., Henry W.L.: Pulsed Doppler echocardiographic study of left ventricular filling in dilated cardiomyopathy. Am J Cardiol *58*:143, 1986.

34. Cogswell, T.L., Sagar, K.B., Wann, L.S.: Left ventricular ejection dynamics in hypertrophic cardiomyopathy and aortic stenosis: Comparison with the use of Doppler echocardiography. Am Heart J *113*:110, 1987.

CHAPTER **4**

DISTURBED FLOW AND PRESSURE DROP

THEORETICAL ASPECTS

This chapter will introduce the concept of flow disturbance and show how computation of pressure drop across an obstructive orifice can be accomplished. Next, this important principle will be applied to the clinical arena.

Brief Review of the History of Flow Disturbance

Prior to 1979, cardiac Doppler was primarily used to detect flow disturbance and flow direction. Virtually all frequency analysis was performed by alinear zero crossing detectors, devices which could analyze only a single frequency during any given time period. The most common display was a time interval histogram. Although a single frequency was correctly plotted by time interval histography, multiple frequencies occurring simultaneously produced a time interval histographic result that was not totally predictable. Flow disturbances always have multiple simultaneous frequencies, thus the unpredictability of plotting by time interval histography actually enhanced the random appearance of a flow disturbance. This random plotting of simultaneous frequencies made time interval histography exquisitely sensitive to detection of flow disturbances. Unfortunately, time interval histography was not a quantitative method.

In 1979, a Fast Fourier Transform (FFT) circuit was first used in a commercial instrument. FFT, a digital analysis method, and a related analog method, Chirp Z, have the capability of displaying all frequencies contained within a time period and, importantly, the signal strength of each velocity may be represented as a scale of gray. Multiple simultaneous velocities are displayed as a frequency spread, but since the points are expressed as velocities, the spread is usually called a velocity spread. An early investigation compared the ability of FFT and time interval histography to detect significant flow disturbance and demonstrated that while both methods record flow disturbances, the disturbance was more apparent by time interval histography.[1] This result occurred because the FFT output was an actual velocity accounting, but the time interval histogram added the additional random factor which resulted from its inability to accurately plot the simultaneous frequencies.

Somewhat later, color-coded Doppler units were used to evaluate disturbed flow. These units introduced still another variable, aliasing at low velocity levels. Aliasing in color-coded units, in some instances, cannot be separated from situations in which cells are flowing at different velocities or in different directions. Color-coded machines display variance as green, white or mosaic. Further, the manufacturer decides what is disturbed and what is not by writing an algorithm based on arbitrary decisions. No documentation for this decision is easily available for the various instruments.

Early Doppler investigators concentrated on detection of flow disturbance and developed a set of observations which permitted a high probability of detecting the anatomic origin of that flow disturbance. Individuals skilled in this technique were able to make diagnoses of congenital and acquired disease,[2-8] but quantitation was not possible. Since the development of quantitative Doppler approaches to flow and flow disturbances, exclusive qualitative detection of a lesion by flow disturbance is rarely, if ever, performed. Quantitative techniques are used to measure velocity in normal laminar flow and in laminar jets, and decisions are based on velocity magnitude and direction. Nonetheless, an understanding of disturbed flow and its effects on the Doppler record is essential. The initial portion of this chapter will detail some characteristics of disturbed flow. Without a background in this information, mistakes can be made even when looking at disturbed flow by color-coded Doppler.

Laminar vs. Disturbed Flow

Although a spectrum exists between laminar and disturbed flow, flow quality assessed by Doppler echocardiography is usually considered to be one or the

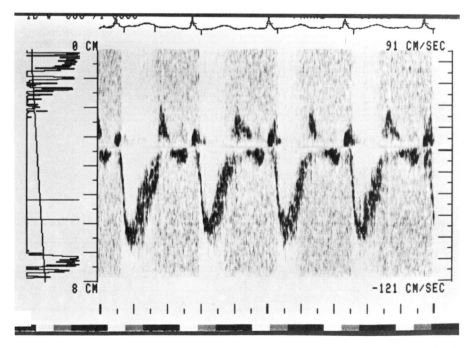

Fig. 4–1. Laminar and disturbed flow in same velocity curve. Although the flow is laminar, technically, the latter portion of each curve represents disturbed flow due to deceleration instability. Flow occurs initially away from the baseline after the QRS complex and is coherent. As flow decelerates, a flow disturbance occurs which has a maximal velocity spread value of approximately 30 cm/sec.

other. The term "disturbed flow" may be preferable to "turbulent flow," because turbulent flow has a mathematical definition. "Disturbed flow," on the other hand, has been used by clinicians and investigators to indicate that flow is not laminar. Laminar, in Doppler echocardiographic terms, means that most of the cell elements move in the same direction and at similar velocities. Disturbed flow, on the other hand, is defined as a situation in which cellular elements are moving at different velocities and/or in different directions. Figure 4–1 shows a pictorial example of disturbed velocities.

Laminar flow may not be uniform throughout the length of a tube or vessel (Fig. 4–1). Lack of uniformity in laminar flow usually is due to velocity profile alterations. Profile refers to the velocity contour of the leading edge of the fluid column (Fig. 4–2). For purposes of Doppler, the ideal profile is flat, a situation that allows the same velocity to be sampled in any part of the profile. Unfortunately, no profile is completely flat since viscous drag slows flow at the interface of the fluid and wall. However, relatively flat profiles occur with pulsatile flows, high flows, during acceleration, and at the inlet to large vessels. These situations are fortunate, because relatively flat profiles occur in the heart and great vessels and provide the Doppler echocardiographer with an opportunity to measure flow. Parabolic profiles occur downstream from the inlet, in small vessels, and at low flow rates. A wide velocity spread is to be expected in parabolic profiles because significant velocity differences are present within the sample volume (Fig. 4–2). Skewed profiles can be found between flat and parabolic profiles. These are flat or slightly parabolic, but skewed across the vessel (Fig. 4–3). In a skewed profile, velocities within the profile may be different, depending on the angle of skew.

Anatomy of a Flow Disturbance

Physical scientists and casual observers have long recognized the anatomy of a flow disturbance. Among examples of flow disturbance are smoke exiting from a chimney or water from a fountain in a plaza (Fig. 4–4). Initially in each, a column exists as smoke from the top of the chimney or as water through a fountain's orifice and assumes a cylindrical appearance. Columnar width is always smaller than the chimney or fountain orifice by a factor called the coefficient of contraction. As this column moves into the atmosphere, as a result of the force of the fire or water pump (pressure), it gradually disperses into a relatively wide, turbulent appearing mass in which particles can be seen to swirl and move laterally from the initial column. This turbulent area smoothes out downstream and particles eventually disappear into the atmosphere, or in the case of the fountain, fall back to earth. Although contained in

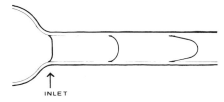

INLET

Fig. 4–2. Flow profile. Flow passes from a main chamber into a channel. The flow profile at the inlet is basically flat, although viscous drag causes slower velocities at the channel edge. As flow passes downstream, the profile becomes more parabolic due to the effects of viscous drag.

FLOW PROFILES

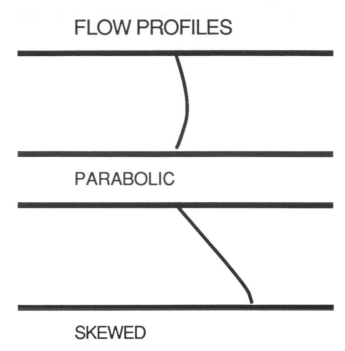

Fig. 4–3.   Flow profiles. The top panel shows a parabolic flow profile and the bottom panel shows a skewed flow profile. See text for details.

tubular structures (vessels), the same phenomenon occurs in the heart and great vessels wherever an obstruction to flow occurs, and the dynamics of the system form the basis of the application of Doppler echocardiography to its detection.

Although the dynamics involved in passage of fluids through orifices have been studied for decades, Kececioglu and co-workers[9] first compared the visual appearance and Doppler output of fluid flow beyond an obstructing orifice. Observations of that study are important for developing an understanding of flow beyond an obstruction. The investigators created an optically clear chamber through which laminar or disturbed flow could pass (Fig. 4–5). An obstructing orifice could be moved to any position within the model so that all areas of flow beyond an obstructing orifice could be investigated. Carbon particles (India ink) were used as Doppler reflectors. A Doppler transducer was mounted at 90° with respect to flow. A transducer in this position would not detect flow moving at exactly 90°, but would detect any radial velocities, i.e., velocities of India ink particles moving at an angle away from the direction of the core flow. The model was exquisitely sensitive to disturbed flow and totally insensitive to normal, laminar flow moving down the axis of the chamber.

When flow moved in a laminar manner, the India ink particles passed in an organized fashion through the observation chamber. However, when an obstruction was placed in the path of flow, a very characteristic pattern, reminiscent of smoke passing from a chimney, was visualized. Figure 4–6 shows that flow beyond an obstruction had several distinct areas; (1) a jet; (2) a parajet; (3) a postjet flow disturbance area, (4) an area of relaminarization, and (5) a boundary layer. Each of these areas could be visualized and each except the

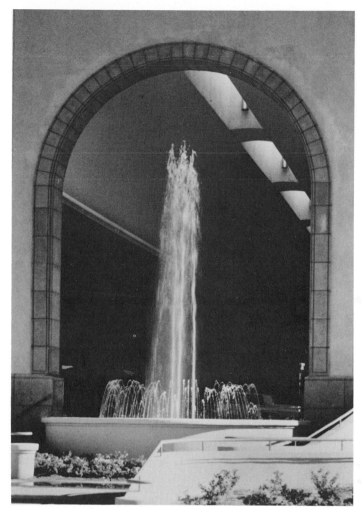

Fig. 4–4. Photograph of a fountain. Note the jet, vortex shed, widening of the jet as it ascends, and turbulence at the end of the jet. Other characteristics of jet formation are described in the text. (Photograph courtesy of Mr. Andrew MacLellan, Tucson Westin La Paloma Hotel).

boundary layer had a character definable by Doppler. A pictorial diagram of these areas is shown in Figure 4–7.[9]

The Jet

The jet could be visualized as a high velocity area that contained dense, particulate matter. No particles passed at an angle away from the jet and no swirling of particles was seen. This is the visual appearance of laminar flow. When the range gate was placed within the jet at a beam-flow intercept angle of 90°, no velocities were detected. Thus, jet flow obeyed the definition of laminar flow, as it should, and was not disturbed, just accelerated.

A visual observation was that jet width, known as the vena contracta, was smaller than the orifice, a principle long understood in hydraulics.[10] The vena

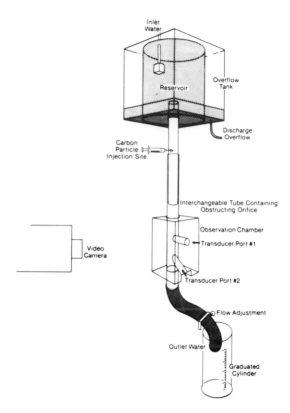

Fig. 4–5. Flow model. The experimental model for studying visual and Doppler flow disturbances. Flow originates in a reservoir and passes through a channel at the base of the reservoir. Carbon particles are injected with a syringe above the obstruction. The obstruction, seen above the observation chamber, could be moved anywhere within the flow system. The observation chamber was made of optically clear lucite and permitted a Doppler transducer to be inserted at port 1, and an imaging transducer to observe for microbubbles at port 2. Port 1 was drilled at 90° with respect to the channel. Flow could be adjusted by a clamp on the outlet of the chamber and the video camera photographed flow in the observation chamber.

contracta, or decrease in jet diameter compared to orifice diameter, results from frictional effects at the orifice edges. The ratio of jet area to obstruction area is the coefficient of contraction. The jet does not remain laminar indefinitely, but after a distance, vortices begin to form. We have termed the distance between the orifice and the point at which these vortices begin to form the "vortex shed distance." The point at which vortices begin to shed is the beginning of the postjet flow disturbance.

Careful evaluation of cineangiograms of valvular stenoses show the same phenomenon, and also demonstrate that jet directivity is quite variable (Fig. 4–8). A similar conclusion can be reached by observing color-coded velocities in patients with obstructive lesions. Jet location becomes quite important when quantitative Doppler approaches to pressure drop estimation are applied.

The laminar jet velocity is evaluated in the calculation of pressure drop across an obstruction. Nevertheless, other aspects of flow are also changed when a pressure drop occurs at an obstruction.

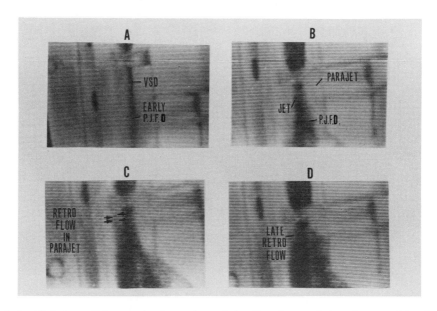

Fig. 4–6. Carbon particles passing beyond an obstruction. In panel *A,* carbon particles form a discrete jet and the distance between the obstruction high in the panel and the early postjet flow disturbance (PJFD) is indicated. That distance is called the "vortex shed distance" (VSD). Later, as indicated in panel *B,* the postjet flow disturbance widens. The site of the parajet is indicated. In panel *C,* some eddies go retrograde from the PJFD into the parajet and eventually fill the parajet. When the Doppler sample volume was placed in the jet, it was found to be laminar. The postjet flow was disturbed. Initially, the parajet was laminar but later demonstrated mild disturbances. Panel *D* shows increased activity in the parajet. (From Kececioglu-Draelos, Z., Goldberg, S.J., Areias, J., Sahn, D.J.: Verification and clinical demonstration of the echo Doppler series effect and vortex shed distance. Circulation *63*:1422, 1981. By permission of the American Heart Association, Inc.)

The Parajet Area

The jet forms immediately distal to the obstruction, does not occupy the entire bore of the chamber, and is even smaller in diameter than orifice diameter. The cylinder of fluid which surrounds the jet is the parajet. In contrast to the high velocity jet, the parajet initially has almost no detectable fluid motion. For this reason, engineers refer to the parajet as the "stagnant area." However, the stagnation is only relative. Shortly after the jet is established, vortices form at the end of the jet and invade the parajet. Although many patterns of vortices were present, the predominant one in the model was retrograde passage of vortices which initially moved near the wall. Many vortices, while losing energy, passed toward the obstruction, turned at the obstruction, and passed along the jet to re-enter the postjet flow disturbance. Range gating into the parajet revealed no initial flow disturbance but later a low level disturbance was detected.[9,11] Color-coded Doppler provides similar information.

The Postjet Flow Disturbance

In the model, the postjet flow disturbance looked much like the billowing of smoke at the end of the jet which emanates from a chimney. The postjet flow disturbance area forms because the jet has lost energy and begins to disperse by casting off swirling downstream vortices. An important difference between the jet and the postjet flow disturbance is velocity magnitude. The jet has high

LAMINAR FLOW

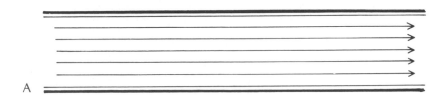

DISTURBED FLOW

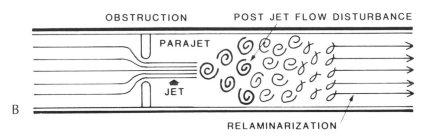

Fig. 4–7. *A,* Laminar flow with all cellular elements outside of the boundary area moving at approximately the same velocity and direction. *B,* The disturbed flow in which the cells are compacted at the obstruction to form the jet, and then break into a postjet flow disturbance with swirling particles. They later undergo relaminarization. The parajet is indicated.

velocity and the postjet flow disturbance has lower velocities. The postjet flow disturbance filled almost the entire bore of the chamber and was much wider than the jet, and, like smoke from the chimney or water from a fountain, would have billowed even further if the chamber wall were not a limiting factor. The postjet flow disturbance did not extend to the chamber wall, and was separated from it by a boundary layer. The energy of the postjet flow disturbance, as judged by the velocity of the swirling, diminished downstream from the obstruction. When the Doppler sample volume was placed within the postjet flow disturbance, marked frequency dispersion was detected because motion of particles was random. The postjet flow disturbance area is thus characterized by a random multidirectional low velocity flow disturbance. Difficulty may be encountered in attempting to display this area by color-coded Doppler because velocities are low and some may be below the color range.

Area of Relaminarization

Vortices within the postjet flow disturbance progressively lost energy as they passed downstream until flow visually again appeared laminar. Hence the term, "area of relaminarization," was coined. If the Doppler sample volume is placed in this area, no significant flow disturbance will be detected.

The Boundary Area

The final area is the boundary layer. The boundary layer lines the inner wall of the tube and represents an area of relatively viscous interface through which

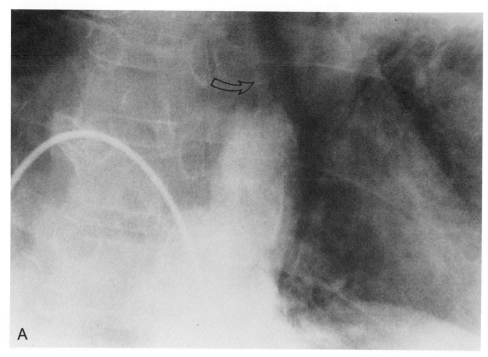

Fig. 4–8. Angiogram and accompanying echo-Doppler examinations from a 68-year-old lady with congenital pulmonary valvular stenosis, tricuspid regurgitation and atrial flutter. On the angiogram, note the eccentricity of the systolic jet across the stenotic valve into the main pulmonary artery. The Doppler examinations show a pre balloon valvuloplasty gradient of over 100 mm Hg, the same as that noted at catheterization, and a post balloon valvuloplasty gradient of 35 mm Hg, also measured at catheterization. Note that pulmonary regurgitation is more prominent after the procedure. Calibration in each Doppler examination is 2 m/sec.
Abbreviations—PS = pulmonary stenosis, PI = pulmonary regurgitation.

fluid moves at a slower rate than in the more central areas of the tube. Kececioglu et al.[9] were unable to make Doppler observations of the characteristics of the boundary layer because the layer had less depth than the sample volume. By visual observation, vortices were separated from the walls of the tube by the boundary layer.

Clinical Equivalent to the Model

An early investigation was performed to determine if the several flow areas could be identified by range-gated Doppler in patients with aortic stenosis.[11] Results indicated that the jet, parajet, and postjet flow disturbance could be identified in almost every patient. As in the Kececioglu model, the jet was laminar, the parajet had little activity but was characterized in some patients by mildly disturbed flow, and the postjet region always contained flow disturbances. In individuals in whom the descending aorta was studied, relaminarization was identified. This type of study could now be much more easily done by using color-coded Doppler.

Doppler Effects Which Cause Interpretation Difficulty

At first evaluation, the result to be expected from Doppler examination of flow disturbances might seem self-evident. However, the clinical situation in

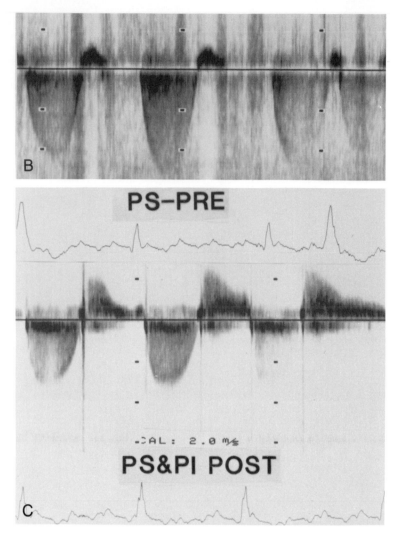

Fig. 4–8 (continued).

man can create some misleading findings which will confuse interpretation of the Doppler observations. Thus, before detailing the Doppler results obtained while studying certain cardiac lesions, some consideration must be given to those effects that may or may not be predicted. These effects include deceleration instability, the series effect, the vortex shed distance, the induction effect, and masking.

Deceleration Instability

Deceleration instability was initially described by McDonald and Helps.[12] From visual observation in a pulsatile flow model, they gave this term to the instability of laminar flow observed at the end of the acceleration phase of flow. This flow disturbance is common in Doppler tracings, occurs at peak deceleration and in some individuals, continues until the velocity waveform reaches baseline (Fig. 4–9). The amplitude of deceleration instability is largely a func-

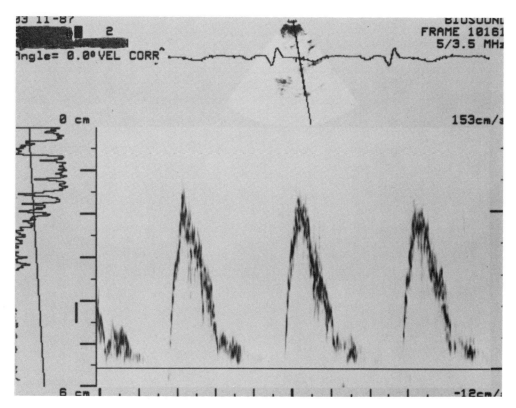

Fig. 4–9. This illustration taken from a suprasternal aortic tracing shows deceleration instability. Note that the initial upstroke of each velocity curve is narrow and laminar. Instability occurs as velocity dispersion after the peak velocities are reached and continues throughout the deceleration phase.

tion of vessel diameter.[13,14] The importance of deceleration instability is that, when detected, it might be confused with a pathologic flow disturbance. Deceleration instability, in quality tracings, is rarely more than 30% of the amplitude of the peak modal velocity.

The Series Effect

Once flow becomes disturbed, it remains disturbed until rheologic factors, such as viscosity or the cardiac cycle, cause it to relaminarize.[7,9] Thus, flow areas which are in circulatory continuity could allow a flow disturbance to pass from one to the other. For example, disturbed flow which results from a ventricular septal defect may pass through the right ventricle and into the pulmonary artery before relaminarization occurs.[9] The diagnostic misinterpretation that may occur as the result of a series effect is that a second cause for a flow disturbance may be postulated to coexist with the first to account for the "extension" of the disturbance. In the ventricular septal defect example, pulmonary stenosis could be suspected as a result of the flow disturbance in the pulmonary artery even though the entire disturbance resulted from the ventricular septal defect and valvar pulmonary stenosis did not coexist. The importance of this factor may be decreasing because we can now follow the jet formation from its origin by color-coded or conventional pulsed Doppler.

The Vortex Shed Distance

The distance from the obstruction to the first evidence of a postjet flow disturbance is the vortex shed distance.[9] If the jet is long and is not detected, the first Doppler evidence of a circulatory problem may be the detection of a distal postjet flow disturbance. The examiner must then decide what obstruction initiated the flow disturbance. An example of the problem of a long vortex shed distance is failure to find a flow disturbance in the left atrium of a patient with an atrioventricular canal, cleft mitral valve and mitral regurgitation.[15] The reason that this may occur is that the high energy jet may be long enough to pass from the mitral valve through the low lying primum atrial defect into the right atrium. Thus, in this instance, the first chamber where a flow disturbance is detected, as a result of mitral insufficiency, would be the right atrium. The jet was simply missed, most likely because it was in a non-interrogated plane. The correct diagnosis could have been suspected by careful echocardiographic demonstration of the defect and properly detecting the jet by Doppler. In pulsed Doppler advantage is taken of the concept that the jet has significant length when attempting to record the jet of aortic stenosis closer to the transducer (i.e., further from the valve). This long jet length allows the operator to measure jet velocity with higher velocity resolution in the near field by pulsed Doppler (Fig. 4–10).

Induction

Induction was an unexpected Doppler finding, although it might have been predicted from a well-known physical finding. In spite of the fact that the transverse aorta lies between the pulmonary artery and the suprasternal notch, patients with pulmonary valvular stenosis frequently have a suprasternal notch thrill. The thrill can be palpated in that location because energy passed through the transverse aortic arch. Thus, in this physical examination instance, a flow disturbance in one area could be detected in another that was not in circulatory continuity but was in physical continuity with the flow disturbance.

In a previous study of children with pulmonary stenosis or other defects that caused a flow disturbance in the pulmonary artery (patent ductus arteriosus, Blalock-Taussig shunts, ventricular septal defects and other lesions) aortic flow disturbances were noted even though the left ventricular outflow tract was entirely normal[16] (Fig. 4–11). A less frequent but equally interesting finding was that patients with aortic flow disturbances arising from left ventricular outflow stenosis has additional flow disturbances found, at times, in the pulmonary artery, even though this set of children had no catheterization evidence of right ventricular outflow tract lesions. Transfer of a flow disturbance from one area that is coupled physically but is not in circulatory continuity with a second area is probably due to some form of physical induction.[16] The flow disturbance that is transferred to the normal outflow tract is weaker and more localized than the primary disturbance. Further, an induced disturbance does not have a jet, parajet, or postjet flow disturbance. The low level flow disturbance in the vessel with initially normal flow is probably due to vibration of that vessel induced by the large flow disturbance in the other vessel (Fig. 4–12).

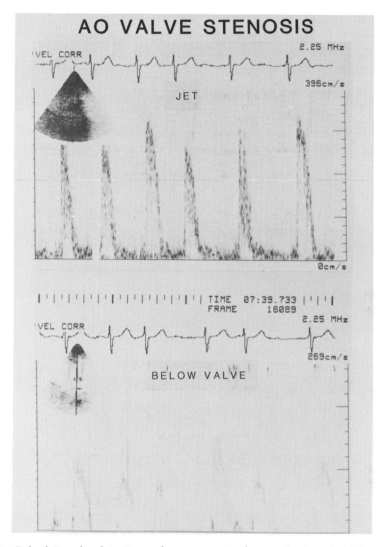

Fig. 4–10. Pulsed Doppler detection and measurement of an aortic stenosis jet (upper panel). Certain patients have jets which are long enough to be interrogated at close range by the pulsed Doppler sample which permits detection of higher velocities. Choice of a low frequency transducer and moving the baseline to the bottom of the trace enhance detection of higher frequencies as well. The lower panel shows V_1, the pre obstructive velocities detected from the suprasternal notch, by passing the sample volume proximal to the aortic valve.

Masking

Masking is related to the concept of the series effect, but describes a different clinical situation. Once flow is disturbed, passage through a second obstruction may not change the character of the disturbance which was initiated by the first obstruction. Thus, the second obstruction, although present, is masked because one disturbance cannot be separated from the other. An example of masking occurs in a patient with subaortic diaphragm and valvar aortic stenosis. The jet is not qualitatively changed by the second obstruction since it is formed

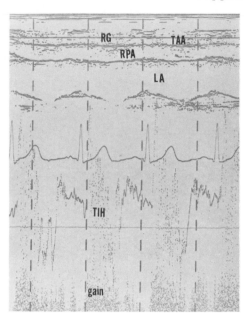

Fig. 4–11. Range gate (RG) is placed in the transverse aortic arch (TAA). The time interval histogram (TIH) is shown below and the EKG is above the TIH. The patient had a ventricular septal defect (VSD). This particular study demonstrated marked systolic frequency dispersion that was not anticipated. There was no abnormality in the aorta. This was due to an induced aortic flow disturbance that originated in the right pulmonary artery (RPA). LA = left atrium.

by the first obstruction and the site of jet contribution from either may be difficult to separate.

Use of an Iatrogenic Flow Disturbance as a Marker of Flow

A major difference between a Doppler echograph and a standard imaging echograph is that the Doppler system is designed to detect weaker signals. This increased sensitivity suggested that Doppler might be superior to standard imaging echo techniques for detecting microbubbles. A simultaneous study of

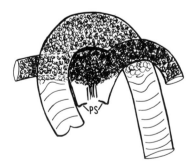

Fig. 4–12. The cause of an induced flow disturbance pictorially demonstrated. Flow passes from the aortic valve in a laminar fashion, and through the pulmonary valve as a jet. The poststenotic (PS) flow disturbance occurs in the pulmonary artery and its branches. Since there is physical contact between the pulmonary artery and aorta, the pulmonary artery causes a vibration in the aorta that induces a flow disturbance. Note that the induced flow disturbance has no jet or parajet, whereas these are present in the area of the true obstruction.

M-mode and Doppler records obtained during injection of saline solution from peripheral and central sites demonstrated that Doppler was far superior for detecting microbubble passage.[1,17] An example of a Doppler contrast study is shown in Figure 4–13. An additional interesting finding of that study was that the time interval histogram was superior to the FFT for detecting microbubbles.[1] The latter result may be due to the fact that the time interval histogram is a nonlinear technique, and when presented with such strong reflectors as microbubbles, the nonlinearity was expressed as a different average velocity at each time period.

QUANTITATION OF FLOW DISTURBANCES

When postjet flow disturbances were studied with time interval histography, an absolute magnitude of more than 1 vertical centimeter of frequency broadening was in excess of any normal value.[5] For FFT records high quality tracings in normals are characterized by velocity spread less than 30% of the true peak amplitude.[13,14,18]

Doppler Estimation of Pressure Drop

INTRODUCTION

In the past, accurate measurement of pressure gradients across intracardiac obstructions required cardiac catheterization with catheter tip manometers.

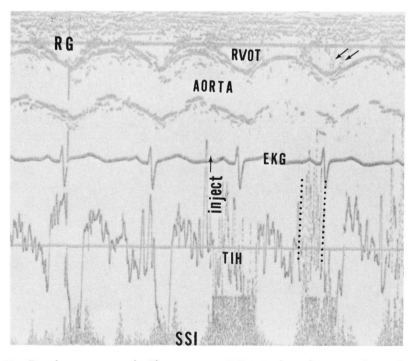

Fig. 4–13. Doppler contrast study. The range gate (RG) is in the right ventricular outflow tract (RVOT). Saline solution injection is performed proximal to the right ventricular outflow tract. A small number of microbubbles can be seen at the arrows in the right ventricular outflow tract. The time interval histogram (TIH) demonstrates a mild flow disturbance, in the beat just after the injection, and a more marked flow disturbance in the subsequent beat (delineated by dotted lines). Note also that the signal-strength indicator (SSI), which is the input signal to the frequency analyzer, demonstrates marked signal strength due to the microbubble passage.

Less accurate measurements could be made with fluid-filled catheters. Indirect implications of the severity of valve stenoses could be obtained from physical examination, electrocardiogram, thoracic roentgenogram, echocardiogram, and systolic time intervals. However, none of these indirect methods allows direct answer to the primary question—what is the pressure drop across the stenotic orifice?

Since cardiac catheterization was required to provide that direct answer, cardiologists were limited by the procedure's expense in finances and time, potential morbidity, and the finite number of times which it could be performed. Thus, the need is evident for an accurate, repeatable, inexpensive, noninvasive method for obtaining the same information. Considerable data are now available which demonstrate that Doppler echocardiography fulfills these criteria.[19–26] This section will be concerned with theoretical and practical considerations for applications of Doppler echocardiography to pressure drop determination. Further, specific applications will be discussed to demonstrate the practical use of Doppler for estimating the pressure drop in common clinical situations.

BACKGROUND

Historically, flow disturbances were studied qualitatively by combined Doppler and M-mode echocardiography. This combination allowed detection of the site of valvar stenosis and regurgitation and suggested the location of shunting lesions.[2–4,6,11,15,16,27–49] Early instruments merely detected the location of jets and flow disturbances. Diagnosis was predicted by the location of various flow phenomena. No quantitative work was possible earlier because spectral analysis was performed by alinear time interval histography (Fig. 4–14). Alinear spectral analysis did not allow measurement of calibrated velocity in flows beyond an obstruction.

Later, when FFT analysis became available, quantitation of normal low flow velocity was possible with pulsed Doppler. Unfortunately, early pulsed systems allowed direct measurement of jet velocities present beyond most obstructive lesions only if the transducer could be placed near the abnormal valve or if the jet had a relatively low velocity. Innovative attempts at overcoming this problem of measuring high velocities included selection of the lowest frequency transducer available, moving the baseline to the top or bottom of the display, cutting and pasting the tops or bottoms of aliased flow velocities to the primary waveform, and creation of large beam-flow intercept angles to reduce the existing velocity to the measurable range. The third technique, cutting and pasting of aliased velocities, is legitimate and can be used in certain circumstances such as quantification of valve insufficiencies, but is usually unnecessary because most instruments now permit movement of the baseline. Most, if not all, Doppler studies are performed with the sample volume aligned with flow as close to 0° or 180° as possible in order to attain the highest amplitude velocity curves. As the beam-flow intercept angle increases, the amplitude of the peak lessens (see Chapter 2). Thus, the last method, increasing the intercept angle to bring the resultant lower velocity into measurement range, can be done, but is hazardous. Both the azimuthal (elevational) angle and the intercept angle in the visualized plane can lead to substantial mismeasurement of spatial angles,

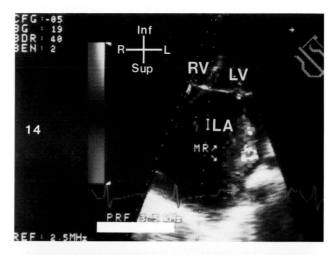

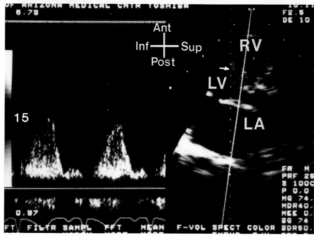

Plate 14. Mitral regurgitation shown on apex 4-chamber view. Note that the aliased flow away from the transducer is encoded in blue. This represents the jet of mitral regurgitation.

Plate 15. Ventricular septal defect. The red jet across the septum in the direction of the transducer represents high velocity flow across a restrictive ventricular septal defect. The continuous wave Doppler beam transects the jet and the velocity curve is enscribed to the right of the figure.

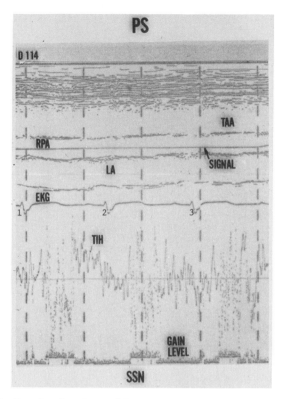

Fig. 4–14. M-mode Doppler time interval histogram in pulmonary stenosis (PS). The sample volume is in the right pulmonary artery. Note the marked frequency dispersion during systole. RPA—right pulmonary artery; TAA—transverse aortic arch; LA—left atrium; TIH—time interval histogram; SSN—suprasternal notch.

a cause of major velocity measurement error. Fortunately, with present technology, use of angle correction is no longer necessary and should be avoided.

Theoretical Considerations

Consider a visual example of a poststenotic jet. To develop a poststenotic jet, a fountain in a plaza requires a pump, adequate flow, and a restrictive orifice through which flow passes. Characteristics of the jet are determined by the force of the pump, degree of obstruction, and flow rate. Jet length, to the point of shedding of vortices, results from these same factors. Directivity of the jet is determined by the position of the orifice. These same situations determine characteristics of a poststenotic jet in the human counterpart. The jet is not disturbed flow; it is a high velocity laminar flow phenomenon. Its velocity measurement requires a Doppler system with the capability of adequate velocity acquisition and resolution for recording jet velocities without ambiguity.

THE EQUATION

The energy balance equation, a common physics equation, takes these factors into account and allows mathematical prediction of the characteristics of the fountain's display. The same equation can be modified to represent a closed system and describe jet flow characteristics in a tube containing a discrete obstruction. In this latter case, the jet passes through a fluid medium instead of air.

The energy balance equation for fluids is:[50]

$$(\Delta P/\rho) + (\tfrac{1}{2}\Delta(V^2)/\alpha) + Ws + \Sigma F + \Delta Zg = 0,$$

where ΔP is the pressure drop across the stenosis, ρ is the density of the fluid, $\Delta(V^2)$ is the change in velocity squared through the area of stenosis, α is a constant which $= 1$ in turbulent flow and $= 0.5$ in laminar flow, Ws is the amount of energy per unit mass put into or removed from a flow system by a pump or generator, $\Sigma F =$ the sum of frictional losses in the system, g is acceleration due to gravity and $\Delta Z =$ the change in height of fluid in the system.

Ordinarily, W and ΔZg are not applicable and may be deleted from the equation, leaving it as;

$$(\Delta P/\rho) + \Delta V^2/2\alpha + \Sigma F = 0$$

The major difference between this equation and the modified Bernoulli equation is that this equation includes ΣF and α. These terms are important for calculation of pressure drops through long segment stenoses as discussed later.

Holen et al. applied a modification of the energy balance equation to an in vitro model and to humans with valvular disease and showed that it could be used to predict gradients across obstructions.[51] Hatle et al. popularized these studies by extensive human investigations and showed that pressure gradients obtained by Doppler application of this formula correlated quite well with those measured at cardiac catheterization.[19]

The equation used by Holen and Hatle is a restatement of the energy balance equation which considers three major factors;[19,50–53] convective acceleration, flow acceleration, and viscous friction,:

$$P_1 - P_2 = \tfrac{1}{2}\rho(V_2^2 - V_1^2) + \rho\, 2dv/dt \times \Delta s + R(v)\ (23),$$

where $P_1 - P_2$ is the pressure pressure drop, ρ expresses mass density of a fluid, $V_2 =$ peak Doppler velocity beyond the obstruction, $V_1 =$ peak Doppler velocity proximal to the obstruction, $dv/dt \times \Delta s =$ rate of velocity change, or acceleration, $\times$ change in distance, and $R(v) =$ viscous resistance of the vessel $\times$ local velocity. Combining ρ for blood with factors which convert the pressure drop to mm/Hg and velocity to m/sec, the coefficient for blood is 3.98. For purposes of computation, most cardiologists round this value to 4.0.

The second term (flow acceleration) applies during valve opening and closing when pressure drop measurement is not clinically relevant. The third term (viscous friction) is thought to be relatively insignificant in most clinical circumstances of short segment stenoses. Thus, the equation can be shortened to:

$$P_2 - P_2 = 4(V_2^2 - V_1^2).$$

HOW ACCURATE IS THE BERNOULLI EQUATION?

Requarth et al.[52] reported an in vitro study which independently compared the pressure drop predicted by the Bernoulli equation, by the continuity equation, and by direct pressure drop measurement. This model allowed passage of water through interchangeable orifices. An in-line Doppler transducer was placed downstream from the orifice. Pressure taps were placed proximal and distal to the obstruction so that the pressure drop could be measured. Doppler-measured velocities correlated closely with those predicted both by the Bernoulli ($r = .99$) and continuity ($r = .99$) equations. (For details about the continuity equation, see Chapter 7.) By plotting measured pressure drop against Doppler-measured jet velocities, the experimental exponent (for water) in the Bernoulli equation was 2.11, whereas theory predicted that it should be 2.0. The coefficient was also close to the theoretical value. This study confirmed that Doppler measurement of velocities in a jet provides results close to those expected in theory.

IS V_1 NECESSARY FOR THE BERNOULLI EQUATION?

In most instances, maximal velocity proximal to a stenotic orifice is less than 1 m/sec. Since 1 m/s represents only 4 mm Hg ($1.0 \times 1.0 \times 4$), this small value can usually be ignored, shortening the equation to $P_1 - P_2 = 4V_2^2$. However, when considering high flow states, or relatively low peak gradients, such as those which occur in atrioventricular valve stenosis, failure to include elevated velocities proximal to the valve may lead to pressure drop overestimation.

WHAT OBSTRUCTIONS OBEY THE MODIFIED BERNOULLI EQUATION?

This modified Bernoulli equation estimates pressure drop across discrete obstructions which allow jet formation. A recent report which evaluated an in vitro model with a tiny opening showed that a spray rather than a focused jet occurs at very small orifices.[53] The equation underestimates pressure drops across these extremely small orifices, probably due to lack of adequate jet formation and orifice friction. An analog of this type of spray formation is a paint aerosol can which has a tiny orifice which produces a spray rather than a jet. The study by Vasko et al.[53] also demonstrated that orifice shape has an effect on maximal velocity. Circular and elliptical orifices allowed more predictable pressure estimates than a triangular orifice. Triangular orifices caused greater than expected pressure drops, probably as a result of viscous friction at the triangular corners.

LONG SEGMENT STENOSES

As discussed above, the terms ΣF and α (the sum of the frictional losses in the system and a constant equal to unity in turbulent flow and equal to 0.5 in laminar flow) are omitted from the modified Bernoulli equation which is applied to discrete stenoses. They do apply, however, to long segment stenoses where frictional losses must be considered.

The sum of frictional losses, ΣF, can be divided into three terms: losses occurring at the contraction site (Fc), losses occurring during passage through the long segment stenosis (Ff), and losses due to subsequent expansion (Fex). Each component must be calculated for estimation of the respective contributions under the various conditions that may be present in the cardiovascular system.

Contraction losses (Fc) can be computed as;

$$Fc = 0.55 \: [1 - (A_2/A_1)]V_2/2\alpha,$$

where A_1 is the area of the precontraction region, A_2 is the area of the contraction, V_2 is the velocity within the contraction, and α is the coefficient for turbulent flow. This equation assumes a reasonably square edge at the contraction site.

Frictional losses at the stenotic area (Ff) can be calculated as;

$$Ff = 2f\ V_2\ L/D$$

In this equation, the Fanning friction factor (f) must be determined. The length and diameter of the obstruction are represented as L and D respectively. The Fanning friction factor is usually determined from a nomogram (Fig. 4–15). In order to use this nomogram, computation of the Reynolds number (Nre) is necessary:

$$Nre = DV\rho/\mu,$$

where D is the diameter of the obstruction in cm., V is the velocity within the stenotic area in m/sec. and ρ is the density of the fluid expressed in g/cm³. The viscosity of the fluid μ, is expressed in g/cm $\times$ sec. The Fanning friction factor can be determined from Fig. 4–15 by assuming a roughness term which is appropriate for the vessel lumen.

Frictional losses at the expension area can be computed as;

$$Fex = [1 - (A_2/A_3)]^2\ V_2/2\alpha,$$

where V, A_2, and α are the same as in the previous equation. The new term A_3 refers to the area of the expansion. This equation also assumes a reasonably square edge at the transition between the long segment stenosis and the expansion.

Computation of the ΣF produces a result in units of N $\times$ m/kg. Density (ρ)

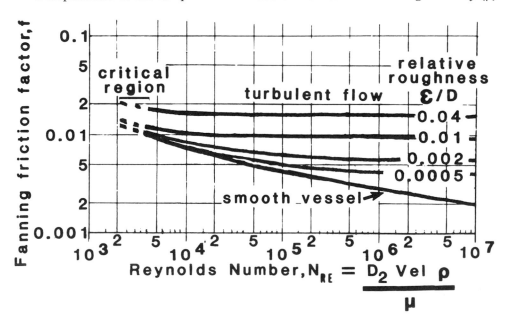

Fig. 4–15. The Fanning friction factor is demonstrated on the vertical axis; the Reynolds number on the horizontal axis. A family of curves relates to the relative roughness of the long segment stenosis. (Reproduced with permission from Goldberg, S.J.[50]).

is in terms of g/cm³. Pressure drop in mm Hg can be computed by using the conversion factor where 1 mm Hg = 133 N/m².

The above terms of ΣF can be simplified if one assumes that frictional losses along the wall are small and that the prestenotic and poststenotic dimensions are generally similar. Using these assumptions, the equation can be simplified to;

$$\Delta P = [4 + 6(1 - A_2/A_1)]/V_2,$$

where ΔP is in mm Hg, V_2 (postobstruction velocity) is in m/sec, and A_1 (prestenotic area) and A_2 (poststenotic area) are in cm².

The above were tested in a model of long-segment stenosis designed by Requarth et al. (Fig. 4–16) and correlated well with measured pressure drops and the simplified equation correlated well with the more complex form of calculation.[50,54]

THE EXAMINATION

The goal of Doppler examination in patients with an obstructive lesion is to accurately record the magnitude of the post obstruction jet velocity. Maximal velocity measurement allows quantification of the pressure drop by the modified Bernoulli equation.

The Velocity Waveform

MORPHOLOGY OF DOPPLER VELOCITY WAVEFORMS IN JETS

The quality and timing of jet velocity waveforms offer insight into the circumstances which create the jet. Misinformation and clinical errors can result by recording and interpreting a poor quality tracing.

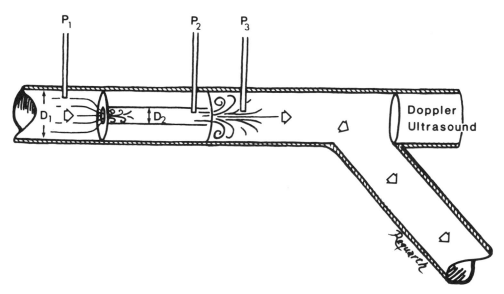

Fig. 4–16. Long segment stenosis model developed by Requarth. Flow (D_1) into the model (left) passes through an area of obstruction (D_2). Pressure ports (P) are inserted before (P_1), within (P_2), and at the end (P_3) of the long segment stenosis. A Doppler transducer is mounted in the direct path of the long segment stenosis for velocity measurement. (Reproduced with permission from Goldberg, S.J.[50]).

A properly inscribed jet Doppler velocity waveform should have a clear origin and termination. The waveform will reflect flow physiology. In most clinical circumstances, the usual appearance of the waveform is rounded with a distinct modal velocity. Invariably, some velocities will exceed the modal waveform, but should not be included in measurements of peak velocity (Fig. 4–17). Instrumentation should have sufficient grey scale capability to display the various velocity inscriptions. If the continuous wave or pulsed beam is not properly aligned with the jet, various inadequate waveforms will result, all of which will underestimate the peak velocity (Fig. 4–18).

Timing of the velocity waveform allows insight into its origin. Since many valves are studied with non-imaging CW Doppler, the examiner may have difficulty in determining whether the jet was due to, for example, mitral regurgitation or aortic stenosis. Jets occur early in systole with mitral regurgitation, tricuspid backflow and ventricular septal defects. Jets which commence later, during the ejection phase of systole, after conclusion of the isovolumic contraction are due to aortic or pulmonary outflow lesions. The more significant semilunar stenoses have not only higher peaks, but also later peaks. If the differential is between aortic or pulmonary stenosis, jet location, direction, and timing are helpful. Pulmonary stenosis jets are found at the left precordium

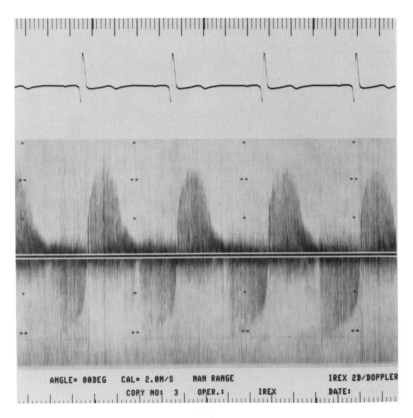

ANGLE= 00DEG   CAL= 2.0M/S   MAN RANGE   IREX 2D/DOPPLER
                           COPY NO: 3   OPER.:   IREX   DATE:

Fig. 4–17. Continuous wave tracing obtained from the right upper sternal border in a patient with aortic stenosis and regurgitation. Note, especially in the second and third full curves that the systolic jet has velocities which exceed the modal velocities. This overshoot should not be measured. Aortic regurgitation is noted and is well demonstrated in the 3rd and 4th beats.

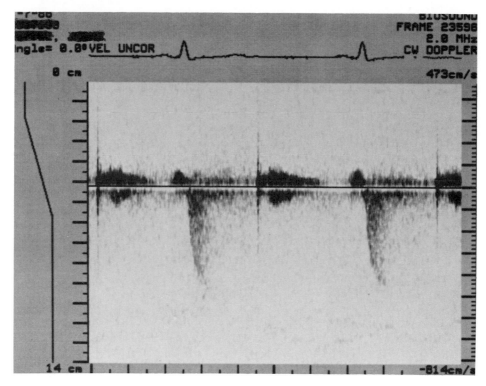

Fig. 4–18. Inadequate jet profile obtained by continuous wave Doppler in a patient with mitral regurgitation. Although the curve could be estimated to have reached its peak, especially in the second beat, underestimation is quite possible. The triangular appearance in the first curve also implies that the jet has only been partially encountered.

and are directed posteriorly. The pulmonary valve usually closes later than the aortic valve.

Early diastolic jets are associated with aortic or pulmonary regurgitation. If ventricular diastolic pressure is elevated, the jet will have an abrupt decline in velocity because of the lessened difference between the vessel's diastolic pressure and that of the ventricle.

Jets which occur after early diastole are due to tricuspid or mitral stenosis. The secondary peak on the velocity waveform will be absent or displaced if the patient is not in sinus rhythm.

For non imaging continuous wave Doppler, further differentiation of the origin of the jet is gained by careful attention to beam direction. For example, differentiation of mitral vs tricuspid regurgitation can be helped by noting that the beam was aimed from the apex toward the left mid-clavicular area for mitral regurgitation and from the apex toward the right lower sternal border for tricuspid regurgitation.

Peak to Peak vs Instantaneous Pressure Drops

Cardiologists who use pressure gradients measured at cardiac catheterization for clinical decision making will be forced by Doppler to reconsider approaches and criteria. Peak-to-peak gradients are commonly obtained by pulling the catheter from one chamber to another and calculating the pressure drop by

subtracting the peak pressure in the distal chamber from the peak in the proximal chamber. Since the peaks occur at different times, these peak-to-peak
gradients are not true measures of physiologic phenomena. A more accurate
method, but one still capable of error, is simultaneous measurement of pressures
on either side of an obstruction by fluid-filled catheters. The problem with this
method is that the fluid filled catheters affect both the amplitude and phase
of the harmonics of pressure and the effects on these two components are not
easily predicted. Accordingly, the magnitude of error is unpredictable. Greatest
accuracy is obtained when dual intravascular or intracavitary transducers are
placed into the areas of interest. Nonetheless, in all of these approaches, a slight
time delay exists between peak pressure development in the chamber or vessel
proximal to the obstruction and in the chamber or vessel distal to the obstruction. The physiologic pressure phase shift is recorded variably by all listed
methods. None compensates for peak-to-peak measurement. Thus, does peak-
to-peak pressure drop reflect the true instantaneous situation which physio-
logically occurs? No, but measurement of the instantaneous pressure differences
generally accomplishes this.

Doppler, like intravascular dual pressure manometry, allows measurement
of instantaneous pressure differences. Accordingly, interpretation of instantaneous pressure differences requires a new set of thoughts for those not accustomed to using them.

Another approach which cardiologists use for clinical assessment of pressure
drop is measurement of mean pressure differences. This approach requires
superimposing R-R matched pullback records and determining the ejection area
by planimerizing or otherwide measuring the difference in pressure and dividing by ejection time (Fig. 4–19). Dual fluid filled catheter techniques or
dual intravascular manometry lessen potential error of R-R matched records
for this measurement.

Most clinical decisions have been made upon the basis of peak-to-peak gra-

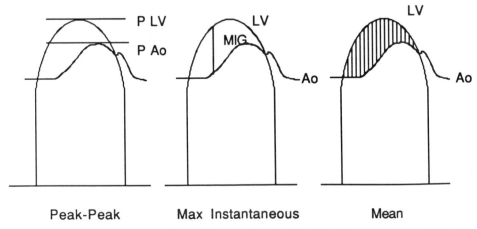

Peak-Peak   **Max Instantaneous**   **Mean**

Fig. 4–19. Gradient information derived from catheterization. The diagrams represent simultaneously obtained left ventricular and aortic pressures in aortic stenosis. Peak to peak gradients are
obtained by measuring the greatest amplitudes of each curve, obtained at different times. Maximal
instantaneous gradient is obtained as the greatest pressure difference at a point in time. Mean
gradient is derived by measuring many instantaneous gradients over equal time segments and
averaging the data. See text for details.

dients, and some incorporate mean pressure drop data. Valve area calculations require mean gradients. To date, no clinical criteria are available which state the meaning of instantaneous gradients in terms of need for operation or effect on ventricles. Unfortunately, even data collected for peak-to-peak gradients are tainted because such gradients often include a greater or lesser degree of artifact created by the recording method. We may thus be pressured by Doppler to rethink our criteria.

Data show that a close correlation exists between gradients calculated from velocities measured by Doppler and gradients measured by manometry at cardiac catheterization. Most of these studies have compared peak velocities with peak-to-peak gradients. As a general rule, with notable exceptions, best correlations occur when the pressure difference across an obstruction is high. When lower peak-to-peak gradients are found, Doppler instantaneous pressure drop will usually exceed the peak-to-peak result. Further, if flow is more than the usual 3.5 to 5.5 L/min/M², V_1 must not be ignored in the equation.

Effect of Flow on a Pressure Drop

Doppler gradients must be evaluated in the same manner as gradients obtained by pressure manometry at cardiac catheterization. Flow affects gradients; therefore, flow through the valve must be measured. Flow cannot be measured by Doppler distal to an obstruction because the area of obstruction is usually unknown. In fact, the most valuable information is the area of the obstruction itself, and pressure drop is used to approximate this area. Flow, however, can usually be measured before the obstruction or in another area. For example, in the absence of a shunt or significant pulmonary regurgitation, pulmonary flow can be measured in a patient with aortic stenosis and this value substituted for systemic flow. If a patient has a ventricular septal defect with a left-to-right shunt, mitral flow may be substituted for pulmonary flow. Examples of substitution of one flow for another are discussed in Chapter 5.

Pressure Drops Measured by Pulsed, High PRF, and CW Doppler

When careful examinations are performed with pulsed, high PRF or CW Doppler systems for the same patients in a constant state, identical or nearly identical data are obtained (Fig. 4–20). High PRF systems are more difficult to use than CW or standard pulsed systems but adequate examinations can be gained from any system. The ease of use of CW probably results from its wider beam and excellent signal to noise ratio.

Examination Technique for Obtaining Pressure Drop Information

Ordinarily, a routine range-gated pulsed Doppler and two-dimensional echocardiographic examination are performed initially. When velocities exceed the Nyquist limit, transducer position is noted. The instrument is then switched to CW Doppler. The examination for measurement of high velocities may be combined with anatomic imaging or performed without imaging. Both the imaging and non-imaging approaches have merit. Imaging with a relatively large dual mode transducer permits the CW cursor to be aligned according to an anatomic frame of reference. Blind transducers are significantly smaller and easier to align with the jet. With either technique, the auditory signal and

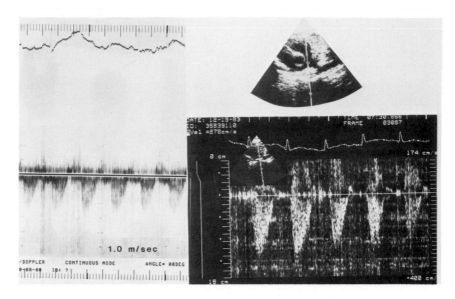

Fig. 4–20. Comparison of continuous wave and high PRF Doppler tracings in a patient with moderate valvar pulmonary stenosis. The calibration scale on the left is 1 m/sec between dots. Thus, peak velocity is 2.75 m/sec. High PRF velocities are shown on the right below the two-dimensional echocardiographic image that shows sample volume locations. On the second velocity curve, the "A" line shows the peak velocity measurement of 2.78 m/sec. Transvalvar gradient is thus predicted at 30 mm Hg. The continuous wave example in this older figure is not ideal, but is used to illustrate the comparison between continuous wave Doppler and high pulse repetition frequency Doppler.

calibrated velocity waveforms are carefully and continuously evaluated until the highest possible velocity occurs coincident with the purest audio signal.

We are frequently asked to teach individuals the audio aspect of the examination and could be criticized for failing to convey the exact sounds. If an individual wishes to hear Beethoven's 5th symphony, no substitute can be found for listening to it. Volumes of written text describing the auditory characteristics of Doppler are inferior to simply listening. On the other hand, listening to Beethoven (or W. Nelson) is much easier than listening to the Doppler output of a stenotic valve jet. Since the audio frequency is different for jets of different velocities, only the principle can be taught. The best beam-jet alignment produces a high, almost pure, tone during peak velocity, but at other times during the cardiac cycle, lower frequencies are present and mix with the higher tones. For very high velocity jets, the audio frequency may be very high, perhaps beyond the audible range. We advise the reader to listen to the Doppler audio output of a few jets; the experience will surpass any of our descriptive capabilities.

Color-coded Doppler has been suggested as useful for aligning with the jet.[55] The high velocity jet is visualized as an aliased signal, and the CW cursor can be aligned with the aliased signal (at least in two dimensions). Fine tuning is still necessary to achieve the highest frequencies and thus the highest velocities. The usefulness of the color-coded Doppler approach has been frequently exaggerated. Most cardiologists and technologists can align with the jet without color-coded Doppler assistance in almost every patient. Further, so many signals, even those of normal velocity, alias on color-coded records that the "assist" can even be a hinderance, and the jet which causes alignment difficulties may also be difficult to align with the aid of color-coded Doppler.

Since the objective is alignment of the transducer and the jet, any transducer position which allows recording of the maximal velocity is the desired position. Since jets vary in length and direction, the examiner must not be lulled into security by seeing the Doppler cursor positioned into the center of a vessel. Jets are frequently eccentric with respect to the vessel walls. Slow and subtle transducer movements are required to be certain that the highest velocity is recorded. Once the maximal jet has been detected, the transducer beam should be in line with the jet and angle correction of velocity magnitude is not necessary or desirable. Further, many jets can be recorded from more than one location. Checking peak velocity magnitude from several locations or in different planes is always safer than accepting the value from the first location or plane tested.

The Doppler examination for maximal jet velocity requires time, patience and experience. Both the patient and the examiner should be comfortable. If a pediatric patient, especially an infant, becomes fussy, combative, and otherwise lacking in the spirit of cooperation, an exercise state has been achieved and the pressure drop, although accurate, certainly does not resemble that of the baseline resting state from which most clinical decision-making is made. However you achieve patient cooperation is up to you. We try feeding, playing, having the mother hold the child, making the room dark and coming back in one-half hour after the child falls asleep (if you have a half hour to wait), or liberal use of chloral hydrate. Adults are not immune to anxiety, discomfort or impatience. In addition to problems similar to those stated above, the adult patient poses all of the other problems which occur in imaging echocardiography. Hyperaeration, small suprasternal notches and thick bones interfere with ultrasonic beam passage and certain cardiac structures may be very distant from the transducer. For a few patients, an adequate Doppler examination may not be possible.

Once a velocity is recorded, it should be examined for trace quality. A semilunar stenosis tracing that shows the highest velocity immediately on the upstroke (Fig. 4–21) is probably a poor tracing as the velocity waveform should be rounded throughout systole. The highest frequencies should create a velocity envelope which appears darker at the periphery than in the central and lower portions, where lower frequencies dominate[19] (Fig. 4–22). If a semilunar valve is severely stenotic, the jet which issues from it will have a velocity peak late in systole. Early peaks in severe semilunar stenosis are probably false. If criteria are met, accurate quantification of the pressure drop is possible, but if they are not achieved, the pressure drop will probably be underestimated.

DETECTION OF LESIONS FROM THE VARIOUS IMAGING PLANES—THE ORGANIZED DOPPLER ECHO EXAMINATION

The sample volume location should be used to greatest advantage in whatever location a jet or flow disturbance is anticipated. Since examiners are accustomed to various imaging planes for the two-dimensional echo examination, this same format is included for the Doppler examination. Some jets and flow disturbances do not follow our conventional imaging planes and thus the examiner should be flexible. Nonetheless, one must start somewhere, and the

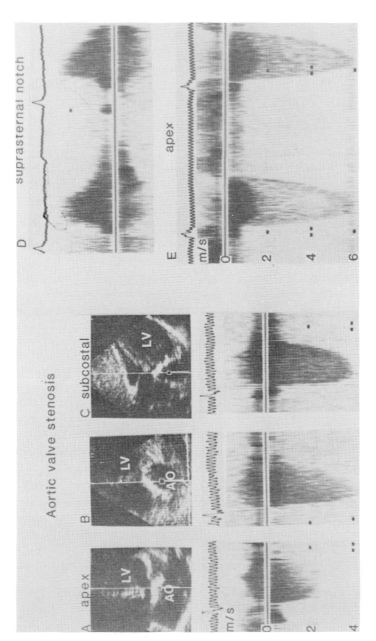

Fig. 4–21. Examples of unacceptable and acceptable velocity curves in aortic stenosis. (From Hatle and Angelson,[19] reprinted with permission). The velocity curve in panel A is incomplete. That in B is triangular and not rounded. The curves in C and E are well rounded and are especially distinct and show both V_1 and V_2 in E. The curve in D is inadequate in that no clear modal velocities are recorded and velocities are seen on both sides of the baseline.

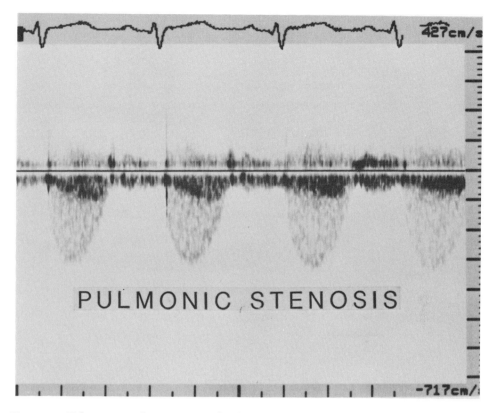

Fig. 4–22. Velocity curve from patient with valvular pulmonary stenosis. Note the darkened outer envelope of modal velocities. These represent where peak velocities should be measured. The darkened inner envelope is from the infundibular area in this patient, and represents V_1. Note also the valve opening and closure spikes in beats 1 and 2.

majority of lesions will be located by using the following format. If color Doppler is incorporated into the examination, detection of flow disturbances may be easier than by conventional examination which requires sweeping the pulsed Doppler sample volume into various cavities and vessels until the disturbance is found. (Whatever instrument is used, some major hints are still gained by starting the examination by palpating the chest and using a stethoscope.)

The Long Axis Plane (Fig. 4–23)

The sample volume is placed in the right ventricle and swept from the apex to the membranous septal area proximal to the septal leaflet of the tricuspid valve. The primary lesion detected by this technique is a ventricular septal defect. If it can be localized by imaging or by color-coded Doppler, the examination is easier. Some defects cannot be imaged and Doppler will confirm their presence. The sample volume should be threaded from the defect to the anterior right ventricular wall. Multiple defects are best detected by use of color-coded Doppler. Once a defect is found, its maximal velocities should be measured, either by pulsed Doppler if the defect is unrestrictive and velocities are low, or by continuous wave Doppler if velocities are high.

The left atrium should be interrogated for presence of the jet of mitral regurgitation. Most of these jets will be off angle from this imaging plane, but

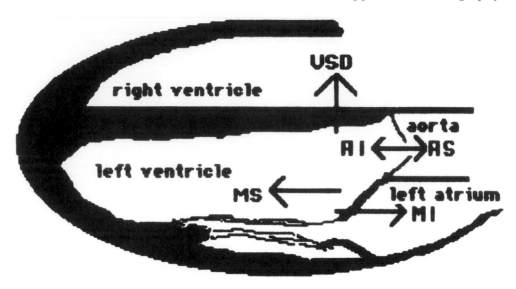

Fig. 4–23. Diagram of two-dimensional echocardiographic long axis view showing possible areas for detection of common sources of jet formation.
Abbreviations; VSD, ventricular septal defect, AI, aortic regurgitation, AS, aortic stenosis, MS, mitral stenosis, MI, mitral regurgitation.

appreciation of the abnormality can still be gained. At times in patients with prosthetic mitral valves, which may interfere with apical imaging and Doppler sampling, the precordial approach may be the only useful examination plane. Additionally, since color-coded Doppler aliases at low velocities, the precordial approach allows introduction of enough angulation to cancel the aliasing effect of normal physiologic flow and thus allows appreciation of flow abnormalities. This application should not be viewed as an advantage of color imaging.

The left ventricle should be interrogated from the mitral outflow area to the subaortic area. Detectable abnormalities include mitral stenosis and aortic regurgitation. Rarely, an aliased signal from a subaortic membrane can be found.

This plane is useful for detection of aortic root flow abnormalities such as found in aortic stenosis or insufficiency. Again, the sample localization is off-angle and quantification is thus invalid from this plane.

Moving the transducer to the right upper sternal border will be useful for demonstration of flow abnormalities associated with aortic stenosis and/or regurgitation. This location is useful in individuals of all ages.

Short Axis Plane

The short axis planes are a series of cuts from the apex of the left ventricle to the aortic root. In Doppler work, two of these planes predominate, the ventricular plane in the mitral-chordal attachment area and the aortic root plane which includes visualization of the pulmonary arteries.

VENTRICULAR PLANE (Fig. 4–24)

The sample volume should be placed into the right atrium proximal to the septal leaflet of the tricuspid valve, near the atrial septum for appreciation of tricuspid backflow. Rarely, flow abnormalities associated with atrial septal

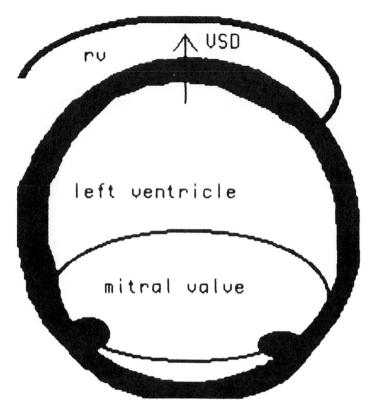

Fig. 4–24. Diagram of two-dimensional echocardiographic short axis ventricular plane view showing possible area for detection of a common source of a jet associated with a restrictive ventricular septal defect. The perpendicularity of Doppler alignment lessens probability of adequately detecting mitral disorders.
Abbreviations; RV, right ventricle, VSD ventricular septal defect.

defects can be detected in the same area. These are usually best seen by color-coded Doppler in this plane.

Next the sample volume should be swept into the right ventricle where flow abnormalities from tricuspid stenosis or ventricular septal defects can be appreciated.

Placing the sample volume into the left ventricle allows detection of abnormal flows due to aortic regurgitation or mitral stenosis. Because of angulation, this is not the best plane of evaluation for either lesion, but the abnormalities are usually detectable.

GREAT VESSEL LEVEL (Fig. 4–25)

This plane is one of the most useful for Doppler evaluation. Either conventional pulsed-Doppler or color-coded Doppler can be used effectively. If imaging is adequate, almost all pulmonary arterial flow disturbances can be evaluated from this plane. The main pulmonary artery should be interrogated for flow disturbances of pulmonary valve stenosis and/or insufficiency. Patent ductus arteriosus with left-to-right shunt is best detected on the lateral main pulmonary artery wall[56] and can also be seen in the right and left pulmonary arteries and on the pulmonary arterial end of the ductus itself. Color-coded Doppler is often

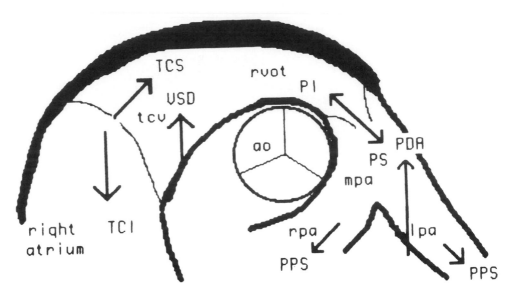

Fig. 4–25. Diagram of two-dimensional echocardiographic short axis great vessel plane view showing possible areas for detection of common sources of jet formation.
Abbreviations; TCI, tricuspid valve regurgitation, TCS, tricuspid stenosis, tcv, tricuspid valve, VSD, ventricular septal defect, rvot, right ventricular outflow tract, PI, pulmonary valve regurgitation, ao, aorta, PS, pulmonary valve stenosis, PDA, patent ductus arteriosus, mpa, rpa, lpa, main, right and left pulmonary arteries, PPS, peripheral pulmonary artery stenosis.

quite useful for detecting ductal shunting where ductal flow appears, usually as red, near the bifurcation of the pulmonary arteries, passes in diastole toward the valve and then turns to flow in the same direction as the normal antegrade pulmonary blood flow.

Moving the sample volume into the left and right branch pulmonary arteries may permit detection of abnormalities due to main-branch pulmonary artery stenosis. The right branch, however, is not well aligned for quantitative Doppler interrogation. This plane is also useful for verification of patency of surgically placed aortic-pulmonary arterial shunts. These produce a flow pattern similar to that seen in patent ductus arteriosus.

Placing the sample volume into the right ventricle just below the pulmonary valve will verify the presence of pulmonary valve regurgitation which is manifest as diastolic flow toward the transducer. The right ventricular body along the septum is then sampled for the presence of a ventricular septal defect. Sampling the right ventricular inflow tract demonstrates high velocity diastolic flow abnormalities due to tricuspid stenosis.

The right atrium can be interrogated for the presence of tricuspid backflow by placing the sample volume or color-coded sample area along the interatrial septum. Occasionally, flow abnormalities due to a left to right shunting atrial septal defect can be detected here as well.

APEX PLANE (Fig. 4–26)

4-CHAMBER

This plane of examination allows evaluation of the four chambers of the heart and is especially useful for sampling on both sides of the atrioventricular valves.

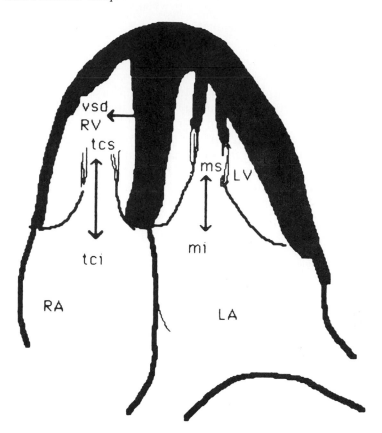

Fig. 4–26. Diagram of two-dimensional echocardiographic apex four chamber view showing possible areas for detection of common sources of jet formation.
Abbreviations; vsd, ventricular septal defect, RV, right ventricle, tcs, tricuspid valve stenosis, tci, tricuspid valve regurgitation, RA, right atrium, ms, mitral valve stenosis, LV, left ventricle, mi, mitral regurgitation, LA, left atrium.

Sampling on the ventricular side of the AV valves allows detection of abnormal flows associated with stenosis. If such abnormalities are present, sampling proximal to the valve for V1 is mandatory. Sampling proximal to atrioventricular valves also allows demonstration of regurgitation. Mitral regurgitation is usually best detected behind the posterior mitral leaflet and tricuspid backflow is detected in most instances along the atrial septal surface proximal to the tricuspid septal leaflet. Color Doppler simplifies this portion of the examination because the direction and extent of AV valve regurgitation can be readily detected (Plate 14).

Other abnormalities which can be detected in this plane in the left atrium include pulmonary vein stenosis and cor triatriatum. The examiner should always practice sampling left atrial inflow for normal pulmonary venous velocities so that their absence can be appreciated in patients with anomalous pulmonary venous return. This manuever is best performed by conventional pulsed Doppler because the signal is far from the transducer and thus weak and because velocity magnitude is frequently low. Color-coded Doppler, at times, does not demonstrate normal pulmonary venous flows.

The right ventricle should be studied along the ventricular septum in the area of the septal leaflet of the tricuspid valve for the presence of disturbed flow from a ventricular septal defect. The beam-jet angle may not be aligned in this plane. Color-coded Doppler may demonstrate a VSD jet without aliasing from this plane because of the beam-jet angle is poorly matched and the result may reduce the apparent jet velocity into the color-coded Doppler range.

By angling the transducer anteriorly, the apex short axis left ventricular outflow plane can be imaged. Here, most of the above findings can be detected, and the left ventricular outflow tract and proximal ascending aorta can be imaged. Aortic regurgitation, subaortic stenosis, and aortic valvular stenosis can be evaluated. The same areas can also be interrogated from the apex long axis left ventricular outflow plane, which is achieved by maintaining the same transducer position and rotating 90° counterclockwise.

The Subcostal Plane

4-CHAMBER (Fig. 4–27)

The subcostal four-chamber view demonstrates all four cardiac chambers with both septae more perpendicular to the transducer. The advantage is that septal defects, if present, will have jets better aligned with the Doppler beam in this plane than in the apex four-chamber plane. A disadvantage is that this plane can not be imaged in some adults. Other abnormalities which can be detected in the various chambers include tricuspid regurgitation and stenosis, mitral regurgitation and stenosis, and various sites of returned anomalous pulmonary venous drainage.

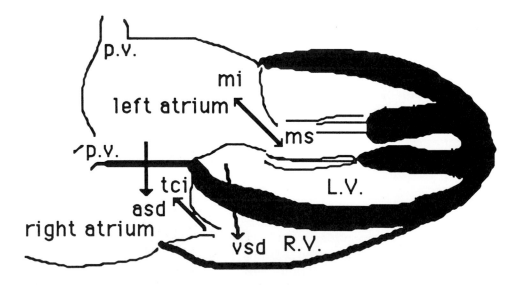

Fig. 4–27. Diagram of "inverted" two-dimensional echocardiographic subcostal 4-chamber view showing possible areas for detection of common sources of jet formation. This view is in anatomic perspective, rather than in the ultrasonic perspective where the right ventricle would appear above the left ventricle.
Abbreviations: p.v., pulmonary veins, mi, mitral regurgitation, ms, mitral stenosis, L.V., left ventricle, asd, atrial septal defect, tci, tricuspid regurgitation, vsd, ventricular septal defect, R.V., right ventricle.

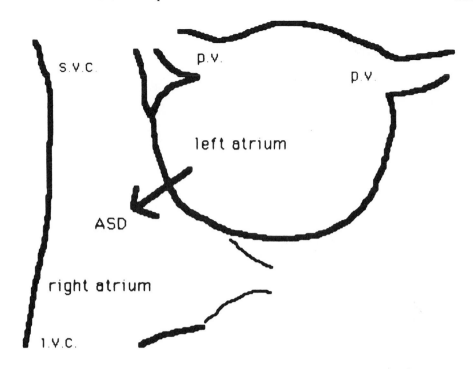

Fig. 4–28. Diagram of "inverted" two-dimensional echocardiographic subcostal short axis atrial plane view showing possible area for detection of a common source of high velocity presence. Venous flow abnormalities can also be detected from this view.
Abbreviations; s.v.c., superior vena cava, i.v.c., inferior vena cava, ASD, atrial septal defect, p.v., pulmonary veins.

SHORT AXIS SUBCOSTAL PLANE

ATRIAL (Fig. 4–28)

The superior and inferior cavae and right atrium can be interrogated for anomalous pulmonary venous drainage. Trans-atrial septal velocities associated with atrial septal defects are best appreciated in this plane. Tricuspid and mitral regurgitation can be noted in their respective atria.

VENTRICULAR (Fig. 4–29)

This valuable examination plane allows demonstration of abnormal right ventricular flows due to tricuspid valve stenosis, ventricular septal defects, anomalous right ventricular muscle bundles, and subpulmonary stenosis. The pulmonary artery can be evaluated for pulmonary valve stenosis and patent ductus arteriosus. Left ventricular abnormalities which can be detected in this plane include mitral stenosis, aortic regurgitation and aortic outflow obstruction. The aorta can be evaluated for stenosis and insufficiency.

The Suprasternal Notch

AORTIC PLANE (Fig. 4–30)

The sample volume or color Doppler window can be moved through the entire aortic arch to detect aortic valvar stenosis, aortic regurgitation, supravalvar aortic stenosis, coarctation of the aorta, and occasionally branch vessel stenosis. The descending aorta-pulmonary artery connection by a ductus can

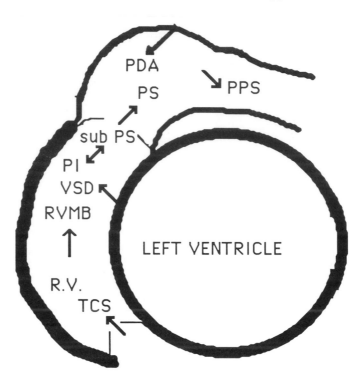

Fig. 4–29. Diagram of "inverted" two-dimensional echocardiographic subcostal short axis ventricular plane view showing possible areas for detection of common sources of jet formation. Abbreviations; TCS, tricuspid valve stenosis, r.v., right ventricle, RVMB, right ventricular muscle bundles, VSD, ventricular septal defect, PI, pulmonary regurgitation, sub PS, sub pulmonary infundibular stenosis, PS, pulmonary valvular stenosis, PDA, patent ductus arteriosus, PPS, branch pulmonary artery stenosis.

be imaged. To some extent the pulmonary artery can be evaluated in this plane for left to right ductal flow, pulmonary valvar stenosis, and branch pulmonary artery stenosis. The left atrium can be interrogated for venous inflow abnormalities and for mitral regurgitation.

CORONAL PLANE (Fig. 4–31)

The inominate and caval veins can be evaluated for the presence of anomalous drainage and for right atrial inflow narrowing. The pulmonary artery can be further evaluated for peripheral branch stenosis. Ductus arteriosus evaluation is often enhanced from this plane because the ductus is more readily visualized.

Other

The examiner can evaluate the areas of the skull and liver for the presence of arteriovenous malformations.

SPECIFIC LESIONS

In this section, the use of Doppler echocardiography will be presented for study of patients with abnormalities of commonly involved cardiac valves, and congenital defects including coarctation of the aorta, abnormal pulmonary valve, and ventricular septal defects.

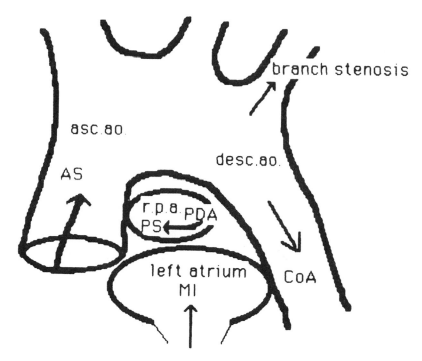

Fig. 4–30. Diagram of two-dimensional echocardiographic suprasternal notch aortic plane view showing possible areas for detection of common sources of jet formation.
Abbreviations; AS, aortic stenosis, asc.ao., ascending aorta, desc.ao., descending aorta, CoA, coarctation of the aorta, r.p.a., right pulmonary artery, PDA, patent ductus arteriosus, PS, pulmonary valve stenosis, MI, mitral regurgitation.

Aortic Valve

STENOSIS

Numerous Doppler studies of aortic valve stenosis have been reported.[11,14,19,22,26,30,38,43,47,57–85] Pressure drop quantification in valvular aortic stenosis requires that the beam be aligned with the maximal jet from whatever position allows detection of the highest velocities. Alignment is usually accomplished from the suprasternal notch, right upper sternal border, apex or subcostal regions. Interrogating from all sites may be necessary to assure recording the maximal velocity. If the transducer location is at the right upper sternal border, rotation of the patient to the right decubitus position may be useful.[19] For all patients, the examination should include interrogation of the left ventricular outflow tract (from apex four chamber planes) to measure V_1. If high, that velocity should be taken into account for pressure drop computation. In CW tracings, the pre-obstruction velocities may be observed frequently within the jet velocity (Fig. 4–32). Pulsed Doppler from the suprasternal notch, right upper sternal border, or apex locations may be used to measure subvalvular velocities. If a velocity pressure drop is not detected between the subvalvar area and the ascending aorta, aortic stenosis is probably not present even if both velocities are elevated above normal. Figure 4–33 shows representative examples of velocities from patients with valvular aortic stenosis.

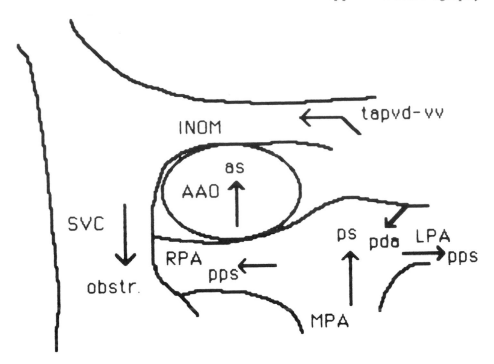

Fig. 4–31. Diagram of two-dimensional echocardiographic suprasternal notch coronal plane view showing possible areas for detection of flow abnormalities.
Abbreviations; SVC, superior vena cava, obstr., obstruction, INOM, inominate vein, tapvd-vv, anomalous pulmonary venous drainage to a vertical vein, AAO, ascending aorta, as, aortic valve stenosis, MPA, RPA, LPA, main, right and left pulmonary arteries, ps, pulmonary valve stenosis, pda, patent ductus arteriosus, pps, branch peripheral pulmonary artery stenosis.

Angle correction should be avoided. Jet direction is too unpredictable and any attempt to correct for an angle may lead to serious pressure drop estimation errors. Angle correction by jet-parajet imaging with color-coded Doppler has been suggested, but the jet-parajet is imaged in only two dimensions. Spatial angular correction is required, not just two dimensional correction. Accordingly, estimation errors may also occur with this approach.

RESULTS OF STUDIES IN AORTIC STENOSIS

Several studies have demonstrated that Doppler-predicted gradients correlated quite well with those measured at cardiac catheterization.[19,22,25,26,57–71] Hatle et al.[22] noted early in their experience that the examination was more difficult in patients over the age of 50 and that children were easiest to examine. However, they later reported that appropriate pressure drop estimation was possible in almost all adults with aortic stenosis. Rare underestimation of the highest gradients was also noted, particularly before they had Doppler analyses by true spectral methods. With spectral analysis, underestimation became uncommon. Other studies have all shown correlation coefficients ranging from .66 to .95[25,26,57,59–71] when catheterization (usually peak-to-peak) and Doppler (usually instantaneous) pressure drops were compared. (Table 4–1)

OTHER TYPES OF AORTIC STENOSIS

Estimates of pressure drop in long segment subaortic obstruction should be approached with caution because the viscous friction component of the Ber-

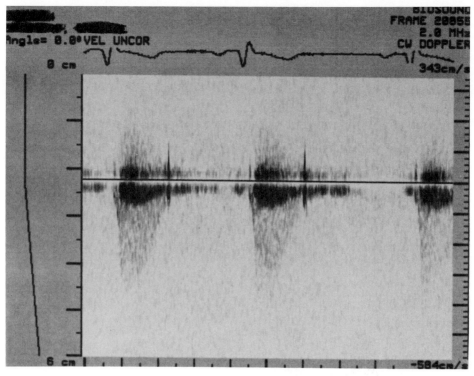

Fig. 4–32. Continuous wave velocity tracings from a patient with valvular aortic stenosis. V_2 is too poorly demonstrated to measure, especially in the last beat which gives the impression of much higher velocities than in the first beat. V_1 is easily seen. Note opening and closing valve spikes.

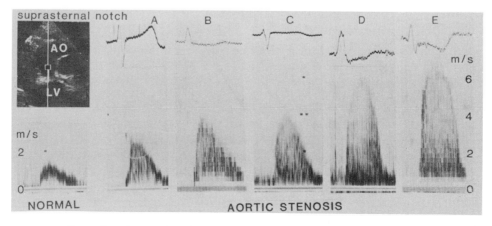

Fig. 4–33. Examples of normal to varying degrees of severity of aortic outflow obstruction (Reprinted with permission from Hatle and Anglesen[19]). All tracings are from the suprasternal notch. Calibration scales are the same in the continuous wave tracings (A though E).

Table 4–1.   Correlation coefficients from various Doppler studies of aortic stenosis. The study from which data are derived is shown in the top column as a reference (ref.). Various gradient measurement techniques are then compared with catheterization data.

Study (Ref.)	60	61	57	62	26	63	59(o)	59>exp	59(nsr)	64	65	67	68	69	70	71
Peak-Peak	.91	.79	.85	.84	.94	—	.68	.78	.85	.85	.95	.85	—	.68	—	.90
Instantaneous	.92	—	—	.87	—	.79	.66	.79	.87	.93	—	—	—	—	.86	—
Mean	.93	—	—	.84	—	.77	.75	.83	.89	.89	.95	—	.92	—	—	—

Abbreviations; o = overall experience in Panidis et al. study,[59] >exp = later data from a greater experience, nsr = normal sinus rhythm.

noulli equation may be significant enough to cause a pressure drop underestimation.[50,54,72] Subaortic stenotic lesions such as hypertrophic obstructive cardiomyopathy with systolic anterior motion of the mitral valve,[86–95] discrete membranous subaortic stenosis (Fig. 4–34) and fibromuscular subaortic stenosis can be evaluated by CW Doppler. However, the examiner must be aware that in patients with hypertrophic obstructive cardiomyopathy, the dominant jet may be one of mitral regurgitation.[19,87,93,95] Separation of the mitral regurgitation jet from the aortic stenotic jet may not be easy without imaging; however, mitral regurgitant begins earlier than ejection in aortic stenosis (Fig. 4–35). In patients with Williams syndrome (supravalvular aortic stenosis), the examination should be performed from the suprasternal notch or from the right upper sternal border. Gradients estimated by Doppler in all these conditions correlated well with gradients found at catheterization, both in terms of pressure drop prediction and localization of the obstructive site.[19,26]

PROSTHETIC AORTIC VALVES

The same methodology used for evaluation of patients with valvar aortic stenosis can be used for those with prosthetic aortic valves. If the valve is bioprosthetic and stenotic, poststenotic jets in the ascending aorta can be detected and measured from the same transducer locations used in patients with native aortic stenosis. If the valve is mechanical, the suprasternal and right precordial locations may be preferable because ultrasound transmitted from an apical and subcostal direction may be attenuated markedly by the mechanical valve.

Studies[96–102] have been performed on patients with aortic valve prostheses. The main conclusions of these studies were that valve obstruction could be detected by high velocities which were closely predictive of pressure drop and that higher than normal velocities were encountered in all prosthetic valves, perhaps related to relatively smaller prosthetic valve annulus size than true annulus size.

CLINICAL APPLICATION OF DOPPLER IN AORTIC STENOSIS

Doppler is useful for following the course of patients with aortic stenosis. Pressure drop alone does not provide enough data for clinical decision-making. Of course, symptoms, clinical examination, electrocardiography, echocardiography, chest x ray, exercise electrocardiography and common sense provide additional data. However, of these several modalities, Doppler permits the most useful evaluation because it provides a transvalve pressure drop which, when combined with other information can be used to estimate the

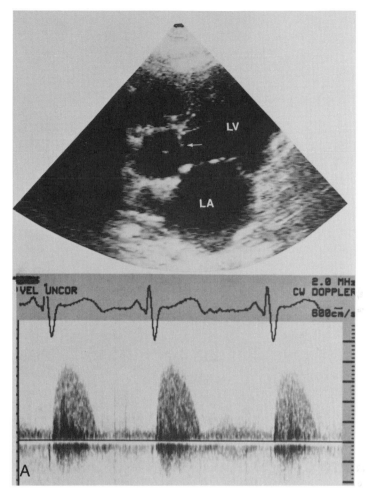

Fig. 4–34. Two examples of subaortic stenosis. The first panel demonstrates the presence of a subaortic membrane in the echo (arrow), and the lower panel shows the continuous wave Doppler tracing obtained from the right upper sternal border. The estimated gradient of 50 mm Hg correlated well with that found at cardiac catheterization. (Reproduced with permission from Hegesh et al. Am Heart J, in press, 1987.)
The second figure was obtained from the right upper sternal border in a patient with idiopathic hypertrophic subaortic stenosis. Note the dense prevalvular velocity envelope due to early obstruction.

valvar area (see Chapter 7). Doppler can be used at the time of initial clinical evaluation, for re-evaluation and serially following operation. The close correlation between Doppler and catheterization-measured gradients is sufficiently accurate that the need for "routine" catheterization for pressure drop measurement must be seriously questioned. However, catheterization may again become important if aortic balloon valvuloplasty proves to have major clinical utility and acceptable risk.

AORTIC REGURGITATION (Fig. 4–36)

Several qualitative and quantitative Doppler studies of aortic regurgitation have been reported.[19,32,34,39,41,45,78,81,103–127] Demonstration of aortic regurgita-

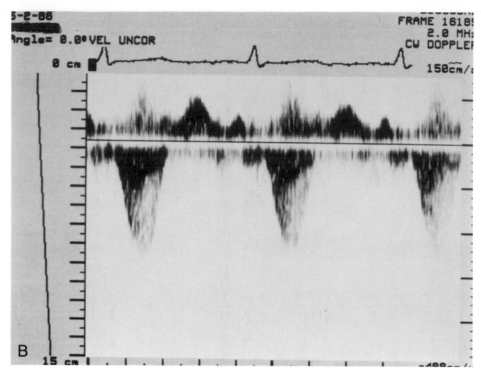

Fig. 4–34 (continued).

tion requires proper alignment of the Doppler beam with the regurgitant jet. Since its location is variable, different transducer locations are required until the examiner is satisfied that the maximal velocities have been obtained. The usual locations which best demonstrate the jet of aortic regurgitation are at the right upper sternal border, the apex, the suprasternal notch, and occasionally the subcostal area. Do not assume that the jet direction for aortic regurgitation is the same as that for any associated aortic stenosis. Precordial locations usually introduce excessive angulation for adequate demonstration of maximal velocities; however, precordial locations are often used for color-coded Doppler analysis[113] since normal flows may cause aliasing and the greater angulation in the precordial position reduces this problem.

Ciobanu et al.[32] showed that approximation of angiographic estimation of the degree of regurgitation was possible by tracing the pulsed Doppler detection of aliased flow into the left ventricle. If aliasing was present only below the aortic cusps, regurgitation was mild. If it extended to mid-septum, it was moderate, and if it extended to the apex it was severe. Hatle and Angelsen[19] also stated that the signal's strength reflected the severity of the regurgitation.

Another estimate of the severity of aortic regurgitation is available by evaluating the pulsed Doppler ascending aortic and descending aortic velocity profiles. If retograde aortic flow is noted, regurgitation is usually at least moderate.[19] Further, the degree of regurgitation can be quantitatively estimated by measuring the area of the velocity waveform[106,107,119,121] (See Chapter 5). If retrograde aortic flow is used to evaluate aortic regurgitation, the examiner is

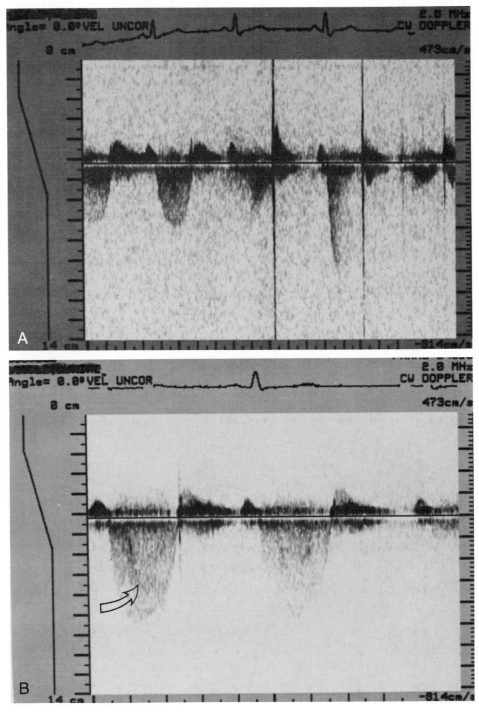

Fig. 4–35. Tracings from a patient with mitral regurgitation and valvular aortic stenosis demonstrating the difference in timing of onset of the two jets. The first panel shows a continuous wave Doppler sweep from the aortic stenosis jet (first 2 beats) to that of mitral regurgitation (4th beat). The tracing in the 4th beat could not be measured however, but does show a definitely different velocity and confirms the diagnosis gained from a separate pulsed Doppler assessment. The second panel, especially in the first beat, shows superimposition of the 2 jet velocity curves. Note the later onset of the aortic stenosis curve (arrow). It also returns to baseline earlier than the mitral regurgitation curve.

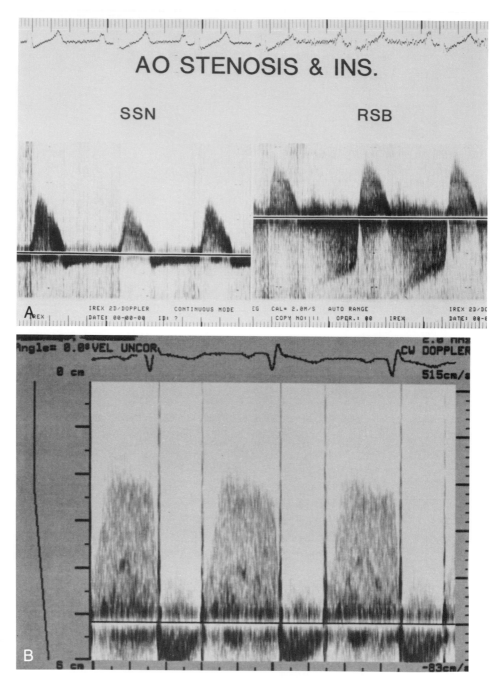

Fig. 4–36. Two examples of aortic regurgitation. The first demonstrates mild aortic stenosis and that the regurgitation jet was not detected from the suprasternal notch view. The aortic regurgitation jet is better demonstrated in the second beat of the second panel, but the tracing is still inadequate. The second figure shows the jet best detected from the apex view in another patient. The examiner should search all possible areas until the best jet is detected.

cautioned to rule out other causes of aortic runoff such as patent ductus arteriosus.

Hatle and Angelsen[19] emphasized timing of diastolic events as a useful means of diagnosing aortic regurgitation, especially when non-echocardiographically guided "blind" continuous wave Doppler transducers are used. The velocity signal of aortic regurgitation begins in early diastole, just after aortic valve closure, whereas mitral events begin slightly later. Regurgitant velocities continue throughout diastole and ordinarily are of greater magnitude than those for mitral stenosis. Insight into the severity of elevation of left ventricular diastolic pressures can be gained by noting the height of the velocity waveform. If the waveform remains significantly elevated at end diastole, the pressure drop between the aorta and the left ventricle is high, indicating more normal left ventricular diastolic pressures. On the other hand, if the waveform tapers and decreases, the pressure gap between aortic and left ventricular diastolic pressures is low. If aortic diastolic pressures are known, the left ventricular diastolic pressure can be estimated grossly by subtracting the predicted pressure drop from the aortic diastolic pressure.

Atrioventricular Valves
STENOSIS

Mitral and tricuspid valve stenoses are most commonly encountered in the adult population. Both may be evaluated by Doppler. The patient is usually examined in a left lateral decubitus position and the transducer is positioned at the cardiac apex. Two-dimensional echocardiography from the apical 4 chamber plane is used to guide the pulsed Doppler sample volume just distal to the respective valve orifice. The velocity baseline should be positioned near the bottom of the display, and if the atrioventricular valve is not too distant from the transducer, most jet velocities across stenotic atrioventricular valves will be in the range of 2.25 MHz pulsed Doppler. If velocity aliasing is encountered, CW Doppler should be used. Small transducer motions are made until the highest velocity jet is detected by both auditory and spectral signals. Next, the examiner should prove that the high velocity jet is due to obstruction and not due to high flow. This is accomplished by moving the sample volume just proximal to the mitral or tricuspid leaflets to allow comparison of velocities on either side of the valve (V_1 and V_2). Care must be used to evaluate the preobstruction velocity in the valve ring area proximal to the leaflets. If the sample volume is positioned more proximally, the flow area rapidly increases and velocities are significantly lower than at the ring (Fig. 4–37). Observations in normals have shown that the maximal transvalve velocity difference is 20 cm/sec.[128] Flows at the upper limits of normal may produce a velocity gradient of about 30 cm/sec. The precise relationship between flow and velocity gradient has not been established, but at present, we consider a velocity gradient in excess of 30 cm/sec indicative of a true pressure drop.

MITRAL STENOSIS

Mitral stenosis has been extensively studied by Doppler.[19–21,23,24,52,78,81,89,113,115,129–182] Hatle et al.[19] and Holen et al.[23,24,52,132] showed that maximal velocity in mitral stenosis is usually obtained after initial opening of the valve. The velocity waveform then decreases slightly and, in sinus rhythm, peaks

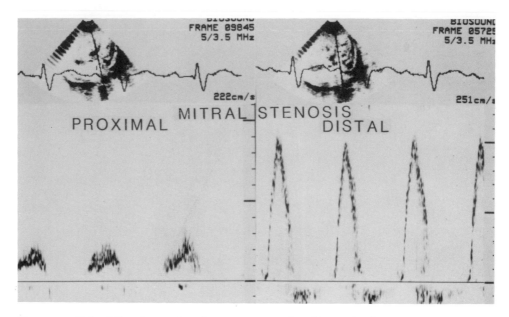

Fig. 4–37. Pulsed Doppler tracings from a patient with mild mitral valve stenosis. The sample volume is located too proximally to gain a valid representation of V_1 (1st panel). It should be placed just before the valve in the area of the annulus.

again following the onset of atrial contraction. Thus, the pressure drop demonstrated by Doppler is not just end diastolic, but represents the entire gamut of transmitral pressure differences at each diastolic instant. Their results in mitral stenosis have been among the best correlation of Doppler and manometry values (Fig. 4–38). The high correlation and accuracy of Doppler estimates raises the question of the value of a catheterization procedure if other issues are not in question (coronary arteries, pulmonary vascular disease, etc.).

Results of other studies have paralleled the experience of Hatle et al.[19] Patients with congenital arcade and parachute malformations,[131] and with stenotic prosthetic valves[144–155] show similar findings to those seen in rheumatic mitral stenosis. Similar findings to those seen in mitral stenosis are noted in high transmitral flow states,[19,128] such as seen in large ventricular septal defects or patent ductus arteriosus. Besides the obvious detection of the primary lesion, sampling before the valve for V_1 helps differentiate the origin of the problem as flow related rather than due to stenosis.

This has been an easy examination to perform. Since maximal resting gradients rarely exceed 36 mm Hg, and since the distance to the jet is short, most patients could be studied with 2.25 MHz pulsed Doppler as well as CW Doppler. At least one word of caution is necessary. The site of obstruction in mitral stenosis is occasionally subvalvar (i.e. chordal). Merely placing the range gate between the cusps may not measure the maximal jet velocity. A Doppler exploration of the entire area is necessary. Doppler measured gradients may also be studied during supine exercise, but the examination is not easy.

Hatle and Angelsen[19] emphasize that the maximal velocity and mean pressure drop across mitral stenosis is affected by heart rate because of different diastolic durations. The higher the heart rate, the greater the pressure drop. They also

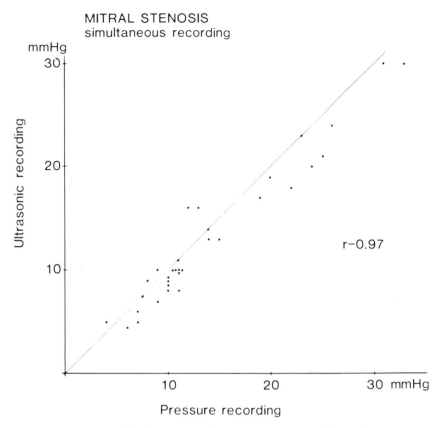

Fig. 4–38. Mean transmitral valve pressure drop in 33 patients with mitral stenosis. Doppler calculated pressure drop is compared with pressure gradient measured simultaneously at cardiac catheterization. An excellent correlation is noted. (From Hatle, L., Angelsen, B.: Doppler Ultrasound in Cardiology. Physical Principles and Clinical Applications. 2nd Ed., Philadelphia, Lea & Febiger, 1985.)

point out that the slope of the velocity waveform is related to the degree of obstruction. This forms the basis of the calculation of the pressure half-time prediction of the mitral valve area, which is discussed in Chapter 7.

TRICUSPID STENOSIS

For patients with tricuspid stenosis,[19,156–158] the approach is similar to that for mitral stenosis, but velocities are frequently lower than those found in mitral stenosis and transducer positions are different. Here, the transducer is located apically or subcostally, but the beam is directed toward the right lower or mid sternal area, and is angulated more anteriorly than the angle used for mitral regurgitation. Greater respiratory variation is present than is seen in normal subjects.[19] Significant pressure drops are usually lower than those across stenotic mitral valves. Hatle makes the point that the diagnosis is made quite easily by Doppler if the examiner is alert to the possibility of the presence of the lesion. The examination is usually successfully performed with a 2.25 MHz pulsed Doppler transducer. CW Doppler examination provides similar information (Fig. 4–39). One aspect that may cause confusion when using non-imaging continuous wave Doppler is that patients with tricuspid stenosis fre-

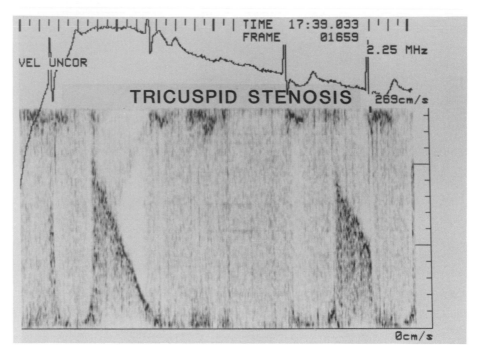

Fig. 4–39. Pulsed Doppler tracing from a patient with tricuspid stenosis and atrial fibrillation. Note that the velocities are much higher than normal, yet can be detected by pulsed wave Doppler.

quently have mitral stenosis as well. Location, velocity amplitude and variation, and timing may help separate the two.

Regurgitation

MITRAL REGURGITATION (Fig. 4–40)

In contrast to tricuspid backflow, mitral regurgitation is seldom seen in normals, and has been the subject of many reports.[3,4,13,19,21,32,39-42,47,78,80,81,89,109,111,113,114,122,125,130,131,133,136,143,159,178] Since flow occurs from a high pressure chamber to a low pressure chamber, the pressure drop is high and continuous wave Doppler is necessary for quantitative examination. Qualitative detection is possible by pulsed or color-coded Doppler. Although jet direction is variable, the regurgitant diastolic jet is often detected proximal to the posterior mitral valve leaflet.

Optimal transducer location for detection of mitral regurgitation is usually apical, either in the two or four chamber views. Color-coded Doppler transducer location may be precordial in order to create an angulation error which reduces aliasing of normal velocities. Occasionally, mitral regurgitation can be detected from the suprasternal notch plane. This signal is occasionally confused with aortic stenosis. Recall that the jet of mitral regurgitation begins earlier than and persists longer than that of aortic stenosis.

Abassi et al.[4] suggest that the severity of mitral regurgitation is reflected by the extent of the Doppler detected jet into the left atrium: the deeper the penetration, the worse the insufficiency. Hatle and Angelsen[19] noted that signal strength is related to the degree of regurgitation.

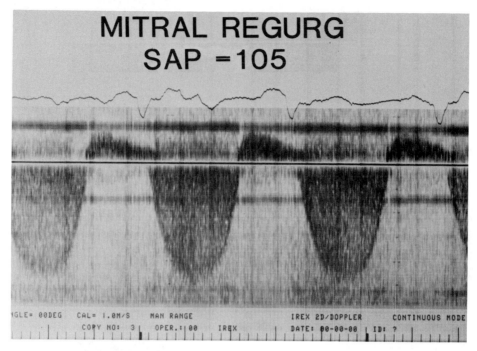

Fig. 4–40. Continuous wave Doppler tracing from a patient with mitral valve regurgitation. Note that the curve starts in early systole and persists throughout. The systolic arterial pressure is 105 mm Hg and the predicted pressure drop is 100 mm Hg, indicating that the systolic pressure drop must be from a chamber with systemic pressures, assuming that the patient does not have aortic stenosis.

Secondary effects of mitral regurgitation include pulmonary hypertension, congestive heart failure, and reversed aortic midsystolic flow. Pulmonary hypertension is reflected by shortened pulmonary artery time to peak velocity and, if present, by increased amplitude of the tricuspid backflow velocity curves. The regurgitant systolic waveform is lower in velocity and longer in duration if the patient has severe congestive heart failure, associated with higher diastolic pressures and lower ventricular systolic pressures. Systolic notching of the aortic forward velocity waveform reflects blood flow dynamics from peaking left ventricular-left atrial backflow velocities.[172] Additionally, if mitral regurgitation is severe, the forward diastolic mitral velocities will be increased because of increased forward flows.

In mitral valve prolapse, the regurgitant jet is usually noted later in systole than the jet of pure mitral regurgitation, and the various maneuvers used to accentuate prolapse will increase the duration of the backflow velocities (Fig. 4–41).

TRICUSPID REGURGITATION (Fig. 4–42)

Tricuspid regurgitation has been the topic of many reports.[19,29,35, 36,43,111,113,114,122,138,157,179-192] Tricuspid regurgitation is a pathologic state in which the Doppler observation of a regurgitant jet is associated with clinical findings, such as presence of a murmur. In contrast, tricuspid backflow is noted in most normals. Whatever the cause, Doppler detection of the jet allows analysis of the pressure drop and prediction of pressures in the right heart.

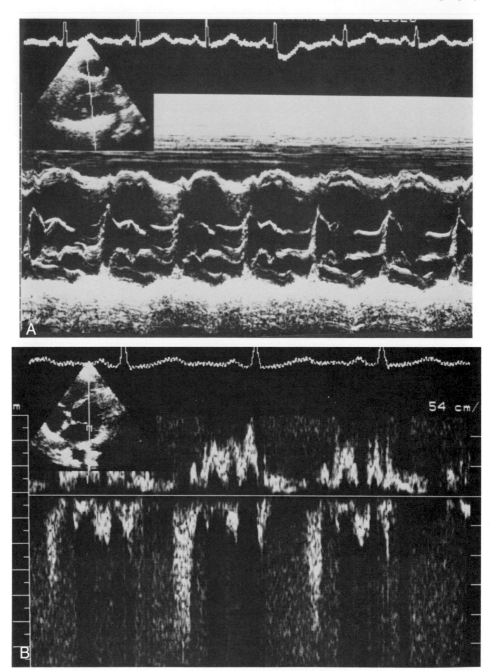

Fig. 4–41. M-mode (1st panel), and pulsed Doppler tracings at rest (2nd) and during isometric exercise (3rd). from a patient with mitral valve prolapse. The prolapse is best demonstrated in the first beat in panel 1. Note the late systolic short duration aliased regurgitant flow signal in panel 2. The sample volume is located just behind the posterior leaflet of the mitral valve (insert). The signal is much broader and more intense during isometric exercise.

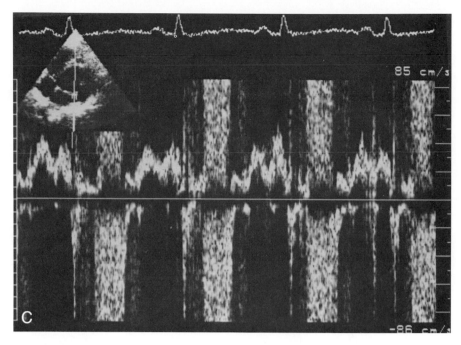

Fig. 4–41 (continued).

Tricuspid backflow is best detected from the same transducer locations used for detection of tricuspid stenosis (see above). The jet is more easily detected by continuous wave Doppler than by pulsed Doppler. Color-coded Doppler usually demonstrates the backflow jet, especially if it is significant. The examination demands subtle and minute angulations of the continuous wave Doppler transducer. The high velocity jet is usually best located along the interatrial septum. Although a generally similar apical position is used for detection of the jet of aortic stenosis, the jet of tricuspid backflow is differentiated from that of aortic stenosis by its timing, since tricuspid flow begins earlier and is longer in duration than the jet of mitral regurgitation. The jet is in a different location, more posterior and lateral than that of aortic stenosis. Last, the jet of mitral regurgitation is generally greater in amplitude than that of aortic stenosis, which, in turn, is generally greater than that of tricuspid backflow. Severity of right ventricular obstruction and pulmonary hypertension certainly alter the latter statement.

Significant tricuspid regurgitation can also be detected in the inferior vena cava and into the hepatic veins mainly in systole and occasionally also in diastole (Fig. 4–43). The retrograde holosystolic wave is greater if the regurgitation is severe.[188] This can be noted by pulsed Doppler or by color-coded Doppler subcostal examinations. Higher velocities could be evaluated by continuous wave Doppler, but this is rarely necessary in the caval and hepatic veins.

The pressure drop calculated as a transtricuspid pressure drop is useful in analysis of right sided pressures and will be discussed in detail later in this chapter.

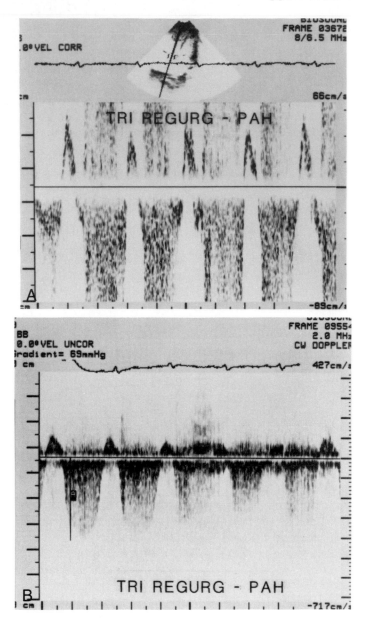

Fig. 4–42. Tricuspid regurgitation in a patient with pulmonary arterial hypertension. The first panel shows the broadened aliased pulsed Doppler signal detected when the sample volume is placed behind the septal leaflet of the tricuspid valve (apex view-insert). The second panel demonstrates the continuous wave high velocity Doppler tracing. The predicted pressure drop is 60 to 70 mm Hg, predicting high right ventricular systolic pressures at approximately 70 mm Hg. The last panel shows a pulmonary artery tracing with markedly shortened time to peak velocities, or acceleration time. Normal is >100 msec. The projected mean pulmonary artery pressure here is 55 mm Hg (80 − 50/2 = 55; see text for details).

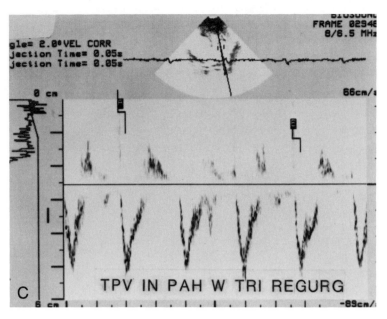

Fig. 4–42 (continued).

Coarctation of the Aorta

Few Doppler studies of coarctation of the aorta have been published.[19,59,193–195] Pressure gradients across an aortic coarctation can usually be determined by subtracting lower extremity blood pressure from upper extremity blood pressure. In most coarctation patients, the Doppler examination for pressure drop is not necessary. Localization of the coarctation can usually be accomplished by barium swallow. The shape and length of the coarctation can sometimes be imaged by echocardiography.[196] Collateral vessels are suggested by rib notching on the chest film in older children, or by digital subtraction angiography, or aortography. Why then use Doppler for evaluation of a patient with coarctation? Some coarctations are missed by barium swallow or are not imaged by two-dimensional echocardiography. In these cases, the pulsed Doppler sample volume can be guided by two-dimensional echocardiography into the descending aorta via the suprasternal notch. If the patient does not have an associated upstream obstruction which creates high velocities, and if the transverse aortic diameter is normal, velocities approximately similar to those in the ascending aorta will usually be encountered proximal to the coarctation (Fig. 4–44). Higher velocities will be encountered distal to the coarctation, thus confirming the site of obstruction. CW Doppler or occasionally, a low frequency pulsed Doppler transducer, allows recording of peak jet velocities and calculation of maximal pressure drop. Pressure drop determination has also been useful for establishing proximal blood pressure in patients who have no upper extremity pulses after axillary cutdowns on the right and subclavian flap procedures on the left. Another situation in which proximal aortic pressure is unobtainable under ordinary circumstances is when the right subclavian artery has aberrant origin at or below the coarctation and the left subclavian artery has been used in flap procedure. Thus, Doppler allows localization of the

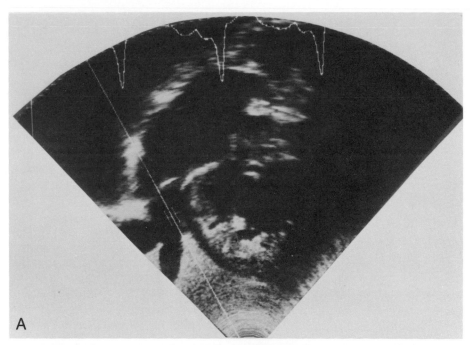

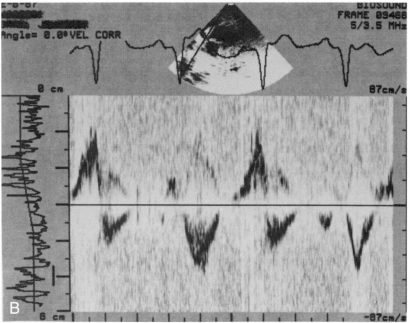

Fig. 4–43. Dilated hepatic veins and inferior vena cava are demonstrated in an inverted subcostal view (first panel) from a patient with severe pulmonary hypertension and tricuspid regurgitation. The second panel shows the inferior caval-hepatic vein velocities recorded from the sample volume location shown in the first panel. Note the systolic velocities away from the transducer, back into the liver (the image in the first panel is inverted, but the Doppler sample is not). The third panel demonstrates the continuous wave Doppler velocities predicting a pressure drop of over 100 mm Hg.

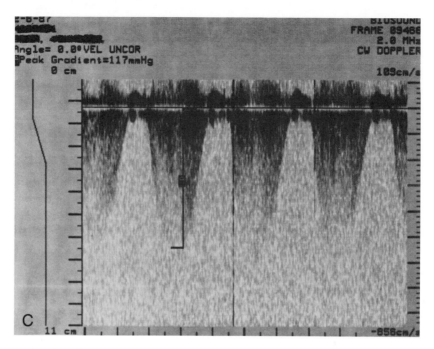

Fig. 4–43 (continued).

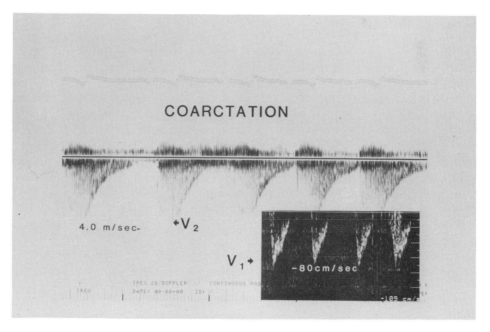

Fig. 4–44. Pre and post velocities in a patient with coarctation of the aorta. The insert is a pulsed Doppler tracing showing V_1 at 80 cm/sec. The peak continuous wave velocities (V_2) predict a pressure drop of 64 mm Hg.

coarctation and estimation of the obstruction. Proximal aortic pressure may be computed by adding the pressure drop to lower extremity pressure. However, Doppler does not provide information about collaterals.

Doppler may be used for pre- and postoperative assessment of coarctation gradients. Restenosis sometimes occurs and Doppler is useful for serial evaluation of postoperative patients. Those with sufficiently high gradients may become balloon angioplasty[197] or reoperative candidates.

We have found color-coded Doppler ineffective for assessing many patients with coarctation. The coarctation sites are far from the transducer and the returning signal is weak. Further, normal velocities and jets of coarctation exceed Nyquist limits, so each aliases the color signal. However, studies show a well-defined jet in some patients.

Pulmonary Valve Stenosis

Doppler echocardiography has been effective in qualitative detection of poststenotic flow disturbances and quantitation of the degree of obstruction in patients with pulmonary valve stenosis.[5,7,19,25,57,59,198-204] The Doppler examination for a patient with pulmonary stenosis is performed from the high parasternal short axis, subcostal or suprasternal location. The short axis examination is accomplished by imaging from the left second or third intercostal space and demonstrating the aortic cross section, high right ventricular outflow tract, pulmonary valve, main pulmonary artery and branching left and right pulmonary arteries (Figs. 4–25 and 4–45). In order to achieve this plane it may be necessary to rotate the transducer somewhat rightward from the classical short axis plane. The patient may often have to lie in an exaggerated left lateral decubitus position which sometimes exceeds 90°. In this position, both walls of the pulmonary artery can usually be imaged and a good quality Doppler signal can be recorded. When the subcostal plane is employed, the transducer is placed in a short axis plane obtained by rotating the transducer clockwise and directing it anteriorly and superiorly with the transducer flat with respect to the patient's abdomen. Imaging from this sagittal position demonstrates the right ventricular body, outflow tract, pulmonary valve, and main pulmonary artery (Figs. 4–29 and 4–46). This examination plane causes discomfort, and places the area of interest at some distance from the transducer. It requires examiner experience and patient compliance or sedation. For patients who have lung covering the pulmonary artery, this plane may present the only possibility for imaging the pulmonary artery and recording pulmonary artery velocities. Sometimes the suprasternal approach is helpful as well.

The Doppler examination is conducted initially by recording velocities in the right ventricular outflow tract proximal to the pulmonary valve. If a high flow state is present, such as occurs in patients with an atrial septal defect, subvalvar velocity (V_1) must be taken into account for it will probably not be negligible. If either the jet or subvalvar velocity exceeds the Nyquist limit, CW Doppler must be employed to accurately record calibrated velocities. If subvalvar velocities are less than 1 m/sec, V_1 can be disregarded for pressure drop measurements. The beam is next directed into the main pulmonary artery. If jet velocities beyond the Nyquist limit are found, CW Doppler must be employed. Once auditory and spectral signal criteria are met, velocities are recorded. Figure 4–46 shows representative velocities from a patient with moderate to severe obstruction.

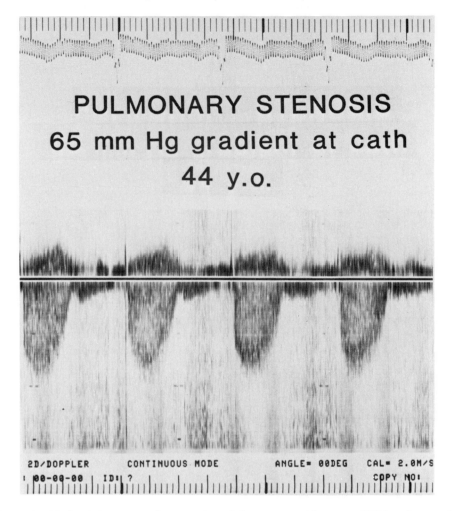

Fig. 4–45. Moderate to severe pulmonary stenosis in a 44-year-old woman. CW Doppler sampling from the left upper precordium was used. The patient had to be rotated to the left nearly onto her abdomen to achieve a proper alignment of jet with beam. Peak velocities are 4 m/sec and the calculated gradient is 64 mm Hg. At cardiac catheterization, peak systolic gradient ranged from 60 to 70 mm Hg.

With CW Doppler, velocities which originate proximal to the valve and higher velocities which originate from the poststenotic jet can frequently be recorded simultaneously if sufficient gray scale is available in the Doppler device (Fig. 4–47). This combination of velocities permits evaluation of the relationship of V_1 and V_2. However, this type of recording is valuable only if the two velocities are in the same alignment with respect to the beam.

Several studies (Table 4–2) have demonstrated that results of the Doppler predicted systolic gradients correlate highly and produce similar absolute magnitude information as compared to gradients measured by manometry at cardiac catheterization. Highest correlations occurred when simultaneous Doppler and pressure manometry results are compared. Figure 4–48 shows our experience for patients with pulmonary valve stenosis with pressure pressure drop determined by Doppler and manometry at catheterization (some measurements were

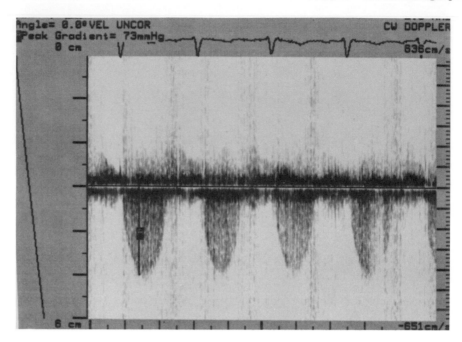

Fig. 4–46. Subcostal plane derived continuous wave Doppler tracings from a 6-week-old child with severe pulmonary valvular stenosis. The peak velocities of >70 mm Hg correlated well with those measured at catheterization prior to balloon valvuloplasty.

not simultaneous). In this study, all Doppler information was recorded from the precordial transducer location. However, the examiner should realize that jet direction will govern the best location for transducer placement. Sometimes the precordial location is best, other times, the subcostal or suprasternal locations are best. Non-angle corrected Doppler-predicted pressure drops closely approximated measurements obtained with fluid-filled catheters.

COMMENT

Doppler pressure drop estimation for patients with pulmonary stenosis appears accurate enough to use primarily, especially for patients with uncomplicated valvar stenosis. Doppler pressure gradients, like invasive gradients, must be evaluated with measured cardiac output. One main reason we still perform catheterization in some patients with valvar stenosis is for therapeutic balloon dilation valvuloplasty. Doppler and echo examination has been valuable for ruling out other problems. Doppler is especially useful for serial post-procedural evaluation of patients who have had balloon valvuloplasty and develop infundibular gradients after the procedure (Figs. 4–47 and 4–49). Here, we use Doppler pressure drop estimates to assess effects of treatment on the muscular component of the stenosis. Doppler pressure drop measurement is also valuable in the postoperative period, both early and late. If a patient has little pressure drop and normal cardiac output, postoperative problems should not be blamed on residual obstruction.

OTHER TYPES OF PULMONARY STENOSIS

The same principles may be applied, generally, to patients with infundibular pulmonary stenosis,[199] tetralogy of Fallot,[19] main pulmonary artery stenosis,

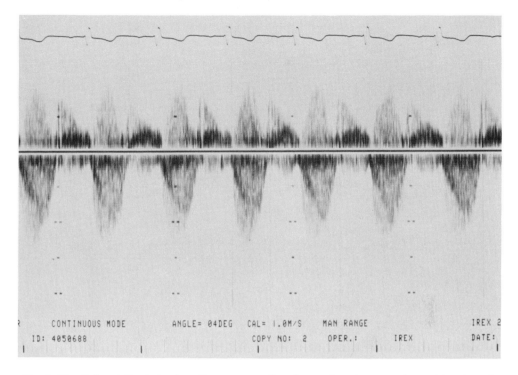

Fig. 4–47. Subcostally derived continuous wave Doppler tracings from a patient with primarily infundibular pulmonary stenosis. The first and fifth through seventh beats best show the superimposition of V_1 (infundibular) with V_2 (total pressure drop) tracings.

pulmonary artery bands[202,203] (Fig. 4–50), extrinsic tumors[204] and stenotic prosthetic valves in conduits.[205,206] The examination for infundibular stenosis is more difficult than for valvar stenosis and may require unusual transducer locations to detect the maximal jet. The subcostal plane usually offers the best information in patients with infundibular stenosis. The jet of infundibular stenosis usually peaks later than the jet of valvular stenosis. The envelope of this jet is frequently superimposed with the jet of the fixed obstruction (Figs. 4–47 and 4–49).

Although branch pulmonary artery stenosis may be detected at the bifurcation of the major pulmonary arteries (Fig. 4–51), vessel angulation, in some instances, may not allow proper alignment with the jet for quantitative purposes. Further, smaller branch pulmonary arteries may normally have some increased velocities over those found in the main pulmonary artery and first branch left and right pulmonary arteries. Distal peripheral pulmonary artery stenoses are embedded in lung tissue and are generally beyond the range of the ultrasonic

Table 4–2. Correlation coefficients and standard error of the estimate (SEE) data from various Doppler and catheterization studies of pulmonary outflow obstructions. Other abbreviations as in Table 4–1.

Investigator (Ref)	198	200	201	25	199	203
r =	.94	.95	.91	.98	.7 to .9	.95
S.E.E. (mm Hg) =	7.9	7.9	8.8	7.0	—	—

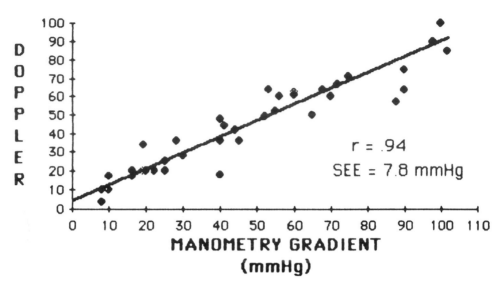

Fig. 4–48. Figure showing comparison of Doppler pressure drop (ordinate) and catheterization pressure drop (abscissa) in patients with pulmonary valvular stenosis. (Reprinted with permission from Goldberg, et al.[198]).

beam. Cardiac catheterization is superior to Doppler for evaluation of peripheral pulmonary artery stenosis.

Another important application of Doppler is serial evaluation of patients who have conduits. Conduits may be used to connect the systemic venous ventricle to the pulmonary artery. Often, conduits contain a bioprosthetic "pulmonary" valve which may calcify and become insufficient or stenotic or both.[205,206] As pressure drops develop and progress, timing of interventional catheterization is augmented by Doppler information. Doppler gradient estimation is similar to that used in evaluation of stenotic native pulmonary valves. The examination is difficult and often requires unusual transducer localization until the maximal jet is detected. Subcostal or superior precordial approaches are usually the most useful. Occasionally a subclavicular approach can be used.

PULMONARY REGURGITATION (Fig. 4–52)

Several Doppler studies regarding pulmonary regurgitation have been published.[19,31,40,44,107,116,207–209] Pulmonary regurgitation is a pathologic state, usually noted postoperatively, but occasionally seen as a congenital problem. It is frequently present when patients have severe pulmonary hypertension and pulmonary artery dilation. Pulmonary arterial backflow, on the other hand is common,[111] and is not a pathologic situation.

The jet from either pulmonary regurgitation or backflow is detected from the precordial short axis plane or from the subcostal plane with the transducer oriented slightly leftward and anteriorly. The pulsed Doppler sample volume should be placed proximal to the pulmonary valve in the right ventricular outflow tract from either location. The continuous wave Doppler transducer is similarly oriented. The signal of pulmonary regurgitation is detected in early

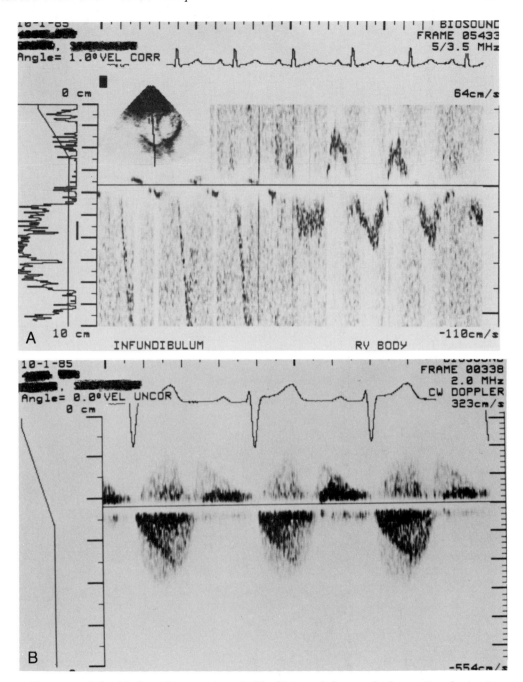

Fig. 4–49. Infundibular pulmonary stenosis. The first panel shows pulsed wave Doppler tracings obtained from the subcostal position. As the sample volume is moved from the right ventricular outflow (infundibulum) to the body, a discrete decrease in velocities is noted. The second panel is from the same patient, and was obtained just after balloon valvuloplasty. The initial pressure drop was 120 mm Hg whereas the total pressure drop is now estimated to be 25 mm Hg. The infundibular component, shown as the darkened inner late peaking envelope, is estimated to be 18 mm Hg. Note that the patient also has slight pulmonary regurgitation which reflects a low pulmonary artery diastolic pressure. This was not audible.

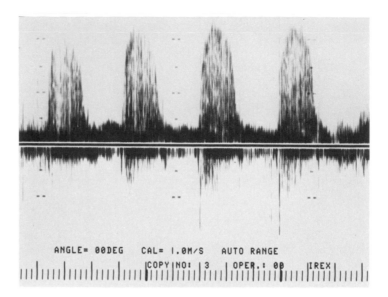

ANGLE= 00DEG   CAL= 1.0M/S   AUTO RANGE

Fig. 4–50. Velocities beyond the site of a pulmonary artery (PA) band. The cursor was located in the pulmonary artery from the suprasternal notch. Note the peak velocities of 4.5 m/sec, translating to a peak gradient of 81 mm Hg. The pulmonary artery distal to a band can also be interrogated from the precordial or subcostal areas or from wherever the jet can be located.

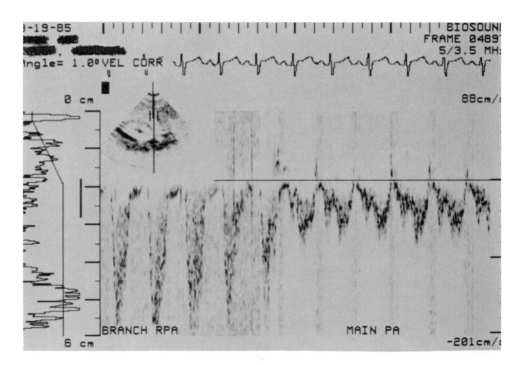

Fig. 4–51. Pulsed wave Doppler tracings from a patient with branch pulmonary artery stenosis. The sample volume was swept from the right pulmonary artery to the main pulmonary artery. Note the sharp drop in velocities, indicating that a mild stenosis is present.

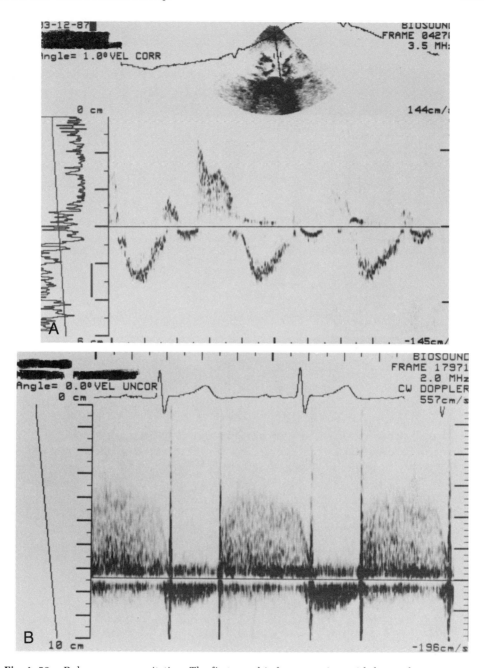

Fig. 4–52. Pulmonary regurgitation. The first panel is from a patient with low pulmonary artery pressures, allowing evaluation with pulsed Doppler (1st beat). The second panel is a continuous wave Doppler tracing from a patient with severe mitral valve stenosis and pulmonary hypertension. The first complex is probably the best but none is perfect. Note that the high velocities reflect a high diastolic pulmonary artery pressure as evidenced by the large pressure drop. The third panel is from a patient who had just undergone a pulmonary balloon valvuloplasty. Note that the pulmonary regurgitation curve reflects a low diastolic pulmonary pressure, similar to that in the patients shown in Figures 4–8 and 4–49.

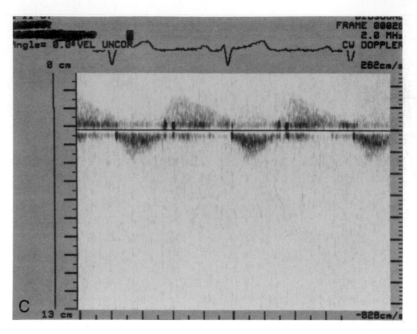

Fig. 4–52 (continued).

diastole and lasts throughout the phase. Hatle and Angelsen[19] state that, similar to aortic regurgitation, the signal strength and the extent of the jet into the right ventricle are reflective of the severity of the regurgitation. Color-coded Doppler will show the depth of penetration of the jet into the right ventricle. In addition to location and magnitude, the jet of pulmonary regurgitation can be separated from that of aortic regurgitation by detecting the characteristic respiratory variation.

Ordinarily, the velocity waveform decreases with atrial contraction, which raises the diastolic ventricular pressure. If pulmonary arterial diastolic pressure is elevated, the velocity waveform will be higher in magnitude.

The pulmonary artery-right ventricular pressure drop can be predicted from the modified Bernoulli equation (see below).

Ventricular Septal Defect (Fig. 4–53)

This lesion is fairly easily evaluated by Doppler and is the subject of many reports.[2,3,19,28,47,49,83,113,116,154,210–222] Ventricular septal defects vary in size and location. Many larger defects can be imaged with two-dimensional echocardiography, but because of lateral resolution physics, their size on the echocardiogram is underestimated. Stevenson et al.[2] have shown that the presence and location of a ventricular septal defect can be detected by Doppler echocardiography. They report "threading" the Doppler sample volume, guided by two-dimensional echocardiography, from the left ventricle through the septum into the right ventricle. They also state that a jet occurs in the septum and can usually be found additionally in the right ventricular cavity. This qualitative technique allowed separation of patients with ventricular septal defects from those with atrioventricular valve insufficiency. The postjet flow disturbance of

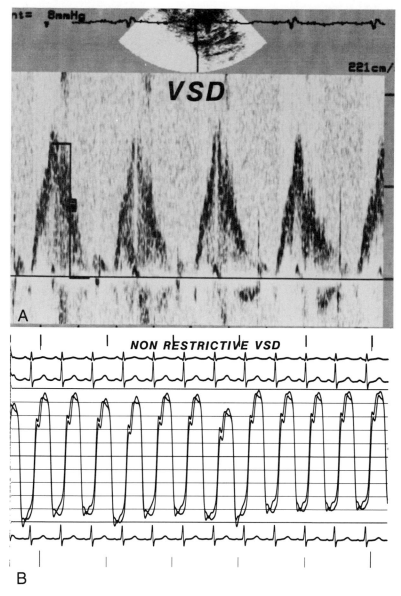

Fig. 4–53. The first panels are from a patient with a non-restrictive ventricular septal defect. Note that the velocity curve peaks at 1.6 m/sec. The accompanying panel are the right and left ventricular pressure tracings obtained at cardiac catheterization. The next panel is from a patient with a restrictive ventricular septal defect. The continuous wave peak velocity is reflective of a pressure drop of 78 mm Hg. This was confirmed at cardiac catheterization.

a ventricular septal defect may be found in the right ventricle and pulmonary artery.

The Doppler examination for presence of a ventricular septal defect should evaluate defect location. The same planes used for general two-dimensional echocardiographic evaluations of ventricular septal defects may be used, sometimes with modification, for the Doppler examination. To inspect the area between the tricuspid and aortic valve, the septum may be interrogated in the

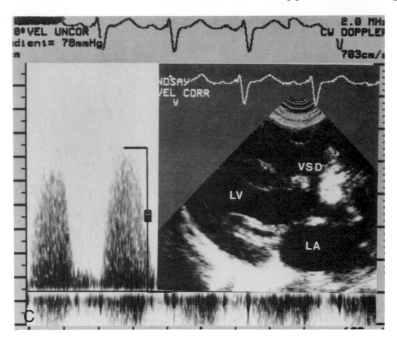

Fig. 4–53 (continued).

long axis plane with the transducer angled medially. A short axis examination may also be performed and the right ventricle can be interrogated from the tricuspid inflow to the right ventricular outflow. Apex long axis, four-chamber and five-chamber views can then be employed with Doppler interrogation of the entire right ventricle. This latter location is more difficult for Doppler because the transducer is almost perpendicular to the jet, but a flow disturbance can often be found. Finally, the subcostal four-chamber and right ventricular outflow planes may be used.

Qualitative color-coded Doppler can be valuable for detection of ventricular septal defects,[113] especially if multiple. The examination is usually accomplished from the precordial long axis plane. The defect(s) is (are) identified as aliased flow from the left ventricle to the right ventricle across the septum in the area of the defect (Plate 15).

If the defect is the size of the aortic root or larger, or if pulmonary resistance is high; little pressure drop should be present between left and right ventricle during systole. However, if the defect is smaller, a pressure difference will occur. Pressure drops across a ventricular septal defect can be approximated by application of the modified Bernoulli equation.[19,212,214,218,222] The pressure drop can be subtracted from the systolic arm blood pressure (in the absence of aortic stenosis) and right ventricular pressure can be predicted (See below).

Use of Doppler for Intracavitary or Intravascular Pressure Estimation

For years, the goal of noninvasive cardiac evaluation has been to determine the anatomy of a cardiac abnormality and then to gain insight into the physiology of intracardiac and great vessel flows, pressures and other functional parameters. Anatomic description of various intracardiac lesions has been achieved by use of two-dimensional echocardiography. Excellent imaging of great vessels is now also possible by nuclear magnetic resonance imaging or by computerized tomography. However, at present images will not provide an insight into intravascular or intracavitary pressures. Doppler now provides much of the remainder of the desired information. In this section, Doppler pressure drop analysis combined with certain clinical pressure measurements will be used to demonstrate how pressures within the heart and great vessels can be predicted (Fig. 4–54).

The Aorta and Left Ventricle

In normal individuals, systolic and diastolic aortic pressures can be closely estimated by routine sphygmomanometry. Descending aortic pressure should be approximately the same as ascending aortic pressure. Left ventricular systolic pressure approximately equals systolic aortic pressure. If the normal left ventricular outflow tract is examined by Doppler, velocities are usually <1.5

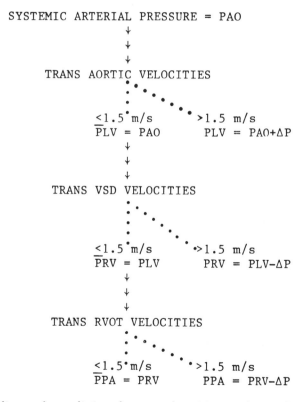

Fig. 4–54. Logic diagram for prediction of pressure drop. Measure the systolic arterial pressure. If no aortic stenosis is noted by Doppler, left ventricular systolic pressure = aortic systolic pressure. If high aortic velocities are encountered, the predicted pressure drop must be added to the aortic pressure to predict systolic left ventricular pressure. The same principle is applied if a ventricular septal defect is present. Pulmonary outflow velocities are similarly considered. See text for details. Abbreviations; PAO = systolic aortic pressure, PLV = left ventricular systolic pressure, ΔP = pressure drop, VSD = ventricular septal defect, PRV = right ventricular systolic pressure, RVOT = right ventricular outflow tract, PPA = systolic pulmonary artery pressure.

m/sec (see Chapter 3). If approximately the same velocity is found in the left ventricular outflow tract and aorta, no pressure drop has occurred.

If the patient has aortic valvular stenosis, the transvalvar pressure drop can be predicted from peak ascending aortic velocities. If peak Doppler velocity (V_2) is 3.5 m/sec, and V_1 = 1 m/sec or less (and thus can be ignored), the pressure drop is 49 mm Hg [$(3.5)^2 \times 4 = 49$]. If systolic arm blood pressure = 100 mm Hg, the left ventricular systolic pressure should be approximately 150 mm Hg (100 + 49 = 149). This example shows how the diagram in Figure 4–54 can be used.

Similarly, if the patient has coarctation of the aorta, the pressure drop across the coarctation can be added to lower extremity sphygmomanometric pressure to calculate the upper extremity pressure. This is a practical problem because some patients have had enough vascular compromise to the arm vessels from catheterizations and surgery that upper pressures cannot be measured. If aortic stenosis coexists, the aortic pressure drop should be added to the derived ascending aortic pressure to predict left ventricular pressure. For example, if the systolic leg pressure is 80 mm Hg, transcoarctation V_2 velocities are 3.0 m/sec and V_1 is 2.0 m/sec, the transcoarctation pressure drop is $((3)^2 - (2)^2) \times 4 = 20$ mm Hg. Thus, the ascending aortic pressure should be 20 + 80 or 100 mg Hg. If transaortic peak velocity, V_2, = 4 m/sec and V_1 = 1 m/sec, the pressure drop is projected at 60 mm Hg. Adding this to ascending aortic pressure allows estimation of systolic left ventricular pressure at 160 mm Hg.

The same concept can be applied to estimation of descending aortic pressure in patients with coarctation when the ascending aortic pressure is known. In this instance, the transcoarctation pressure drop is subtracted from the systolic arm blood pressure (Fig. 4–55).

The Right Ventricle and Pulmonary Artery

Right ventricular pressure in normal and abnormal states can be approximated from Doppler data combined with physiologic information. If pulmonary valve stenosis is not present, systolic right ventricular pressure equals systolic pulmonary artery pressure.

Tricuspid backflow is a physiologic phenomenon which occurs in most normals.[19,111,181,191,192] The observation of tricuspid backflow is so common in normal people that the term, "tricuspid insufficiency," should probably be reserved for pathologic states. The systolic jet of tricuspid backflow can be interrogated best by CW Doppler and the result permits estimation of the systolic pressure drop between right ventricle and right atrium. Right ventricular systolic pressure can be approximated by adding right atrial pressure to the pressure drop. Right atrial pressure, in normal situations, can be approximated at 5 mm Hg in infants and children and from 5 to 10 mm Hg in adults. Another method of estimating right atrial pressure in adults is analysis of the height above the heart at which neck vein distention occurs.[192] Postoperatively and in patients with indwelling central venous lines, right atrial pressure can be directly measured. In the latter instance, be certain that pressure is measured in mm Hg. If it is measured in cm H_2O, convert the value to mm Hg (1 mm Hg = 1.3 cm H_2O).

The following is an example of right ventricular peak systolic pressure prediction. A postoperative patient had a valve replacement for valvular mitral

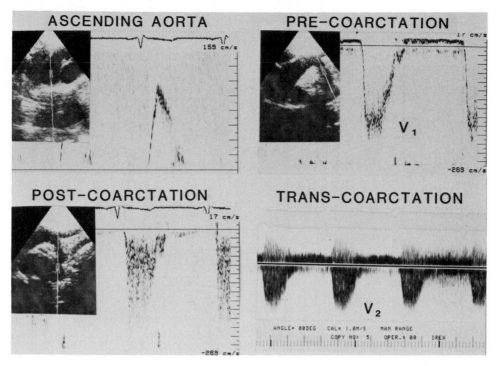

Fig. 4–55. Residual gradient in a patient who is postoperative for repair of coarctation of the aorta. The first panel shows normal ascending aortic velocities indicating no aortic stenosis. The second (upper right) panel shows the pre-coarctation (V_1) velocities. The pulsed signal is weak distal to the location of the coarctation (3rd panel). Continuous wave Doppler (4th panel) shows peak velocities (V_2) of 2.5 M/sec, translating to a pressure drop of 25 mm Hg (Reprinted with permission from Marx and Allen[193]).

stenosis. Right atrial pressure from the central venous line measures 12 mm Hg. Peak tricuspid backflow velocity is 3.5 m/sec. What is the right ventricular (and thus pulmonary arterial) systolic pressure? Adding the predicted pressure drop ($3.5^2 \times 4$) or 49 mm Hg to measured right atrial pressure of 12 mm Hg yields an estimated right ventricular peak systolic pressure of 61 mm Hg.

Right ventricular pressure can also be predicted in patients with cardiac abnormalities such as valvular pulmonary stenosis or ventricular septal defects. For a patient with valvular pulmonary stenosis, the pressure drop across the pulmonary valve can be added to a presumed systolic pulmonary arterial pressure of 15 to 20 mm Hg to yield an estimation of right ventricular pressure. For example, if the peak transvalvar velocity were 4.0 m/sec, the projected right ventricular pressure should be ($4.0^2 \times 4$) or 64 mm Hg + 15 to 20 mm Hg (estimated pulmonary arterial pressure) = 80 to 85 mm Hg.

Ventricular septal defects can be large and unrestrictive, or small and restrictive. The term restrictive implies that the defect creates a pressure drop from the left ventricle to the right ventricle. If no pressure drop is present as evidenced by right ventricular jet V_2 value of 1.5 m/sec or less, systolic right ventricular pressure will approximate the left ventricular systolic pressure. Left ventricular peak systolic pressure in the absence of aortic stenosis = aortic peak systolic pressure and aortic systolic pressure can be approximated by cuff arm pressure.[212,214,218,222] Further, if no pulmonary stenosis is present, pulmonary arterial pressure will be the same as the right ventricular pressure and will thus be predicted by the arm systolic pressure. In Figure 4–56, the patient with an endocardial cushion defect has systemic pulmonary arterial systolic pressures on the basis of a non-restrictive ventricular septal defect and the absence of stenosis of either semilunar valve.

If a ventricular septal defect is restrictive, pressure drop across the defect should be subtracted from peak systolic left ventricular pressure which is derived from the cuff arm pressure. Assume that peak Doppler velocities (V_2) across a ventricular septal defect are 3.0 m/sec. Peak velocity is 3.0 m/sec. Peak ascending aortic velocities are 1.0 m/sec, thus, no aortic stenosis is present. Transpulmonary velocities are 0.8 m/sec. Arm blood pressure was 90 mm Hg. What is pulmonary arterial pressure? Arm systolic blood pressure = left ventricular systolic pressure. Right ventricular systolic pressure is derived by subtracting the pressure drop from the left ventricular systolic pressure (90 mm Hg) − (3.0² × 4, or 36 mm Hg) = 54 mm Hg. Systolic pulmonary artery pressure = right ventricular systolic pressure = 54 mm Hg.

Similarly, Marx et al.[223] have shown that pulmonary arterial pressures can be predicted from intravascular pressure drops across aorticopulmonary shunts. If the patient has a systemic arterial-pulmonary arterial shunt (patent ductus

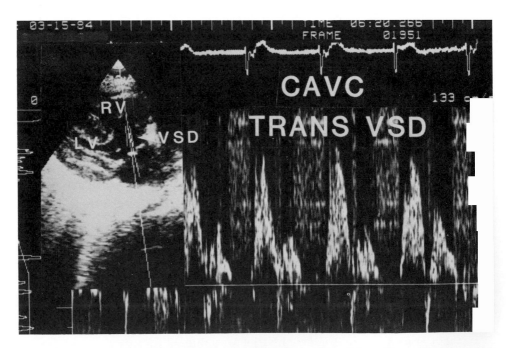

Fig. 4–56. Tracing from a patient with an endocardial cushion defect. The ventricular septal defect is not restrictive. Thus, right ventricular pressure = left ventricular pressure. Since the patient had no pulmonary outflow obstruction, the pulmonary artery systolic pressure is systemic. This was proven at cardiac catheterization.

arteriosus, Blalock-Taussig shunt, Waterston shunt, Gortex® interposition graft shunt, or Potts shunt), pressure drop across that shunt can be subtracted from ascending aortic (arm) blood pressure to predict pulmonary arterial systolic pressure. Recording these transobstructive jet velocities often requires innovative transducer locations (such as in the right mid-clavicular line or even in the clavicular fossa) but can usually be successfully measured. Figure 4–57 compares pulmonary arterial pressures measured at catheterization with those predicted by Doppler.[223]

Peak pulmonary arterial pressure has also been predicted by combining noninvasive modalities which measure the time interval from pulmonary valve closure to tricuspid valve opening. Burstin[224] used the jugular phlebogram (tricuspid opening) and a phonocardiogram (pulmonary valve closure) and developed a nomogram which related heart rate and time interval from pulmonary closure to tricuspid opening to peak pulmonary arterial pressure. Hatle[224] used Doppler to record pulmonary and tricuspid velocities. The interval from the end of pulmonary systolic flow to the onset of tricuspid flow was measured. Stevenson et al.[225] used M-mode echo tracings of pulmonary valve closure and tricuspid opening to define the closing-opening interval and demonstrated a reasonable prediction of mean pulmonary artery pressure. The major contribution from these studies was to extrapolate the data developed by Burstin et al. to include higher heart rates (Fig. 4–58).

Mean and peak systolic pulmonary arterial pressure have also been dem-

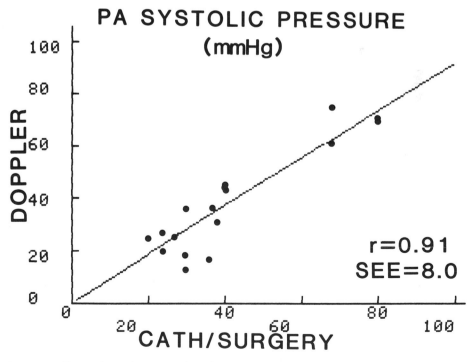

Fig. 4–57. Comparison of pressure drop from aorta to pulmonary artery measured at catheterization (abscissa) with that estimated by Doppler (ordinate). See text for details. (Reproduced with permission from Marx et al.[223]).

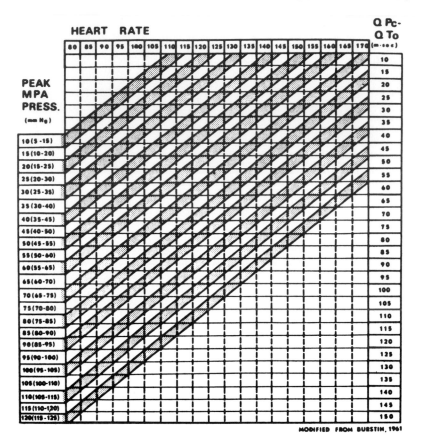

Fig. 4–58. Burstin diagram modified by Stevenson et al.[225] and reprinted with permission. Peak pulmonary artery pressure (left column) is predicted from the pulmonary closure-tricuspid opening times in msec (right column), and is heart rate corrected (top).

onstrated to correlate with the time to peak velocity (also known as acceleration time) of non-jet laminar pulmonary arterial velocity waveforms (Fig. 4–42). Several groups[19,227–235] have reported reasonable (r≈.8 to .95) correlations of mean or systolic pulmonary arterial pressures and acceleration time. In general terms, time to peak velocity is >100 m/sec in subjects with normal pulmonary arterial pressures if subjects are not infants (see Table 3–1, Chapter 3). The slope of regression lines in reported studies is quite similar. A simplification shows that mean pulmonary arterial pressures can be estimated as MPAP ≈ 90 − .6*TPV.[235] One major problem with the use of time to peak pulmonary velocity as an indicator of pulmonary arterial pressure is that the resolution is low. The time interval difference between normal and severe pulmonary hypertension is only 50 milliseconds. Since the regression is imperfect and the standard error of the estimate is not zero, prediction of the exact pressure for a patient within such narrow confines can be difficult.

Diastolic pulmonary arterial pressures can be predicted[19,207–209] if the patient has pulmonary valvar backflow, a normal phenomenon for many people.[111] In this situation, the end diastolic pressure drop, added to a presumed normal right ventricular end diastolic pressure of 5 mm Hg yields an approximation of the diastolic pulmonary arterial pressure (Fig. 4–52).

REFERENCES

1. Goldberg, S.J., Valdez-Cruz, L.M., Carnahan, Y., Hoenecke, H., Allen, H.D., Sahn, D.J.: Comparison of microbubble detection by M-mode echocardiography and two-dimensional echo/Doppler techniques. *In* Echocardiology. Edited by Rijsterborgh H. The Hague, Martinus Nijhoff, 1981, p. 263.
2. Stevenson, J.G., Kawabori, I., Dooley, T., Guntheroth, W.G.: Diagnosis of ventricular septal defect by pulsed Doppler echocardiography. Sensitivity, specificity and limitations. Circulation *58*:322, 1979.
3. Stevenson, J.G., Kawabori, I., Guntheroth, W.G.: Differentiation of ventricular septal defect from mitral regurgitation by pulsed Doppler echocardiography. Circulation *56*:14, 1977.
4. Abbasi, A.S., Allen, M.W., DeCristofaro, D., Ungar, I.: Detection and estimation of the degree of mitral regurgitation by range gated pulsed Doppler echocardiography. Circulation *61*:143, 1980.
5. Areias, J.C., Goldberg, S.J., Spitaels, S.E.C., de Villeneuve, V.H.: An evaluation of range gated pulsed Doppler echocardiography for detecting pulmonary outflow tract obstruction in d-transposition of the great vessels. Am Heart J *96*:467, 1978.
6. Goldberg, S.J., Areias, J.C., Spitaels, S.E.C., de Villeneuve, V.H.: Use of time interval histographic output from echo Doppler to detect left-to-right atrial shunts. Circulation *58*:147, 1978.
7. Goldberg, S.J., Areias, J.C., Spitaels, S.E.C., de Villeneuve, V.H.: Echo Doppler detection of pulmonary stenosis by time-interval histogram analysis. J Clin Ultrasound *7*:183, 1979.
8. Allen, H.D., Sahn, D.J., Lange, L., Goldberg, S.J.: Noninvasive assessment of surgical systemic-to-pulmonary artery shunts by range-gated pulsed Doppler echocardiography. J Pediatr *94*:395, 1979.
9. Kececioglu-Draelos, Z., Goldberg, S.J., Areias, J., Sahn, D.J.: Verification and clinical demonstration of the echo Doppler series effect and vortex shed distance. Circulation *63*:1422, 1981.
10. Pai, S.: Fluid Dynamics of Jets. New York, D. van Nostrand, 1954.
11. Goldberg, S.J., Kececioglu-Draelos, Z., Sahn, D.J., Valdes-Cruz, L.M., Allen, H.D.: Range gated echo Doppler velocity and turbulence mapping in patients with valvular aortic stenosis. Am Heart J *103*:858, 1982.
12. MacDonald, D.A., Helps, E.P.W.: Streamline flow in veins. London, Wellcome Foundation Film Library, 1959.
13. Hegesh, J.T., Goldberg, S.J., Schwartz, M.L.: Analysis of causes of velocity spread during initial deceleration in the ascending aorta in children and young adults. Am J Cardiol *59*:967, 1987.
14. Schwartz, M., Goldberg, S., Wilson, N., Allen H., Marx, G.: Relation of Still's murmur, small aortic diameter and high aortic velocity. Am J Cardiol *57*:1344, 1986.
15. Areias, J.C., Goldberg, S.J., de Villeneuve, V.H.: Use and limitations of time interval histogram output from echo Doppler to detect mitral regurgitation. Am Heart J *101*:805, 1981.
16. Goldberg, S.J., Areias, J., Feldman, L., Sahn, D.J., Allen, H.D.: Lesions that cause aortic flow disturbance. Circulation *60*:1539, 1979.
17. Goldberg, S.J., Valdes-Cruz, L.M., Feldman, L., Sahn, D.J., Allen, H.D.: Range gated ultrasound detection of contrast echographic microbubbles for cardiac and great vessel blood flow patterns. Am Heart J *101*:793, 1981.
18. Grenadier, E., Lima, C.O., Allen, H.D., Sahn, D.J., Barron, J.V., Valdes-Cruz, L.M., Goldberg, S.J.: Normal intracardiac and great vessel Doppler flow velocities in infants and children. J Am Coll Cardiol *4*:34, 1984.
19. Hatle, L., Angelsen, B.: Doppler Ultrasound in Cardiology, 2nd Ed., Lea & Febiger, Philadelphia, 1985.
20. Hatle, L., Brubakk, A., Tromsdal, A., Angelsen, B.: Noninvasive assessment of pressure drop in mitral stenosis by Doppler ultrasound. Br. Heart J *40*:131, 1978.
21. Hatle, L., Angelsen B., Tromsdal, A.: Noninvasive assessment of atrioventricular pressure half-time by Doppler ultrasound. Circulation *60*:1096, 1979.
22. Hatle, L., Angelsen, B.A.J., Tromsdal, A.: Noninvasive assessment of aortic stenosis by Doppler ultrasound. Br Heart J *43*:284, 1980.
23. Holen, J., Aaslid, R., Landmark, K., Simonsen, S.: Determination of pressure gradient in mitral stenosis with a noninvasive ultrasound Doppler technique. Acta Med Scand *199*:455, 1976.
24. Holen, J., Simonsen, S.: Determination of pressure gradient in mitral stenosis with Doppler echocardiography. Br Heart J *41*:529, 1979.
25. Lima, C.O., Sahn, D.J., Valdes-Cruz, L.M., Goldberg, S.J., Barron, J.V., Allen, H.D., Grenadier,

E.: Noninvasive prediction of transvalvular pressure gradient in patients with pulmonary stenosis by quantitative two-dimensional echocardiographic Doppler studies. Circulation *67*:866, 1983.

26. Lima, C.O., Sahn, D.J., Valdes-Cruz, L.M., Allen, H.D., Goldberg, S.J., Grenadier, E.: Prediction and severity of left ventricular outflow tract obstruction by quantitative two-dimensional echocardiographic Doppler studies. Circulation *68*:348, 1983.
27. Goldberg, S.J., Allen, H.D., Sahn, D.J.: Pediatric and Adolescent Echocardiography: A Handbook. 2nd Ed., Chicago, Year Book Medical Publishers, 1980.
28. Johnson, S.L., Baker, D.W., Lute, R.A., Kawabori, I.: Detection of small ventricular septal defects by Doppler flowmeter. (abstr) Circulation *50*(III):142, 1974.
29. Brubakk, A.O., Angelsen, B.A.J., Hatle, J.: Diagnoses of valvular heart disease using transcutaneous Doppler ultrasound. Cardiovasc Res *11*:461, 1977.
30. Young, J.B., Quinones, M.A., Waggoner, A.D., Miller, R.R.: Diagnosis and quantification of aortic stenosis with pulsed Doppler echocardiography. Am J Cardiol *45*:987, 1980.
31. Cheatham, J.P., Latson, L.A., Gutgesell, H.P.: Echocardiographic pulsed Doppler features of absent pulmonary valve syndrome in the neonate. Am J Cardiol *49*:1773, 1982.
32. Ciobanu, M., Abbasi, A.S., Allen, M., Hermer, A., Spellberg, R.: Pulsed Doppler echocardiography in the diagnosis and estimation of severity of aortic insufficiency. Am J Cardiol *49*:339, 1982.
33. Dooley, T.K., Rubenstein, S.A., Stevenson, J.G.: Pulsed Doppler echocardiography: The detection of mitral regurgitation. *In* Ultrasound in Med. Vol. 4. Edited by White, D., Lyons, E.A. New York, Plenum Press, 1978, p. 383.
34. Esper, R.J.: Detection of mild aortic regurgitation by range gated pulsed Doppler echocardiography. Am J Cardiol *50*:1037, 1982.
35. Farthing, S., Peronneau, P.: Flow in the thoracic aorta. Cardiovasc Res *13*:607, 1979.
36. Garcia-Dorado, D., Falzgraf, S., Almazan, A., Delcan, J., Lopez-Bescos, L., Menarguez, L.: Diagnosis of functional tricuspid insufficiency by pulsed wave Doppler ultrasound. Circulation *66*:1315, 1982.
37. Kalmanson, D., Veyrat, C., Abitbol, G., Farjon, M.: Doppler echocardiography and valvular regurgitation with special emphasis on mitral insufficiency. Advantages of two-dimensional echocardiography with real-time spectral analysis. *In* Echocardiology. Edited by Rijsterborgh, H. The Hague, Martinus Nijhoff, 1981, p. 279.
38. Lange, L., Allen, H.D., Goldberg, S.J., Sahn, D.J.: The usefulness of range gated pulsed Doppler echocardiography. A review. Z Kardiol *68*:158, 1979.
39. Magherini, A., Azzolina, G.: Pulsed Doppler echocardiography in the diagnosis of mitral and aortic valve insufficiency. Boll Soc Ital Cardiol *26*:1817, 1981.
40. Patel, A.K., Rowe, G.G., Dhanani, S.P., Kosolcharoen, P., Lyle, L.E., Thomsen, J.H.: Pulsed Doppler echocardiography in diagnosis of pulmonary regurgitation: Its value and limitations. Am J Cardiol *49*:1801, 1982.
41. Quinones, M.A., Young, J.B., Waggoner, A.D., Ostojic, M.C., Riberio, L.G.T., Miller, R.R.: Assessment of pulsed Doppler echocardiography in detection and quantification of aortic and mitral regurgitation. Br Heart J *44*:612, 1980.
42. Stevenson, J.G., Kawabori, I., Brandestini, M.A.: a twenty-month experience comparing conventional pulsed Doppler echocardiography and color-coded digital multigate Doppler for detection of atrioventricular valve regurgitation and its severity. *In* Echocardiology. Edited by Rijsterborgh, H. The Hague, Martinus Nijhofh, 1981, p. 399.
43. Veyrat, C., Cholot, N., Abitbol, G., Kalmanson, D.: Noninvasive diagnosis and assessment of aortic valve disease and evaluation of aortic prosthesis function using echo pulsed Doppler velocimetry. Br Heart J *43*:393, 1980.
44. Waggoner, A.D., Quinones, M.A., Young, J.B., Brandon, T.A., Shah, A.A., Verani, M.S., Miller, R.R.: Pulsed Doppler echocardiographic detection of right-sided valve regurgitation. Experimental results and clinical significance. Am J Cardiol *47*:279, 1981.
45. Ward, J.M., Baker, D.W., Rubenstein, S.A., Johnson, S.L.: Detection of aortic insufficiency by pulsed Doppler echocardiography. J Clin Ultrasound *5*:5, 1977.
46. Allen, H.D., Goldberg, S.J., Valdes-Cruz, L.M., Sahn, D.J.: Use of echocardiography in newborns with patent ductus arteriosus: A review. Pediatr Cardiol *3*:65, 1982.
47. Allen, H.D., Sahn, D.J., Goldberg, S.J., Valdes-Cruz, L.M.: Doppler echocardiography: An Overview. Indian Pediatr *19*:79, 1982.
48. Allen, H.D., Sahn, D.J., Lange, L., Goldberg, S.J.: Noninvasive assessment of surgical systemic-to-pulmonary artery shunts by range-gated pulsed Doppler echocardiography. J Pediatr *94*:395, 1979.
49. Stevenson, J.G.: Echo Doppler analysis of septal defects. *In* Proceedings of Cardiovascular Application of Doppler Echography. Edited by Peronneau, P. Paris, Colloque Inserm III: Editions Inserm, 1983.
50. Goldberg, S.J.: The principles of pressure drop in long segment stenosis. Herz *11*:291, 1986.

51. Holen, J., Aaslid, R., Landmark, K., Simonsen, S., Ostrem, T.: Determination of effective orifice area in mitral stenosis from noninvasive ultrasound Doppler data and mitral flow rate. Acta Med Scand *201*:83, 1977.

52. Requarth, J.A., Goldberg, S.J., Vasko, S.D., Allen, H.D.: In vitro verification of Doppler prediction of transvalve pressure gradient and orifice area in stenosis. Am J Cardiol *53*:1369, 1984.

53. Vasko, S.D., Goldberg, S.J., Requarth, J.A., Allen, H.D.: Factors affecting accuracy of in vitro valvar pressure gradient estimates by Doppler ultrasound. Am J Cardiol *54*:893, 1984

54. Requarth, J.A., Marx, G.R., Goldberg, S.J., Allen, H.D.: Is the modified Bernoulli equation accurate for estimating pressure drop in long segment stenosis? (abstr). Circulation *79*:435, 1985.

55. Sahn, D.J.: Real-time two-dimensional Doppler echocardiographic flow mapping. Circulation *71*:849, 1985.

56. Stevenson, J.G.: Experience with qualitative and quantitative applications of Doppler echocardiography in congenital heart disease. Ultrasound Med Biol *10*:771, 1984.

57. Hatle, L.: Noninvasive assessment and differentiation of left ventricular outflow obstruction with Doppler ultrasound. Circulation *64*:381, 1981.

58. Hagler, D.J., Tajik, A.J., Seward, J.B., Ritter, D.G.: Noninvasive assessment of pulmonary valve stenosis, aortic valve stenosis and coarctation of the aorta in critically ill neonates. Am J Cardiol *57*:369, 1986.

59. Panidis, J., Mintz, J., Ross, J.: Value and limitations of Doppler ultrasound in the evaluation of aortic stenosis: A statistical analysis of 70 consecutive patients. Am Heart J *112*:150, 1986.

60. Currie, P.J., Hagler, D.J., Seward J.B., Reeder, G.S., Fyfe, D.A., Bove, A.A., Tajik, A.J.: Instantaneous pressure gradient: A simultaneous Doppler and dual catheter correlative study. J Am Coll Cardiol *7*:800–6, 1986.

61. Berger, M., Berdoff, R.L., Gallerstein, P.E., Goldberg, E.: Evaluation of aortic stenosis by continuous wave Doppler ultrasound. J Am Coll Cardiol *3*:150, 1984.

62. Krafchek, J., Robertson, J.H., Radford, M., Adams, D., Kisslo, J.: A reconsideration of Doppler assessed gradients in suspected aortic stenosis. Am Heart J *110*:765, 1985.

63. Otto, C.M., Pearlman, A.S., Comess, K.A., Reamer, R.P., Janko, C.L., Huntsman, L.L.: Determination of the stenotic aortic valve area in adults using Doppler echocardiography. J Am Coll Cardiol *7*:509, 1986.

64. Smith, M.D., Dawson, P.L., Elion, J.L., Wisenbaugh, T., Kwan, O.L., Handshoe, S., DeMaria, A.N.: Systematic correlation of continuous-wave Doppler and hemodynamic measurements in patients with aortic stenosis. Am Heart J *111*:245, 1986.

65. Stevenson, J.G., Kawabori, I.: Noninvasive determination of pressure gradients in children: Two methods employing pulsed Doppler echocardiography. J Am Coll Cardiol *3*(III):179, 1984.

66. Yeager, M., Yock, P.G., Popp, R.L.: Comparison of Doppler-derived pressure gradient to that determined at cardiac catheterization in adults with aortic valve stenosis: Implications for management. Am J Cardiol *57*:644, 1986.

67. Teien, D., Eriksson, P.: Quantification of transvalvular pressure differences in aortic stenosis by Doppler ultrasound. Int J Cardiol *7*:121, 1985.

68. Teirstein, P., Yeager, M., Yock, P.G., Popp, R.L.: Doppler echocardiographic measurement of aortic valve area in aortic stenosis: A noninvasive application of the Gorlin formula. J Am Coll Cardid *8*:1059, 1986.

69. Warth, D.C., Stewart, W.J., Block, P.C., Weyman, A.E.: A new method to calculate aortic valve area without left heart catheterization. Circulation *70*:978, 1984.

70. Williams, G.A., Labovitz, A.J., Nelson, J.G., Kennedy, H.L.: Value of multiple echocardiographic views in the evaluation of aortic stenosis in adults by continuous wave Doppler. Am J Cardiol *55*:445, 1985.

71. Zoghbi, W., Farmer, K., Soto, J., Nelson, J., Quinones, M.: Accurate noninvasive quantification of stenotic aortic valve area by Doppler echocardiography. Circulation *73*:452, 1986.

72. Teirstein, P.S., Yock, P.G., and Popp, R.L.: The accuracy of Doppler ultrasound measurement of pressure gradients across irregular, dual, and tunnellike obstructions to blood flow. Circulation *72*:577, 1985.

73. Agatston, A.S.: Doppler diagnosis of valvular aortic stenosis. Echocardiography *3*:3, 1986.

74. Barnes, R.W., Rittenhouse, E.A., Miller, E.V.: Doppler ultrasonic assessment of aortic stenosis by analysis of axillary arterial blood velocity upstroke time. Chest *70*:48, 1976.

75. Bass, J., Berry, J., Einzig, S.: Flow in the aorta and patent ductus arteriosus in infants with aortic atresia or aortic stenosis: a pulsed Doppler ultrasound study. Circulation *74*:315, 1986.

76. Cannon, S.R., Richards, R.L., Rollwitz, W.T.: Digital Fourier techniques in the diagnosis and quantification of aortic stenosis with pulsed Doppler echocardiography. J Clin Ultrasound *10*:101, 1982.

77. Huhta, J.C., Latson, L.A., Gutgesell, H.P., Cooley, D.A., Kearney, D.L.: Echocardiography in the diagnosis and management of symptomatic aortic valve stenosis in infants. Circulation *70*:438, 1984.

78. Johnson, S.L., Baker, D.W., Lute, R.A., Dodge, H.T.: Doppler echocardiography. The localization of cardiac murmurs. Circulation *48*:810, 1973.

79. Kawabori, I., Stevenson, J.G., Dooley, T.K., Guntheroth, W.G.: Evaluation of ejection murmurs by pulsed Doppler echocardiography. Br Heart J *43*:623, 1980.

80. Oh, J.K., Nishimura, R.A., Seward, J.B., Tajik, A.J.: Differentiation of the aortic stenosis jet from mitral regurgitation by analysis of continuous wave Doppler spectrum: Illustrative cases. Echocardiography. *3*:55, 1986.

81. Richards, K.L., Cannon, S.R., Crawford, M.H., Sorensen, S.J.: Noninvasive diagnosis of aortic and mitral valve disease with pulsed Doppler spectral analysis. Am J Cardiol *51*:1122, 1983.

82. Robinson, P.J., Wyse, R.K., Deanfield, J.E., Franklin, R., Macartney, F.J.: Continuous wave Doppler velocimetry as an adjunct to cross-sectional echocardiography in the diagnosis of critical left heart obstruction in neonates. Br Heart J *52*:552, 1984.

83. Stevenson, J.G.: Experience with qualitative and quantitative applications of Doppler echocardiography in congenital heart disease. Ultrasound Med Biol *10*:771, 1984.

84. Stamm, R.B., Martin, R.P.: Quantification of pressure gradients across stenotic valves by Doppler ultrasound. J Am Coll Cardiol *2*:707, 1983.

85. Voelkel, A.G., Kendrick, M., Pietro, D.A., Parisi, A.F., Voelkel, V. Greenfield, D., Askenazi, J., Folland, E.D.: Noninvasive tests to evaluate the severity of aortic stenosis: Limitations and reliability. Chest *77*:153, 1980.

86. Boughner, D.R., Schuld, R.L., Persaud, J.A.: Hypertrophic obstructive cardiomyopathy. Assessment by echocardiographic and Doppler ultrasound techniques. Br Heart J *37*:917, 1975.

87. Chandraratna, P.A., Aronow, W.S.: Genesis of the systolic murmur of idiopathic hypertrophic subaortic stenosis. Phonocardiographic, echocardiographic, and pulsed Doppler ultrasound correlations. Chest *83*:638, 1983.

88. Gidding, S., Snider, A.R., Rocchini, A., Peters, J., Farnsworth, R.: Left ventricular diastolic filling in children with hypertrophic cardiomyopathy: assessment with pulsed Doppler echocardiography. J Am Coll Cardiol *8*:310, 1986.

89. Kalmanson, D., Veyrat, C., Bouchareine, F., Degroote, A.: Noninvasive recording of mitral valve flow velocity patterns using pulsed Doppler echocardiography. Application to diagnosis and evaluation of mitral valve disease. Br Heart J *39*:517, 1977.

90. Joyner, C.R., Harrison, F.S., Gruber, J.W.: Diagnosis of hypertrophic subaortic stenosis with Doppler velocity flow detector. Ann Intern Med *74*:692, 1971.

91. Jenni, R., Ruffman, K., Vieli, A., Anliker, M., Krayenbuehl, H.P.: Dynamics of aortic flow in hypertrophic cardiomyopathy. Eur Heart J *6*:391, 1985.

92. Keren, G., Belhassen, B., Sherez, J., Miller, H.I., Megidish, R., Berenfeld, D., Laniado, S.: Apical hypertrophic cardiomyopathy: Evaluation by noninvasive and invasive techniques in 23 patients. Circulation *71*:45, 1985.

93. Kinoshita, N., Nimura, Y., Okamoto, M., Miyatake, K., Nagata, S., Sakakibara, H.: Mitral regurgitation in hypertrophic cardiomyopathy. Noninvasive study by two-dimensional Doppler echocardiography. Br Heart J *49*:574, 1983.

94. Kitabatake, A., Inoue, M., Asao, M., Tanouchi, J., Masuyama, T., Abe, H., Morita, H., Senda, S., Matsuo, H.: Transmitral blood flow reflecting diastolic behavior of the left ventricle in health and disease—a study by pulsed Doppler technique. Jpn Circ J *46*:92, 1982.

95. Yock, P.G., Hatle, L., Popp, R.L.: Patterns and timing of Doppler-detected intracavitary and aortic flow in hypertrophic cardiomyopathy. J Am Coll Cardiol *8*:1047, 1986.

96. Mehlman, D., Kramer, B., Talano, J.: Doppler-echocardiographic evaluation of aortic ball-in-cage prostheses: hemodynamic correlations. Echocardiography *3*:253, 1986.

97. Panidis, J., Ross, J., Mintz, G.S.: Normal and Abnormal Prosthetic Valve Function as Assessed by Doppler Echocardiography. J Am Coll Cardiol *8*:317–326, 1986.

98. Ramirez, M.L., Wong, M.: Reproducibility of stand-alone continuous-wave Doppler recording of aortic flow velocity across bioprosthetic valves. Am J Cardiol *55*:1197, 1985.

99. Veyrat, C., Cholot, N., Abitbol, G., Kalmanson, D.: Noninvasive diagnosis and assessment of aortic valve disease and evaluation of aortic prosthesis function using echo pulsed Doppler velocimetry. Br. Heart J *43*:393, 1980.

100. Weinstein, I.R., Marbarger, J.P. Perez, J.E.: Ultrasonic assessment of the St. Jude prosthetic valve: M-mode, two-dimensional and Doppler echocardiography. Circulation *68*:897, 1983.

101. Sagar, K.B., Wann, L.S., Paulsen, W.H.J., Romhilt, D.W.: Doppler echocardiographic evaluation of Hancock and Bjork-Shiley prosthetic valves. J Am Coll Cardiol *7*:681, 1986.

102. Hoffman, A., Amann, F.W., Gradel, E., Burkhardt, D.: Noninvasive determination of pressure gradients of heart valve prostheses using Doppler ultrasound. Schweiz Med Wochenschr *112*:1600, 1982.

103. Bierman, F.Z., Yeh, M., Swersky, S., Martin, E., Wigger J.H., Fox, H.: Absence of aortic valve: Antenatal and postnatal two-dimensional and Doppler echocardiographic features. J Am Coll Cardiol *3*:833, 1984.

104. Bommer, W.J., Mapes, R., Miller, L., Mason, D.T., DeMaria, A.N.: Quantitation of aortic regurgitation with two-dimensional Doppler echocardiography. (abstr) Am J Cardiol *47*:412, 1981.

105. Diebold, B., Blanchard, D., Nee, M., Colonna, G., Peronneau, P., Guermonprez, J.L., Forman, J., Sellier, P., Maurice, P.: Noninvasive study of aortic insufficiency by Doppler echocardiography. Arch Mal Coeur *75*:1259, 1982.

106. Fukushima, M., Hiramatsu, M., Yoshima, H., Yamada, M., Ohkubo, N., Matsuwaka, R., Yoshii, Y., Ohgidani, N., Hoki, N., Hata, S., Onishi, K., Kobayashi, Y.: Quantitative assessment of regurgitant fraction in aortic regurgitation: Comparision of two-dimensional Doppler echocardiography with other methods. J Cardiogr *15*:483, 1985.

107. Goldberg, S.J., Allen, H.D.: Quantitative assessment by Doppler echocardiography of pulmonary or aortic regurgitation. Am J Cardiol *56*:131, 1985.

108. Hatteland, K., Semb, B.: Assessment of aortic regurgitation by means of pulsed Doppler ultrasound. Ultrasound Med Biol. *8*:1, 1982.

109. Hatle, L.: Maximal blood flow velocities—hemodynamic data obtained noninvasively with CW Doppler. Ultrasound Med Biol *10*:225, 1984.

110. Hoffmann, A., Pfisterer, M., Stulz, P., Schmitt, H.E., Burkart, F., Burckhardt, D.: Noninvasive grading of aortic regurgitation by Doppler ultrasonography. Br Heart J, *55*:283, 1986.

111. Kostucki, W., Vandenbossche, J., Friart, A., Englert, M.: Pulsed Doppler regurgitant flow patterns of normal valves. Am J Cardiol *58*:309, 1986.

112. Nakayama, N., Yoshimura, S., Hara, M.,Teruya, H., Nakasuka, T., Furuhata, H.: Noninvasive quantitative evaluation of aortic regurgitation using an ultrasonic pulsed Doppler flowmeter. Jpn Circ J *47*:641, 1983.

113. Omoto, R.: Color Atlas of Real-Time Two-Dimensional Doppler Echocardiography. 2nd Ed., Tokyo, Shindan-To-Chiryo Co., Ltd., 1984.

114. Omoto, R., Yokote, Y., Takamoto, S., Kyo, S., Ueda, K., Asano, H., Namekawa, K., Kasai, C., Kondo, Y.: The development of real-time two-dimensional Doppler echocardiography and its clinical significance in acquired valvular diseases. With special reference to the evaluation of valvular regurgitation. Jpn Heart J *25*:325, 1984.

115. Saal, A.K., Gross, B.W., Franklin, D.W., Pearlman, A.S.: Noninvasive detection of aortic insufficiency in patients with mitral stenosis by pulsed Doppler echocardiography. J Am Coll Cardiol *5*:176, 1985.

116. Sato, Y., Okoshima, T., Matsuoka, Y., Yamamoto, K., Sennari, E., Hayakawa K.: A study of aortic regurgitation with conal ventricular septal defect by means of pulsed Doppler echocardiography. J Cardiogr *12*:257, 1982.

117. Sequeira, R.F., Watt, J.: Assessment of aortic regurgitation by transcutaneous aortovelography. Br Heart J *39*:929, 1977.

118. Takahashi, H., Sakamoto, T., Hada, Y., Amano, K., Yamaguchi, T., Ishimitsu, T., Takikawa, R., Hasegawa, I., Takahashi, T.: Pulsed Doppler echocardiography and pharmacodynamic phonocardiography in the diagnosis of silent aortic regurgitation: A correlative study. J Cardiogr *15*:495, 1985.

119. Takenaka, K., Dabestani, A., Gardin, J., Russell, D., Clark, S., Allfie, A., Henry, W.: A simple Doppler echocardiographic method for estimating severity of aortic regurgitation. Am J Cardiol. *57*:1340, 1986.

120. Teague, S.M., Sublett, K.L., Andersen, J., Olson, E.G., Thadani, U.: Doppler half-time index correlates with the severity of aortic regurgitation. (abstr) Circulation *70*:(II):394, 1984.

121. Toguchi, M., Ichimiya, S., Yokoi, K., Hibi, N., Kambe, T.: Clinical investigation of aortic insufficiency by means of pulsed Doppler echocardiography. Jpn Heart J *22*:537, 1981.

122. Veyrat, C., Abitbol, G., Bas, S., Manin, J.P., Kalmanson, D.: Quantitative assessment of valvular regurgitations using the pulsed Doppler technique. Approach to the regurgitant lesion. Ultrasound Med Biol *10*:201, 1984.

123. Veyrat, C., Ameur, A., Gourtchiglouian, C., Lessana, A., Abitbol, G., Kalmanson, G.: Calculation of pulsed Doppler left ventricular outflow tract regurgitant index for grading the severity of aortic regurgitation. Am Heart J *108*:507, 1984.

124. Veyrat, C., Lessana, A., Abitbol, G., Ameur, A., Benaim, R., Kalmanson, D.: New indexes for assessing aortic regurgitation with two-dimensional Doppler echocardiographic measurement of the regurgitant aortic valvular area. Circulation *83*:998, 1983.

125. Wautrecht, J.C., Vandenbossche, J.L., Englert, M.: Sensitivity and specificity of pulsed Doppler echocardiography in detection of aortic and mitral regurgitation. Eur Heart J *5*:404, 1984.

126. Zabalgoitta-Reyes, M.: Aortic regurgitation: utility of continuous and pulsed wave Doppler in assessing severity. Echocardiography *3*:119, 1986.

127. Zhang, Y., Nitter-Hauge, S., Ihlen, H., Rootwelt, K., Myhre, E.: Measurement of aortic regurgitation by Doppler echocardiography. Br Heart J *55*:32, 1986.

128. Goldberg, S.J., Wilson, N., Dickinson, D.F.: Increased blood velocities in the heart and great

vessels of patients with congenital heart disease. An assessment of their significance in the absence of valvar stenosis. Br Heart J *53*:640, 1985.

129. Chuwa, T., Akira, K., Shinichi, A., Kiyotake, A., Yutaka, O., Kumiko, N., Hiromitsu, T.: Continuous wave Doppler measurement of transmitral pressure gradients in mitral stenosis: Comparisons with simultaneous catheterization measurements. J Cardiogr *15*:1097, 1985.

130. Diebold, B., Theroux, P., Bourassa, M.G., Thuillez, C., Peronneau, P., Guermonprez, J.L., Xhaard, M., Waters, D.D.: Noninvasive pulsed Doppler Study of mitral stenosis and mitral regurgitation. Preliminary study. Br Heart J *42*:168, 1979.

131. Grenadier, E., Sahn, D.J., Valdes-Cruz, L.M., Allen, H.D., Lima, C.O., Goldberg, S.J.: Two-dimensional echo Doppler study of congenital disorders of the mitral valve. Am Heart J *107*:319, 1984.

132. Holen, J., Hoie, J., Froysaker, T.: Determination of pre- and postoperative flow obstruction in patients undergoing closed mitral commissurotomy from noninvasive ultrasound Doppler data and cardiac output. Am Heart J *97*:499, 1979.

133. Kalmanson, D., Veyrat, C., Bernier, A., Savier, C.H., Chiche, P., Witchitz, S.: Diagnosis and evaluation of mitral valve disease using transseptal ultrasound catheterization. Br Heart J *37*:257, 1975.

134. Kalmanson, D., Veyrat C., Bernier, A., Witchitz, S., Chiche, P.: Opening snap and isovolumic relaxation period in relation to mitral valve in patients with mitral stenosis. Significance of A2-OS interval. Br. Heart J *38*:135, 1976.

135. Knutsen, K.M., Bae, E.A., Sivertssen, E., Grendahl, H.: Doppler ultrasound in mitral stenosis. Assessment of pressure gradient and atrioventricular pressure half-time. Acta Med Scand *211*:433, 1982.

136. Labovitz, A.J., Nelson, J.G., Windhorst, D.M., Kennedy, H.L., Williams, G.A.: Frequency of mitral valve dysfunction from mitral annular calcium as detected by Doppler echocardiography. Am J Cardiol *55*:133, 1985.

137. Mehlman, D.J.: Doppler and 2-dimensional echocardiographic assessment of mitral stenosis. Echocardiography. *3*:109, 1986.

138. Miyatake, K., Okamoto, M., Kinoshita, N., Izumi, S., Owa, M., Takao, S., Sakakibara, H., Nimura, Y.: Clinical applications of a new type of real-time two-dimensional Doppler flow imaging system. Am J Cardiol *54*:857, 1984.

139. Robson, D.J., Flaxman, J.C.: Measurement of the end diastolic pressure gradient and mitral valve area in mitral stenosis by Doppler ultrasound. Eur Heart J *5*:660, 1984.

140. Taeymans, Y., Goldstein, M., Vandenbossche, J.L., Englert: Evaluation of mitral stenosis by the study of the left ventricular diastolic phase. Acta Cardiol (Brus) *37*:357, 1982.

141. Thuillez, C., Theroux, P., Bourassa, M.G., Blanchard, D., Peronneau, P., Guermonprez, J.L., Diebold, B., Waters, D.D., Maurice, P.: Pulsed Doppler echocardiographic study of mitral stenosis. Circulation *61*:381, 1980.

142. Tei, C., Kisanuki, A., Arima, S., Arikawa, K., Otsuji, Y., Natsugoe, K., Tanaka, H.: Continuous wave Doppler measurement of transmitral pressure gradients in mitral stenosis: Comparisons with simultaneous catheterization measurements. J Cardiogr *14*:1097, 1985.

143. Ferrara, R.P., Labovitz, A.J., Wiens, R.D., Kennedy, H.L., Williams, G.A.: Prosthetic mitral regurgitation detected by Doppler echocardiography. Am J Cardiol *55*:229, 1985.

144. Wilkins, G.T., Gillam, L.D., Kritzer, G.L., Levine, R.A., Palacios, I.F., Weyman, A.E.: Validation of continuous-wave Doppler echocardiographic measurements of mitral and tricuspid prosthetic valve gradients: A simultaneous Doppler-catheter study. Circulation *74*:786, 1986.

145. Holen, J., Hoie, J., Semb, B.: Obstructive characteristics of Bjork-Shiley, Hancock, and Lillehei-Kaster prosthetic mitral valves in the immediate postoperative period. Acta Med Scand *204*:5, 1978.

146. Holen, J., Nitter-Hauge, S.: Evaluation of obstructive characteristics of mitral disc valve implants with ultrasound Doppler techniques. Acta Med Scand *201*:429, 1977.

147. Holen, J., Simonsen, S., Froysaker, T.: An ultrasound Doppler technique for the noninvasive determination of the pressure gradient in the Bjork-Shiley mitral valve. Circulation *59*:436, 1979.

148. Holen, J., Simonsen, S, Froysaker, T.: Determination of pressure gradient in Hancock mitral valve from noninvasive ultrasound Doppler data. Scand J Clin Lab Invest *41*:177, 1981.

149. Kitabake, A., Tanouchi, J., Asao, M., Mishima, M., Ishihara, K., Inoue, M., Abe, H., Matsuo, H., Morita, H.: Intracardiac flow dynamic alterations with a prosthetic mitral valve studied by pulsed Doppler technique. J Cardiogr *15*:469, 1985.

150. Kisanuki, A., Tei, C., Arikawa, K., Natsugoe, K., Otsuji, Y., Kawazoe, Y., Tanaka, H., Morishita, M., Taira, A.: Continuous wave Doppler assessment of prosthetic valves in the mitral position: Comparison of the St. Jude Medical Mechanical valve and the porcine xenograft valve. J Cardiogr *15*:1119, 1986.

151. Mann, D., Gillam, L., Marshall, J., King, M., Weyman, A.E.: Doppler and two-dimensional echocardiographic diagnosis of Bjork-Shiley prosthetic valve malfunction: importance of

interventricular septal motion and the timing of onset of valve flow. J Am Coll Cardiol *8*:971, 1986.

152. Raizada, V., Hoyt, T.W., Corlew, S., Abrams, J.: A study of the diastolic flow velocity profile of the clinically uncomplicated mitral porcine bioprosthesis using an echo-Doppler technique. Jpn Heart J *24*:59, 1983.
153. Ryan, T., Armstrong, W.F., Dillon, J.C., Feigenbaum, H.: Doppler echocardiographic evaluation of patients with porcine mitral valves. Am Heart J *111*:237, 1986.
154. Sagar, K.B., Wann, L.S., Paulsen, W.H.J., Romhilt, D.W.: Doppler echocardiographic evaluation of Hancock and Bjork-Shiley prosthetic valves. J Am Coll Cardiol *7*:681, 1986.
155. Weinstein, I.R., Marbarger, J.P., Perez, J.E.: Ultrasonic assessment of the St. Jude prosthetic valve: M-mode, two-dimensional and Doppler echocardiography. Circulation *68*:897, 1983.
156. Perez, J.E., Ludbrook, P.A., Ahumada, G.G.: Usefulness of Doppler echocardiography in detecting tricuspid valve stenosis. Am J Cardiol *55*:601, 1985.
157. Veyrat, C., Kalmanson, D., Farjon, M., Manin, J.P., Abitbol, G.: Noninvasive diagnosis and assessment of tricuspid regurgitation and stenosis using one and two-dimensional echo pulsed Doppler. Br Heart J *47*:596, 1982.
158. Kalmanson, D., Veyrat, C., Witchitz, S., Derai, C., Chiche, P.: Les dysfontionnements tricuspidiens: Une nouvelle entité physiopathologique. Etude par velocimetrie Doppler. Ann Cardiol Angeiol *21*:433, 1972.
159. Kalmanson, D., Bernier, A., Veyrat, C., Witchitz, S., Savier, C.H., Chiche, P.: Normal pattern and physiological significance of mitral valve flow velocity recorded using transseptal directional Doppler ultrasound catheterization. Br Heart J *37*:249, 1975.
160. Keren, G., LeJemtel, T., Zelcer, A., Meisner, J.S., Bier, A., Yellin, E.: Time variation of mitral regurgitant flow in patients with dilated cardiomyopathy. Circulation *74*:684, 1986.
161. Houda, N., Takeuchi, M., Morita, N., Nakano, T., Takezawa, H.: Diagnosis and estimation of mitral regurgitation by two-dimensional pulsed Doppler echocardiography. J. Cardiogr. *15*:449, 1985.
162. Johnson, S.L., Baker, D.W., Lute, R.A., Murray, J.A.: Detection of mitral regurgitation by Doppler echocardiography. (abstr) Am J Cardiol *33*:146, 1974.
163. Kinney, E., Machado, H., Cortado, X.: Cooing intracardiac sound in a perforated porcine mitral valve detected by pulsed Doppler echocardiography. Am Heart J *112*:420, 1986.
164. Kronzon, I., Mercurio, P., Winer, H.E., Colvin, S.: Echocardiographic evaluation of Carpentier mitral valvuloplasty. Am Heart J *106*:362, 1983.
165. Loperfido, F., Biasucci, L., Pennestri, F., Laurenzi, F., Gimigliano, F., Vigna, C., Rossi, E., Favuzzi, A., Santarelli, P.: Pulsed Doppler echocardiographic analysis of mitral regurgitation after myocardial infarction. Am J Cardiol *58*:692, 1986.
166. Matsuo, H., Morita, H., Senda, S., Kitabatake, A., Asao, M., Tanouchi, J., Michima, M., Abe, H.: Detection and visualization of regurgitant flow in valvular diseases by pulsed Doppler technique. Jpn Circulation J *46*:377, 1982.
167. Mehlman, D.J.: Utility of two-dimensional and Doppler echocardiography in assessing the etiology and severity of mitral regurgitation. Echocardiography *3*:97, 1986.
168. Meijboom, E.J., Ebels, T., Anderson, R.H., Schasfoort-van Leeuwen, J.M., Deanfield, J.E., Eijgelaar, A., Homan van der Heide, J.N.: Left atrioventricular valve after surgical repair in atrioventricular septal defect with separate valve orifices ("ostium primum atrial septal defect"): An echo-Doppler study. Am J Cardiol *57*:433, 1986.
169. Miyatake, K, Izumi, S., Okamoto, M., Kinoshita, N., Asonuma, H., Nakagawa, H., Yamamoto, K., Takamiya, M., Sakakibara, H., Nimura, Y.: Semiquantitative grading of severity of mitral regurgitation by real-time two-dimensional Doppler flow imaging technique. J Am Coll Cardiol *7*:82, 1986.
170. Miyatake, K., Nimura, Y., Sakakibara, H., Kinoshita, N., Okamoto, M., Nagata, S., Kawazoe, K., Fujita, T.: Localization and direction of mitral regurgitant flow in mitral orifice studied with combined use of ultrasonic pulsed Doppler technique and two-dimensional echocardiography. Br Heart J *48*:449, 1982.
171. Miyatake, K., Kinoshita, N., Nagata, S., Beppu, S., Park, Y., Sakakibara, H., Nimura, Y.: Intracardiac flow pattern in mitral regurgitation studied with combined use of the ultrasonic pulsed Doppler technique and cross-sectional echocardiography. Am J Cardiol *45*:155, 1980.
172. Nichol, P.M., Boughner, D.R., Persaud, J.A.: Noninvasive assessment of mitral insufficiency by transcutaneous Doppler ultrasound. Circulation *54*:656, 1976.
173. Ohwa, M., Sakakibara, H., Mijatake, K., Okamoto, M., Kinoshita, N., Ueda, E., Funahashi, T., Nakasone, I., Nimura, Y.: Mitral regurgitation: detection and quantitative evaluation by two-dimensional Doppler echocardiography. J Cardiogr *15*:807, 1986.
174. O'Rourke, R.A., Crawford, M.H.: Mitral valve regurgitation. *In* Current Problems in Cardiology. Chicago, Year Book Medical Publishers, 1984.
175. Patel, A.K., Rowe, G.G., Thomsen, J.H., Dhanani, S.P., Kosolcharoen, P., Lyle, L E.: Detection and estimation of rheumatic mitral regurgitation in the presence of mitral stenosis by pulsed Doppler echocardiography. Am J Cardiol *51*:986, 1983.

176. Schluter, M., Langenstein, B.A., Hanrath, P., Kremer, P., Bleifeld, W.: Assessment of trans-esophageal pulsed Doppler echocardiography in the detection of mitral regurgitation. Circulation *66*:784, 1982.
177. Shah, A.A., Quinones, M.A., Waggoner, A.D., Barndt, R, Miller, R.R.: Pulsed Doppler echocardiographic detection of mitral regurgitation in mitral valve prolapse; Correlation with cardiac arrhythmias. Cathet Cardiovasc Diagn *8*:437, 1982.
178. Veyrat, C., Ameur, A., Bas, S., Lessana, A., Abitbol, G., Kalmanson, D.: Pulsed Doppler echocardiographic indices for assessing mitral regurgitaiton. Br Heart J *51*:130, 1984.
179. Benchimol, A., Harris, C.L., Desser, K.B.: Noninvasive diagnosis of tricuspid insufficiency utilizing the external Doppler flowmeter probe. Am J Cardiol *32*:868, 1973.
180. DePace, N.L., Ross, J., Iskandrian, A.S., Nestico, P.F., Kotler, M.N., Mintz, G.S., Segal, B.L., Hakki, A.H., Morganroth, J.: Tricuspid regurgitation: Noninvasive techniques for determining causes and severity. J Am Coll Cardiol *3*:1540, 1984.
181. Diebold, B., Touati, R., Blanchard, D., Colonna, G., Guermonprez, J.L., Peronneau, R., Forman, J., Maurice: Quantitative assessment of tricuspid regurgitation using pulsed Doppler echocardiography. Br Heart J *50*:443, 1983.
182. Friedman, G., Kronzin, I., Nobile, J., Cohen, M.L., Winer, H.E.: Echocardiographic findings after tricuspid valvectomy. Chest *87*::668, 1985.
183. Limacher, M.C., Ware, J.A., O'Meara, M.E., Fernandez, G.C., Young, J.B.: Tricuspid regurgitation during pregnancy: Two-dimensional and pulsed Doppler echocardiographic observations. Am J Cardiol. *55*:1059, 1985.
184. Miyatake, K., Okamoto, M., Kinoshita, N., Ohta, M., Kozuka, T., Sakakibara, H., Nimura, Y.: Evaluation of tricuspid regurgitation by pulsed Doppler and two-dimensional echocardiography. Circulation *66*:777, 1982.
185. Mikami, T., Kudo, T., Sakurai, N., Sakamoto, S., Tanabe, Y., Yasuda, H.: Mechanisms for development of functional tricuspid regurgitation determined by pulsed Doppler and two-dimensional echocardiography. Am J Cardiol *53*:160, 1984.
186. Nimura, Y., Miyatake, K., Okamoto, M., Beppu, S. Kinoshita, N., Sakakibara, H.: Pulsed Doppler echocardiography in the assessment of tricuspid regurgitation. Ultrasound Med Biol *10*:239, 1984.
187. Novack, H., Machac, J., Horowitz, S.F.: Inversion of the radionuclide regurgitant index in right sided valvular regurgitation. Eur Nucl Med *11*:205, 1985.
188. Pennestri, F., Loperfido, F., Salvatori, M.P., Mongiardo, R., Ferrazza, A., Guccione, P., Manzoli, U.: Assessment of tricuspid regurgitation by pulsed Doppler ultrasonography of the hepatic vein. Am J Cardiol *54*:363, 1984.
189. Sakai, K., Nakamura, K., Satomi, G., Kondo, M., Hirosawa, K.: Evaluation of tricuspid regurgitation by blood flow pattern in the hepatic vein using pulsed Doppler technique. Am Heart J *108*:516, 1984.
190. Skjaerpe, T., Hatle, L.: Diagnosis of tricuspid regurgitation. Sensitivity of Doppler ultrasound compared with contrast echocardiography. European Heart J *6*:429,1985.
191. Yock, P., Naasz, C., Hill, S., Popp, R.: Doppler evaluation of valvular regurgitation. Echocardiography *3*:157, 1986.
192. Yock, P.G., Popp, R.L.: Noninvasive estimation of right ventricular systolic pressure by Doppler ultrasound in patients with tricuspid regurgitation. Circulation *70*:657, 1984.
193. Marx, G., Allen, H.D.: Accuracy and pitfalls of Doppler evaluation of the pressure gradient in aortic coarctation. J Am Coll Cardiol *7*:1379, 1986.
194. Sanders, S.P., MacPherson, D., Yeager, S.B.: Temporal flow velocity profile in the descending aorta in coarctation. J Am Coll Cardiol *7*:603, 1986.
195. Wyse, R.K., Robinson, P.J., Deanfield J.E., Tunstall-Pedoe, D.S., Macartney, F.J.: Use of continuous wave Doppler ultrasound velocimetry to assess the severity of coarctation of the aorta by measurement of aortic flow velocities. Br Heart J *52*:278, 1984.
196. Sahn, D.J., Allen, H.D., McDonald, G., Goldberg, S.J.: Real-time cross-sectional echocardiographic diagnosis of coarctation of the aorta: A prospective study of echocardiographic-angiographic correlations. Circulation *52*:762, 1977.
197. Allen, H.D., Marx, G.R., Ovitt, T.W., Goldberg, S.J.: Balloon dilation angioplasty for coarctation of the aorta. Am J Cardiol *57*:731, 1986.
198. Goldberg, S.J., Vasko, S.D., Allen, H.D., Marx, G.R.: Can the technique for Doppler estimate of pulmonary stenosis gradient be simplified? Am Heart J *111*:709, 1986.
199. Houston, A.B., Simpson, I.A., Sheldon, C.D., Doig, W.B., Coleman, E.N.: Doppler ultrasound in the estimation of the severity of pulmonary infundibular stenosis in infants and children. Br Heart J *55*:381, 1986.
200. Johnson, G.L., Kwan, O.L., Handshoe, S., Noonan, J.A., DeMaria, A.N.: Accuracy of combined two-dimensional echocardiography and continuous wave Doppler recordings in the estimation of pressure gradient in right ventricular outlet obstruction. J Am Coll Cardiol. *3*:1013, 1984.

201. Kosturakis, D., Allen, H.D., Goldberg, S.J., Sahn, D.J., Valdes-Cruz, L.M.: Noninvasive quantification of stenotic semilunar valve areas by Doppler echocardiography. J Am Coll Cardiol *3*:1256, 1984.
202. Fyfe, D.A., Currie, P.J., Seward, J.B., Tajik, A.J., Reeder, G.S., Mair, D.D., Hagler, D.J.: Continuous-wave Doppler determination of the pressure gradient across pulmonary artery bands: Hemodynamic correlation of 20 patients. Mayo Clin Proc *59*:744, 1984.
203. Valdes-Cruz, L.M., Horowitz, S., Sahn, D.J., Larson, D., Lima, C.O., Mesel, E.: Validation of a Doppler echocardiographic method for calculating severity of discrete stenotic obstructions in a canine preparation with a pulmonary artery band. Circulation *69*:1177, 1984.
204. Fox, R., Panidis, I.P., Kotler, M.N., Mintz, G.S., Ross, J.: Detection by Doppler echocardiography of acquired pulmonic stenosis due to extrinsic tumor compression. Am J Cardiol *53*:1475, 1984.
205. Canale, J.M., Sahn, D.J., Copeland, J.G., Goldberg, S.J., Valdes-Cruz, L.M., Salomon, N., Allen, H.D.: Two-dimensional Doppler echocardiographic/M-mode echocardiographic and phonocardiographic method for study of extracardiac heterograft valved conduits in the right ventricular outflow tract position. Am J Cardiol *49*:100, 1982.
206. Reeder, G.S., Currie, P.J., Fyfe, D.A., Hagler, D.J., Seward, J.B., Tajik, A.J.: Extracardiac conduit obstruction: Initial experience in the use of Doppler echocardiography for noninvasive estimation of pressure gradient. J Am Coll Cardiol *4*:1006, 1984.
207. Masuyama, T., Kodama, K., Kitabatake, A., Sato, H., Nanto, S., Inoue, M.: Continuous-wave Doppler echocardiographic detection of pulmonary regurgitation and its application to noninvasive estimation of pulmonary artery pressure. Circulation *74*:484, 1986.
208. Miyatake, K., Okamoto, M., Kinoshita, N., Matsuhisa, M., Nagata, S., Beppu, S., Park, Y., Sakakibara, H., Nimura, Y.: Pulmonary regurgitation studied with the ultrasonic pulsed Doppler technique. Circulation *65*:969, 1982.
209. Chandraratna, P.A., Wilson, D., Imaizumi, T., Ritter, W.S., Aronow, W.S.: Invasive and noninvasive assessment of pulmonic regurgitation: Clinical, angiographic, phonocardiographic, echocardiographic, and Doppler ultrasound correlations. Clin Cardiol *5*:360, 1982.
210. Hatle, L., Rokseth, R.: Noninvasive diagnosis and assessment of ventricular septal defect by Doppler ultrasound. Acta Med Scand *645*:47, 1981.
211. Magherini, A., Azzolina, G., Wiechman, V., Fantini, F.: Pulsed Doppler echocardiography for diagnosis of ventricular septal defects. Br Heart J *43*:143, 1980.
212. Marx, G.R., Allen, H.D., Goldberg, S.J.: Doppler echocardiographic estimation of systolic pulmonary artery pressure in pediatric patients with interventricular communications. J Am Coll Cardiol *6*:1132, 1985.
213. Miyatake, K., Okamoto, M., Kinoshita, N., Park, Y., Nagata, S., Izumi, S., Fusejima, K., Sakakibara, H., Nimura, Y.: Doppler echocardiographic features of ventricular septal rupture in myocardial infarction. J Am Coll Cardiol *5*:182, 1985.
214. Otterstad, J.E., Simonsen, S., Vatne, K., Myhre, E.: Doppler echocardiography in adults with isolated ventricular septal defect. Eur Heart J *5*:332, 1984.
215. Panidis, I., Mintz, G., Goel, I., McAllister, M., Ross, J.: Acquired ventricular septal defect after myocardial infarction: Detection by combined two-dimensional and Doppler echocardiography. Am Heart J *111*:427, 1986.
216. Recusani, F., Raisaro, A., Sgalambro, A., Tronconi, L., Venco, A., Salerno, J., Ardissino, D.: Ventricular septal rupture after myocardial infarction: Diagnosis by two-dimensional and pulsed Doppler echocardiography. Am J Cardiol *54*:277, 1984.
217. Richards, K.L., Hoekenga, D.E., Leach, J.K., Blaustein, J.C.: Dopplercardiographic diagnosis of interventricular septal rupture. Chest *76*:101, 1979.
218. Silbert, D., Brunson, S., Schiff, R., Diamant, S.: Determination of right ventricular pressure in the presence of a ventricular septal defect using continuous wave Doppler ultrasound. J Am Coll Cardiol *8*:379, 1986.
219. Stevenson, J.G., Kawabori, I., Stamm, S.J., Bailey, W.W., Hall, D.G., Mansfield, P.B., Rittenhouse, E.A.: Pulsed Doppler echocardiographic evaluation of ventricular septal defect patches. Circulation *70*:138, 1984.
220. Veyrat, C., Abitbol, G., Berkmann, M., Malergue, M.C., Kalmanson, D.: Pulsed echo Doppler diagnosis and evaluation of tricuspid valve, and interventricular and interatrial communication insufficiencies. Flowmeter study of shunts. Arch Mal Coeur *73*:1037, 1980.
221. Veyrat, C., Cholot, N., Berkmann, M.: Diagnostic non-traumatique des communications interventricularies par la velocimetrie Doppler-pulse. Acta Cardiol (Brus) *34*:401, 1979.
222. Murphy, D.J., Ludomirsky, A., Huhta, J.C.: Continuous-wave Doppler in children with ventricular septal defect: Noninvasive estimation of interventricular pressure gradient. Am J Cardiol *57*:428, 1986.
223. Marx, G.R., Allen, H.D., Goldberg, S.J.: Doppler estimation of systolic pulmonary artery pressure in patients with aortic-pulmonary shunts. J Am Coll Cardiol *7*:880, 1986.

224. Burstin, L.: Determination of pressure in the pulmonary artery by external graphic recordings. Br Heart J *29*:396, 1967.

225. Hatle, L., Angelsen, B.A.J., Tromsdal, A.: Noninvasive estimation of pulmonary artery systolic pressure with Doppler ultrasound. Br Heart J *45*:157, 1981.

226. Stevenson, J.G., Kawabori, I., Guntheroth, W.G.: Noninvasive estimation of peak pulmonary artery pressure by M-Mode echocardiography. (abstr) Am J Cardiol *5*:1021, 1984.

227. Friedman, D., Bierman, F., Barst, R.: Gated pulsed Doppler evaluation of idiopathic pulmonary artery hypertension in children. Am J Cardiol *58*:369, 1986.

228. Hsieh, K., Sanders, S., Colan, S., MacPherson, D., Holland C: Right ventricular systolic time intervals: Comparison of echocardiographic and Doppler-derived values. Am Heart J *112*:103, 1986.

229. Isobe, M., Yazaki, Y., Takaku, F., Koizumi, K., Hara, K., Tsuneyoshi, H., Yamaguchi, T., Machii, K.: Prediction of pulmonary arterial pressure in adults by pulsed Doppler echocardiography. Am J Cardiol *57*:316, 1986.

230. Kitabatake, A., Inoue, M., Asao, M., Masuyama, T., Tanouchi, J., Morita, T., Mishima, M., Uematsu, M., Shimazu, T., Hori, M., Abe, H.: Noninvasive evaluation of pulmonary hypertension by a pulsed Doppler technique. Circulation *68*:302, 1983.

231. Kosturakis, D., Goldberg, S.J., Allen, H.D., Loeber, C.: Doppler echocardiographic prediction of pulmonary arterial hypertension in congenital heart disease. Am J Cardiol *53*:1110, 1984.

232. Matsuda, M., Sekiguchi, T., Sugishita, Y., Kuwako, K., Iida, K., Ito, I.: Reliability of noninvasive estimates of pulmonary hypertension by pulsed Doppler echocardiography. Br Heart J *56*:158, 1986.

233. Okamoto, M., Miyatake, K., Kinoshita, N., Sakakibara, H., Nimura, Y.: Analysis of blood flow in pulmonary hypertension with the pulsed Doppler flowmeter combined with cross-sectional echocardiography. Br Heart J *51*:407, 1984.

234. Serwer, G., Cougle, A., Eckerd, J., Armstrong, B.: Factors affecting use of the Doppler-determined time from flow onset to maximal pulmonary artery velocity for measurement of pulmonary artery in children. Am J Cardiol *58*:352, 1986.

235. Dabestani, A., Mahan, G., Gardin, J.M., Takenaka, K., Burn, C., Allfie, A., Henry, W.L.: Evaluation of pulmonary artery pressure and resistance by pulsed Doppler echocardiography. Am J Cardiol *59*:662, 1987.

CHAPTER **5**

FLOW COMPUTATION

Flow computation is one of the major capabilities of Doppler echocardiography. Constant flow through a rigid tube can be computed as the product of mean flow velocity determined over time and the area through which flow passes. Units of area are cm² and units of velocity are cm/sec. Accordingly,

$$\text{cm}^2 \times \text{cm/sec} = \text{cm}^3/\text{sec} = \text{ml/sec (flow)}$$

Flow through circulatory structures may differ in important ways from constant flow through a rigid tube. First, circulatory flow is usually pulsatile, or at least variable throughout a cardiac cycle. Secondly, a rigid tube does not change area significantly during constant flow, but a vessel or cardiac location probably changes dimension.

Velocity, measured by Doppler, will be recorded as a lower value if the Doppler beam is not aligned with the flow path. If non-alignment occurs, velocity magnitude may be adjusted to true magnitude by dividing measured velocity by the cosine of the intercept angle (COS Θ). Thus, the final formula becomes:

$$\text{Flow} = \text{flow area} \times \text{velocity/COS } \Theta$$

ASSUMPTIONS FOR DOPPLER CARDIAC OUTPUT

The most precise application of this relationship requires that instantaneous velocity be multiplied by instantaneous area to determine instantaneous flow. To achieve flow over a complete cardiac cycle, all of these instantaneous products must be summed. The mathematical term for this process is "integration." Clearly, the process, as outlined, is beyond the scope of an ultrasonic examination because of the requirement of measuring instantaneous flow area. Accordingly, certain compromises are necessary, the greatest of which is the assumption that flow area does not change significantly during the flow period. A second assumption, probably of a lower order of importance, is that mean velocity/cycle is an adequate descriptor of the velocity factor. The third assumption is that alignment with flow is sufficiently accurate to eliminate the cosine factor or that the appropriate beam-flow intercept angle can be computed. The fourth assumption is that, in normals, the volume of flow during the opposite phase of the cardiac cycle is negligible. These several assumptions will be discussed in some detail and their application to various areas of the heart will be addressed.

153

Assumption: Flow Area Does Not Change Significantly During the Cardiac Cycle

The most direct assessment of this proposition would be to evaluate flow area continuously during the cardiac cycle in each patient. This is not a practical solution since it would require continuous measurements as well as imaging and resolution capability not available with present instrumentation. A second possibility would be to make the assumption that flow area remains constant during the cardiac cycle. This proposition has been evaluated in the great vessels of dogs, but no comparable human data are available. Loeber et al.[1] demonstrated in a canine preparation that aortic and pulmonary artery area varied by a mean of 6 and 12% respectively under conditions of marked changes in preload and afterload. At baseline flow, maximal variation in vessel area was approximately half this value. This area change was measured by recording the circumferential length of a sensitive, non-restrictive mercury strain gauge manometer which was fixed around the great vessel. No similar study has been performed on humans. Although a human study of great vessel diameter change could be proposed using ultrasonic imaging, a major problem is evident which can be best understood by substituting numbers for concepts. If an aortic diameter changed from 24 to 25 mm during the cardiac cycle, that area change would be greater than the baseline change for dogs. A change of 1 mm in 25 is difficult to appreciate on most human studies. For atrioventricular valve flow areas the problem is even greater because flow area change would be difficult to confirm. Accordingly, an indirect method has been used to assess flow area. This method is to compare flow derived by another method, usually invasive, to flow determined by Doppler. This is an indirect use of the continuity equation which states that flow measured at one area is equal to flow measured at another if no loss or gain of fluid occurs between the two (Fig. 5–1.) If the two flows are quite similar over a range of subjects, possible conclusions are that flow area was correctly computed or that the velocity term consistently corrected

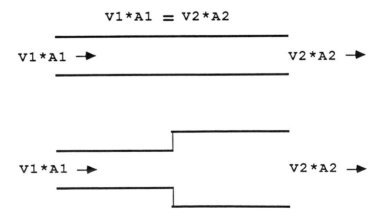

Fig. 5–1. Continuity equation. The product of velocity and area at the entrance of the tube equals the product of velocity and area at the exit of the tube. The lower panel shows that the same relationship holds even if the exit area is different from the entrance area.

for any error in flow area. One note of caution is that invasive methods for measuring flow are also suspect for accuracy.[2]

Assumption: Mean Velocity is an Adequate Descriptor of the Velocity Factor

Mean velocity refers to the integral of velocity with respect to time (i.e., the area of the curve) divided by cardiac cycle length. This method for computing the velocity factor obscures instantaneous changes. A corollary of this assumption is that velocity is uniform across the vessel. The corollary is not entirely true because of viscous drag at the walls. However, the sample volume is wide and probably samples most of the vessel.

The ideal method for computation would determine the instantaneous relationship between velocity and area because it is possible that the early and late phase of the flow cycle occur at a different flow area than does the peak velocity. However, if all contributions of velocity are included, and if the time over which flow occurred is accurate, mean velocity should properly represent velocity. One likely error to be made in this aspect will probably occur in time determination; however, the magnitude of this error is likely to be small. Further, the magnitude of the error can be reduced by determining the total time for several cardiac cycles.

Assumption: Alignment of the Beam and Flow Path is Possible

Measured velocity is recorded at full amplitude only if the beam is spatially aligned with the flow path. Failure to align will cause an amplitude reduction equal to the product of true amplitude and the cosine of the intercept angle (Fig. 5–2). The process is not linear with respect to the angle since a 20° intercept angle will reduce amplitude by only 6%. However, beyond 20° the error quickly increases (Fig. 5–3). Methods used to interrogate the various cardiac and great vessel areas are detailed in Chapter 3. Although an early

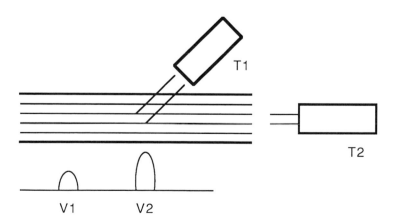

Fig. 5–2. Two transducers (T1 and T2) are interrogating flow through a vessel. T2 measures full velocity amplitude (V2) because the transducer beam is parallel to flow. T1 measures a lower amplitude of velocity (V1) because of the beam-flow intercept angle. The decrease in amplitude is a function of the cosine of the intercept angle.

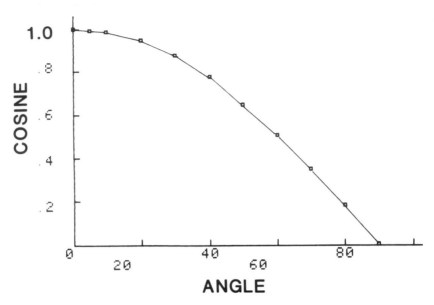

Fig. 5–3. Relationship of the value of the cosine (vertical axis) and the angle in degrees (horizontal axis). Note that if the angle is zero, the value of the cosine is +1. If the angle is 20°, the value of the cosine is still 94%. As the angle increases beyond 20°, however, the value of the cosine drops rapidly. Negative cosines are not shown.

concept was that alignment might be a difficult problem, experience has failed to confirm this hypothesis. In some instances special transducers and maneuvers are required. Proof that alignment is not a significant problem came indirectly in the form that cardiac output measured by simultaneous Doppler and invasive methods provided similar values.[3-5]

Assumption: Forward Flow During the Opposite Part of the Cardiac Cycle is Negligible

This proposition has not been studied. As indicated in Chapter 3, diastolic forward flow occurs in the pulmonary artery and is not taken into account by present Doppler flow methods. This flow appears to very small in volume. Forward flow through other valves during the opposite portion of the cardiac cycle is not reported.

GENERAL PRINCIPLES FOR FLOW MEASUREMENT

Determination of Mean Velocity

The method for determination of a mean velocity requires measurement of the area between the curve and the zero velocity line (Fig. 5–4). The procedure for determination of area is relatively uniform for all cardiac and great vessel areas. Since velocities change with respiration and rhythm, mean velocity of a number of beats are usually averaged. We utilize a microcomputer for this purpose. A dedicated program controls an Apple II computer. Data are entered from a digitizing pad by tracing the modal velocity of 4 to 8 beats. The digitizing process requires less than a minute, and mean velocity is immediately obtained after digitization. The curve is replotted on a video monitor so that the examiner

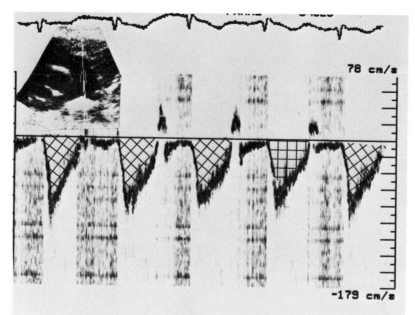

Fig. 5–4. The area to be planimetered between the baseline and the curve is shown crosshatched. Digitization is performed of the several areas. Note that each area differs a bit from the next. When digitization reaches the baseline at the end of systole, we trace along the baseline until the next downstroke.

can be certain that no extraneous points were entered or detected by the computer. Recently, numerous commercial computer programs have been developed to accomplish this same goal.

Modal velocity refers to that instantaneous velocity which has the most frequent occurrence level. Determining modal velocity is important because at any point in time a number of different velocities are present. Since occurrence amplitude is depicted as gray scale, the most common velocity is represented by the blackest or whitest portion of the tracing (Fig. 5–5). Occasionally an entire band of velocities have approximately the same shade of gray. In that

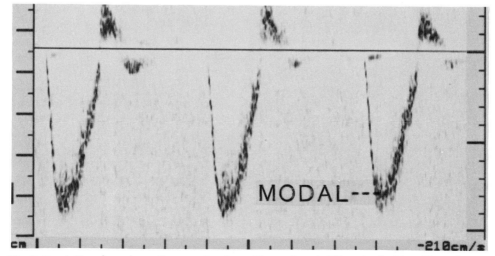

Fig. 5–5. A Doppler echocardiogram showing cells moving at different velocities. The velocity at which most cells move is marked "modal." Note, however, that some cells are moving at greater or lesser velocities than the modal and are depicted in less intense shades of gray.

instance, we digitize through the middle of the velocity spectrum. The modal velocity, rather than some other velocity, was selected intuitively,[3] and results so closely approximated measurements of cardiac output by invasive techniques that we and others have continued to use this method.

At the present time on-line methods for determination of mean velocity have not become a suitable substitute for manual digitization of modal velocity because the simple programs written to date have failed to identify the modal velocity of interest. The problem appears to be that a second stronger intensity modal signal usually exists near the zero velocity baseline. Presently, no program has adequately separated this baseline signal from the velocity signal of interest. Most present programs cycle between the baseline or other artifact and the signal of interest, but better programming in the future will probably allow an on-line mean velocity program to be developed. Use of the average velocity has not fared much better because low and high frequency noise is averaged with true signals, and the result of this misidentification makes the computed mean inaccurate. The human eye and mind, today, are the most accurate and reliable instruments for determining modal occurrence.

Figure 5–4 demonstrates pictorially the digitizing technique. The cross-hatched area represents the area to be integrated. Notice that velocity is digitized beginning with the downstroke until the velocity again reaches baseline. It must be emphasized that zero baseline is then digitized until the next downstroke and this process is repeated. Zero baseline is digitized even though obvious velocities may be recorded in diastole (for the great vessels). The only time that flow has been reported to have been digitized throughout the cardiac cycle is when flow is usually proceeding continuously, such as across the atrial septum in patients with atrial septal defects.[6]

The question may arise regarding digitizing velocities in the opposite part of the cardiac cycle. A small amount of pulmonary flow occurs in diastole[7] and pulmonary regurgitation of minor degree occurs in almost all normals and patients with cardiac disease.[8] Further, trivial regurgitation at other valves may occur. To date these minor out of usual cycle flows have not been added to or subtracted from the in cycle flow for two reasons. First the flow area through which out of phase velocities pass is almost certainly different than the area through which in cycle flow passes. Secondly, the absolute magnitude of out of phase velocity is very small.

Mean velocity is determined by dividing area under the curve by distance along the time axis. Division converts area into mean amplitude. Two methods, both of which give identical answers, are in current use. The first method requires digitization of only forward velocity phases and multiplication of this integral of velocity by flow area. This method computes stroke volume. Cardiac output may be computed as the product of average stroke volume and heart rate. The second method requires continuous digitizaton of forward velocity of each beat and digitization of the baseline between complexes. The computer then sums the area of each velocity and divides by the total time base. This method computes mean velocity per second. Multiplication of the mean velocity per second by 60 (sec/min) provides mean velocity per minute. The product of mean velocity/minute and flow area is cardiac output expressed as ml/min. We have used both methods and find that the latter is faster because the digitizing pen does not have to be raised from the digitizer pad between complexes. Results for the two methods are essentially identical.

Digitization of good velocity curves by either technique has an intraobserver and interobserver variability of 6%.[9] However, poor records (which probably should not be digitized in the first place) provide variability up to 15%. Accordingly, repeatability is dependent upon record quality and we advise digitizing only appropriate tracings. Our definition of an appropriate tracing is one that has a maximal velocity dispersion of less than 30%. Tracings with wider velocity dispersions usually are recorded (1) in disturbed flow, (2) at an intercept angle greater than 20°,[10] or (3) in a very large vessel.[11] We digitize traces that we record because this requirement forces us to strive for the highest quality original record. Low quality records will not provide good data and are difficult to digitize.

Digitization of a tracing is not the only method for determining mean velocity. Gardin et al.[12] has proposed a simplified method for determining the area of an aortic velocity. They proposed that a peak velocity measurement and an ejection time can be converted into an area according to the following formula:

$$FVI = 1.14 (PFV \times .5ET) + .3$$

where FVI = flow velocity integral, PFV = peak flow velocity, and ET = ejection time.

Donnerstein[13] observed that great vessel waveforms look like half of an inverted parabola and studied the difference in area between digitization and use of a parabola equation. His results indicate that the area under the velocity curve can be approximated by: area = 2/3 (peak velocity) × ejection time

Correction of Velocity Amplitude by Beam-Flow Intercept Angle

The cosine of the beam-flow intercept angle can be used to adjust amplitude of mean velocity to its true value. If possible, the spatial beam intercept angle should be parallel to flow. If the angle exceeds 20°, velocity magnitude will be diminished by more than 6%. Figure 5–3 shows the relationship of magnitude and cosine of the angle.

The method for proper alignment of the beam with flow is discussed in detail in Chapter 3 and will be discussed only briefly subsequently in this chapter for each flow measurement location. The fundamental problem for determination of the beam-flow intercept angle is estimation of the proper spatial angle. In clinical situations estimation of the proper spatial angle is usually not possible. Accordingly, most Doppler echocardiographers attempt to align with flow. If the beam can be maintained parallel to flow in two dimensions, the transducer can be moved slightly in the third dimension to achieve the highest velocity. If highest velocity is achieved by third dimension transducer angulation, and if the Doppler beam is parallel to flow in the visualized plane, spatial alignment in all three dimensions can be reasonably assumed.

If an angle must be computed in the two visualized dimensions, some structure must serve as a general guide for establishment of a parallel flow path. For great vessel flow, walls of great vessels, and for atrioventricular valve flows the ventricular septum and left free wave have been used.

Flow Area Measurement for Great Vessels

Velocity is a direct function of flow area at the site of velocity measurement. Thus, flow area must be measured *at the point of sampling.* Neither an upstream nor a downstream position is appropriate because caliber of the flow channel may change. Identical locations for vessel diameter and sample volume are possible for great vessels.

A protocol is necessary for measuring diameter. Studies by Loeber et al. show that vessel diameter changes during the cardiac cycle and maximal area occurs in mid to late systole.[1] However, diameter measurement for area computation at maximal size is not important because the maximal area occurs only transiently. Further, area change in proximal great vessels during systole is small. Maximal area change during the entire cardiac cycle in a canine preparation was only 6% for the aorta and 12% for the pulmonary artery. Human data are unavailable and will be difficult to obtain under a protocol that is appropriate to answer the question. In view of these data, a pragmatic approach seems reasonable. The approach that we have adopted is to record the velocity tracing first. Next the vessel image is recorded on videotape. On stop frames selected from slow tape replay, several (usually 5) measurements of vessel diameter are made through the middle of the sample volume. These diameter measurements are selected from random cycle time images of different cycles and all must demonstrate vessel dimension clearly. Measurements are made with a hand caliper by the lateral resolution method (i.e. from the middle of the image of one wall to the middle of the image of the other wall). Measurement of a single vessel dimension, particularly one caught by arbitrarily pressing the "freeze frame" switch without respect to image quality, is an inappropriate substitute. Electronic calipers could be used, but the measurement cursor is invariably large and covers the image to be measured. Further, electronic calipers are seldom easily moved from pixel to pixel. Hand calipers are an inexpensive, low-tech solution which works well. Marx and co-workers[14] compared the recommended method for measuring ascending aortic diameter with the diameter found on angiography and found a correlation coefficient of .89 for precordial imaging and a correlation coefficient of .97 for suprasternal imaging with an off axis transducer. More importantly, the regression for the precordial method had a standard error of the estimate of 2.7 mm, whereas the suprasternal method had a standard error of the estimate of only 0.7 mm. These data show that the suprasternal method for measuring ascending aortic diameter is superior to the precordial method. Some investigators have proposed measuring aortic ring diameter,[4] but no data are available to determine if this method is as accurate as the suprasternal method for measuring ascending aortic diameter. Further, this method requires velocity measurement within the ring.

Flow Profile

Flows are best calculated from areas which have flat flow profiles. Flat profiles occur at inlets, during acceleration, and in large vessels.[8] Fortunately, these are areas that are convenient for measurement of flow. Profiles are considered flat even if they are a bit rounded at the wall and/or skewed across the lumen. Clearly, no velocity pattern is totally flat. Parabolic profiles with greater drag at vessel walls occur at slow flows, in small vessels, and at locations far from the inlet. For accurate flow measurements, velocities in the sample volume should be representative of those across the lumen. This situation is most true for flat velocity profiles. When a parabolic profile exists (Fig. 5–6), numerous velocities will be sampled within the sample volume.

A flat profile will gradually become a parabolic profile as flow progresses

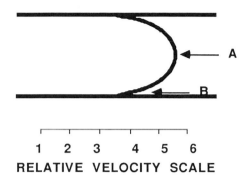

1   2   3   4   5   6

RELATIVE VELOCITY SCALE

Fig. 5–6. Velocity profile in a vessel. Note that the velocity is considerably faster in the center of the vessel (A) than near the wall (B). A relative velocity scale is shown only as a reference and to indicate that velocity is scaled on the X-axis in this illustration.

downstream. In order to understand this transformation, conceptualize flow as composed of numerous circular lamellae of molecules. Consider the rings of lamellae to simulate the concentric rings of a cut onion. Each ring of fluid must slip on the next ring. The degree of slippage is a function of viscosity. Highest viscous resistance occurs at the interface of the vessel wall and the first lamella of fluid. Thus, this layer moves much more slowly than the centrally located lamellae. This difference in slippage rate always causes a slightly rounded profile at the vessel wall. The further that flow passes downstream, the greater the effect of the wall. Central proximal great vessel flow has the most uniform profile within the length of the great vessel. These same factors are also operative at inlets of atrioventricular valves. Accordingly, locations in which parabolic flow occurs are areas of enhanced probability for making an error in velocity measurement as a result of the multiplicity of velocities present simultaneously within the sample volume.

AREAS FOR DOPPLER FLOW MEASUREMENT

Ascending Aorta

The ascending aorta can be imaged from the precordium, suprasternal notch or subcostal position. From the precordium, the intercept angle with aortic flow is always large. Most investigators have studied flow in the ascending aorta[3,4,15–17] from a suprasternal notch transducer location which permits imaging of the ascending aorta parallel to flow. From the subcostal position, it is difficult to be certain that the beam and flow are parallel. Nonetheless, aortic flow has been measured from the subcostal position.[18] Further, both pulsed[3,5,15,18] and CW[4,16] Doppler have been used to measure aortic flow.

VELOCITIES

Alignment with the axis of the ascending aorta is usually difficult with standard two-dimensional imaging transducers because they are physically large and because crystals are mainly in-line with the transducer handle. The ascending aorta, on the other hand, angles somewhat anteriorly from the aortic valve. These physical considerations cause in-line transducers, in most instances, to image the junction of the ascending aorta and transverse arch, and parallel interrogation of the posteriorly angled retrosternal ascending aorta is not possible.[10] Thus, standard transducers frequently provide velocities which are reduced by the cosine of the spatial intercept angle. Further, velocity broadening of the waveform is common because the beam cuts across the flow profile at a steep angle and because cells in the junction of the ascending and transverse aorta move in different directions within the sample volume.[10] Some cells are moving mainly toward the transducer, while others are beginning to turn around the arch. These factors account for the velocity broadening.

Two types of transducers are available for imaging ascending aortic velocities with the beam parallel to flow. One is a two-dimensional off-axis imaging transducer, and the other is a previously designed M-mode suprasternal probe. One two-dimensional imaging transducer is designed to image 25 degrees from the in-line axis (Fig. 5–7). This angle permits retrosternal imaging and alignment of the beam and the central axis of the ascending aorta. Of the first 53 individuals studied with this transducer, we were able to obtain high quality velocity traces and aortic diameters in 47. Two children struggled too much to obtain satisfactory results, and two adults had sternocleidomastoid muscles which inserted on the contralateral side of the superior portion of the sternum, thus effectively eliminating the suprasternal notch. We were not able to image the ascending aorta in two other adults. In the years following cataloguing of results in these 53 patients, we found a number of other individuals in whom we could not obtain suprasternal notch velocities from the ascending aorta. These patients had certain profiles. The first profile consisted of patients who had no depression of the tissues in the suprasternal notch. In these individuals the transducer could not be placed into the notch and rotated anteriorly and inferiorly enough to image the ascending aorta. The second profile consisted of patients whose trachea, in the supine position, appeared to bulge from the notch. Some, but not all, of these individuals experienced paroxysms of coughing when the transducer put pressure on the trachea. Finally, some individuals had an ascending aorta which passed much more posteriorly than most. No transducer that we have found permits consistent alignment with this kind of aorta from the suprasternal notch. These factors occur most commonly but not exclusively in adults, particularly older ones. While studying 830 unselected consecutive subjects, we found that alignment with the aorta from the suprasternal notch can be accomplished in about 96% of children and 73% of adults.

The other transducer that we have used to image ascending aortic velocities

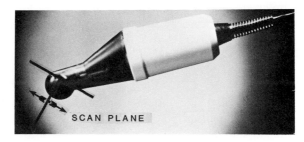

Fig. 5–7.   Off-axis imaging suprasternal notch transducer. The direction of the scan plane is marked with arrows.

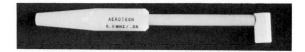

Fig. 5–8. Right-angle transducer that does not produce a sectoring image. We have found this transducer useful for obtaining velocities from the suprasternal notch in line with the mid-ascending aorta. We usually use a low-frequency transducer for high velocities.

parallel to flow was originally developed for M-mode suprasternal notch echocardiography (Fig. 5–8). This transducer is somewhat similar in shape to a commercially available continuous wave transducer. It is manufactured in two crystal sizes, 6 and 12 mm. The small size is most useful for babies and the larger crystal is most useful for larger children and adults. These transducers increase the yield in the adult population by about 8% over the 25° off-axis imaging transducer. This transducer is, however, used without two-dimensional imaging. The range gate is set at approximately 5 to 8 cm in an adult or 3 to 6 cm in a small child. The transducer is angled until an appropriate appearing ascending aortic velocity is achieved. Then experimentation in depth can be employed to record the best quality velocity.

CW Doppler has also been used for computation of aortic flow.[4,16,17] This method also employs an off-axis transducer placed in the suprasternal notch. The beam is directed into the ascending aorta until highest available velocities are recorded. Where these velocities originated is uncertain, but one general rule is that the highest velocity probably came from the narowest point in the circulation. In the absence of a specific left ventricular outflow tract obstruction, the narrowest location in the left ventricular outflow tract is at or just below the aortic annulus. Accordingly, CW velocities are usually paired with aortic annular measurements for computation of cardiac output.

An acceptable ascending aortic velocity has very little frequency dispersion on the upstroke, slight deceleration instability at the peak, and minimal decelerating frequency dispersion. As a general rule for pulsed Doppler, maximal velocity broadening should be less than 30% of the total amplitude of the velocity tracing.[10,19] We are able to achieve this objective in almost all individuals in whom we are able to image the ascending aorta parallel to flow[19] except those with aortas larger than 2.5 cm in diameter. Individuals with aortae >2.5 cm in diameter and normal hematocrits almost always have excessive velocity broadening because their aortic diameters are so wide that the wall has little influence on central core velocities.[11] Velocities recorded using CW almost always have a much wider velocity dispersion[10] and no rules are available to judge the adequacy of CW tracings.

FLOW AREA

Measurement of aortic flow area can be performed in a number of ways. When utilizing the 25° off-axis pulsed imaging transducer, both walls of the aorta at the location of sample volume can be imaged by lateral resolution (Fig. 5–9). Since both walls are imaged with lateral resolution, measurement is performed from center to center of the aortic wall image. Another technique for diameter measurement is to image the ascending aorta above the sinuses of Valsalva from the precordium. In this instance, imaging is possible with axial resolution and, therefore, diameter measurement is made from leading

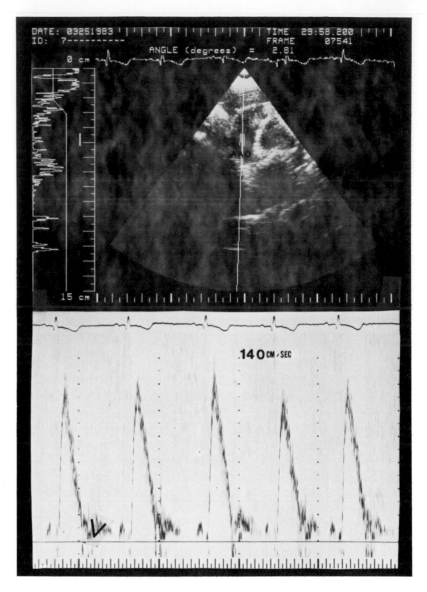

Fig. 5–9. A high-quality trace of ascending aortic velocities. The ascending aortic sample volume position is shown. Aortic diameter should be measured in the middle of the sample volume, which is demonstrated as two lines flanking the cursor line and located just above the A in the ascending aorta (A AO). The bottom panel demonstrates aortic velocities that must be integrated to compute cardiac output. Pointer markers show where the digitization should return to the baseline during diastole on the first two complexes.

edge to leading edge of the ascending aortic wall. Several problems occur with the precordial measurement. First, imaging superior to the sinuses is not always possible. Secondly, when velocity is recorded from the suprasternal notch and diameter is measured from the precordium, confirmation that the sample volume was placed in exactly the same location as the diameter was measured is not possible. This could be a major source of error if the diameter changes at any point superior to the sinuses, and it frequently does. Another major problem is that the accuracy of ascending aortic diameter measurement is reduced when measuring from the precordium even though axial resolution methodology is possible. The reason for this possibly unexpected finding was the difficulty of confirmation that imaging was accomplished above the sinuses of Valsalva. The usual superior limit of precordial imaging of the aorta occurs at or slightly above the sinuses of Valsalva. Accordingly, sometimes the correct measurement is made and sometimes the wider sinus of Valsalva is measured inadvertently.

Aortic diameter can be measured by lateral resolution from a subcostal approach. Sanders et al.[18] used this method. The aorta is far from the transducer in this plane for all except small infants. Far field imaging causes walls to be somewhat less than discrete. Subcostal aortic diameter measurement will probably remain a secondary method.

INTERCEPT ANGLE

The only other major consideration for computation of aortic flow is the beam-flow intercept angle. Few Doppler echocardiographers use intercept angle corrections since ways to achieve parallel beam-flow intercept are now relatively simple and since large errors can be made by assuming the ability to predict these angles. One important caution is that images may be deceiving. As a result of the elevational angle, the cursor may appear to be perfectly aligned with the aorta, but no velocity or only a poor velocity record may be obtained. The transducer must be angled in the elevational plane to obtain the most representative record. Color-coded Doppler has been touted to improve accuracy of velocity measurements by showing the position of the jet within the chamber and allowing angle correction. However, alignment with the jets has rarely presented a significant problem. Further, color-coded Doppler is a two-dimensional imaging system and three-dimensional (spatial angle) is required for angle correction. It seems doubtful that angle correction by color-coded Doppler will add much to flow measurement in individuals with hearts in a usual location. For others, the possibility of assistance exists but no careful study of the problem has been reported.

HOW ACCURATE IS AORTIC FLOW MEASURED BY DOPPLER?

Investigations before incorporation of FFT circuitry into Doppler equipment showed promise for quantitation of aortic flow.[20–21] Magnin and co-workers,[21] using a nonlinear zero crossing analyzer, demonstrated a relatively strong correlation between ascending aortic flow and invasively measured flow, but the slope of the relationship was relatively flat and the intercept was large, findings which suggest systematic error. These problems were most likely due to the spectral analysis technique. Early investigators, utilizing continuous wave equipment, found strong correlations with flow measured by invasive methods and velocity integrals.[22–24] The first study which compared simultaneous invasive and Doppler measurements of flow with spectral analysis by FFT demonstrated a high correlation with a slope approaching 1 (Fig. 5–10).[3] Subsequent studies have confirmed this relationship.[4–5,15–18,25–29] Reports of aortic flow measurement by CW are now available and results suggest that their

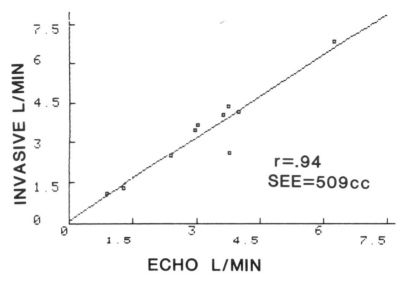

Fig. 5–10. Comparison of aortic flow by indicator dilution and Doppler echocardiography. Indicator dilution data are plotted on the vertical axis and Doppler echo flow data (echo) are plotted on the horizontal axis.[3]

correlation is similar to that found with pulsed Doppler.[4,16,17] Many studies were performed with an in-line pulsed transducer, a configuration which would significantly reduce ability to record aortic velocities accurately, but even those studies provided a reasonable correlation of Doppler and invasive measurements of aortic flow. Table 5–1 shows results of numerous studies in tabular form. Aortic flow measurement has now been extensively studied and, when properly performed, is considered to be a reliable technique.

Descending Aortic Flow

Cardiac output has been measured by continuous wave Doppler interrogation of the descending aorta. From the suprasternal notch, it is possible to place the sample volume generally parallel to flow in the junctional portion of the distal transverse aortic arch and proximal descending aorta. In fewer individuals, it is also possible to position the sample volume along the axis of flow in the more distal descending aorta (Fig. 5–11). The diameter of the descending aorta can be measured with reasonable ease by the lateral resolution method from the suprasternal notch. Unfortunately, relatively wide spectral dispersion occurs in the junction of the aorta because some cells are moving leftward, while others within the same sample volume are moving inferiorly.[10] This spectral dispersion reduces ability to accurately digitize the main velocity. It has been suggested that velocity in the entire aortic arch is constant and that flow diminishes merely due to reduction of caliber of the vessel as it proceeds distally.[30] Accordingly, these authors suggested that mean velocity in the most proximal descending aorta, which is relatively easy to image parallel to flow, can be substituted for mean velocity in the ascending aorta. If this is done, ascending aortic flow area would be substituted for descending aorta because coupling descending aortic area and mean velocity would measure flow after the arm and head vessels had exited the aorta.

Table 5–1. **Aortic or LVOT Flow**

First Author	r =	SEE	Slope	Y-intercept	Comparison
Sanders[18]	.78	810	0.81	900	Fick
Touche[30]	.94	560	0.75	1130	Indicator D.
Alverson[27]	.98	220	1.07	−4	Fick
Goldberg[3]	.91	600	0.86	700	Indicator D.
Chandraratna[4]	.97	420	0.96	410	Thermal
Dickinson[5]	.94	470	0.94	260	Fick
Huntsman[17]	.94	580	0.95	380	Thermal
Ihlen[26]	.96	700	0.81	1080	Thermal
Ihlen[26]	.90	700	0.82	270	Thermal
Labovitz[28]	.85	990	NA	NA	Thermal
Lewis[29]	.91	630	0.85	1100	Thermal
Magnin[21]*	.83	NA	0.60	3300	Thermal
Kosturakis[15]	.88	560	0.70	470	Thermal
Nishimura[16]	.94	780	1.00	−130	Thermal
Loeppky[25]	.84	610	0.84	440	Fick
Average	.90	616	.85	736	

Results of numerous reports of aortic or left ventricular outflow (LVOT) Doppler measurements of flow. Abbreviations: r = correlation coefficient value, SEE = standard error of the estimate, NA = not available. If certain data in the table were not presented by the authors, and if raw data were available, the appropriate statistic was computed and entered in the table. Comparison refers to the reference technique that was used as a comparison for Doppler flow measurement. The * after the data of Magnin refers to the fact that an alinear analysis technique was used. This technique substantially affected data. The reader is advised that different methodologies were used in the various studies. Although an average value is reported for r, SEE, slope and Y-intercept, this average is only conceptual and not intended to provide more information than is contained in individual studies.

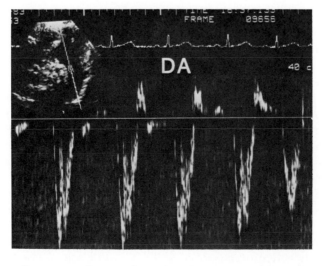

Fig. 5–11. Descending aortic velocity and sample volume position. DA – descending aorta.

We have confirmed, for a population, that mean ascending aorta velocity is similar to mean velocity in the descending aorta.[10] However, when paired data of individuals were analyzed, considerable discrepancy for individual measurements was noted. Thus substitution of an individual's mean descending aortic velocity for mean ascending aortic velocity is hazardous. One main reason for the discrepancy in mean velocities for an individual is that velocity spread made digitization of descending aortic velocity a speculative task. In view of the excellent results obtained from the ascending aorta via the suprasternal notch, with CW, and pulsed methods, descending aortic velocities will probably not find favor in the future for measurement of aortic flow.

Pulmonary Artery Flow

Pulmonary artery flow can be computed in most young individuals and in many older ones. The pulmonary artery is best imaged from a modified parasternal short axis location in children and adults, but in infants and toddlers it can also be imaged from the subcostal approach. The modification of the parasternal short axis that we use is a plane about halfway between the parasternal short axis and the plane of the long axis of the left ventricle. This plane was one that was originally called the long axis of the right ventricular outflow tract.[31] It is used because it allows a better alignment with the main pulmonary artery in some individuals than a standard high short axis. Unfortunately, the position of the pulmonary artery is closely related to that of the left lung, and this relationship often causes the lateral border of the pulmonary artery to be obscured. In order to reduce this problem and to allow improved pulmonary artery imaging and velocity recording, the patient can be placed in an extreme (90° or more) left decubitus position. This position, for many individuals, allows the pulmonary artery to be imaged separately from the lung and rib cage.[32] Subcostal pulmonary artery imaging is possible in the young and in occasional older individuals. Imaging from this position is explained in depth in the text by Williams and co-workers.[33]

MEASUREMENT OF PULMONARY ARTERY FLOW AREA

Pulmonary artery diameter is measured according to lateral resolution methods in both the parasternal short axis (Fig. 5–12) and subcostal planes (Fig. 5–13). We use hand calipers to measure the diameter at least in triplicate on stop frames obtained by slow videotape replay while the patient is still on the examining table. If images are inadequate, the imaging portion of the examination is repeated. No effort is made to select a timed measurement because the single time most representative of "the true measurement" is unknown. Accordingly, an effort is made to obtain an averaged value by measuring at random cardiac cycle times. An effort, however, is made to obtain frames showing the widest dimensions.

One problem that bears comment is that imaging of the pulmonary artery suggests that it markedly changes size between systole and diastole. This apparent change is principally due to a fixed transducer imaging a moving pulmonary artery. The apparent diameter decreases as the vessel moves out of field. The situation is shown pictorially in Figure 5–14. Study of cyclic change in canine pulmonary artery area showed that the maximal change was of the

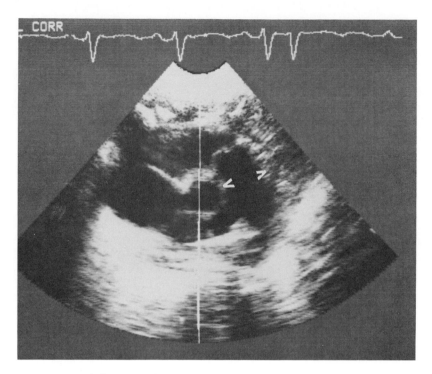

Fig. 5–12. Parasternal short axis plane showing pulmonary artery dimension. The < > markers indicate the diameter.

order of 12% under worst case circumstances (i.e. massive alterations in circulating volume), whereas changes at rest were less than half this value.[1]

RECORDING PULMONARY VELOCITIES

Initially, the sample volume is placed in the distal main pulmonary artery and the Doppler cursor is aligned with the pulmonary artery walls (Fig. 5–12). Next small motions of the transducer in the visual plane are made to record the highest velocity and least spectral broadening. Once alignment in these two axes is achieved, alignment in the third axis can be sought by moving the transducer in small increments in the superior inferior axis. The record containing the highest velocity and least spectral broadening is then recorded for digitization. An example is shown in Figure 5–15. Pulmonary velocities should not be angle corrected. This view on angle correction stems from several bases: (1) non-corrected flows generally match simultaneous invasively measured flows, (2) the alignment technique generally corrects for any initial beam-flow malalignment, (3) if malalignment occurs, the spatial value of the malalignment is totally speculative, since the walls, which themselves do not define flow direction, can be seen in only two axes at a time, and (4) pulmonary flow is imaged from either parasternal short axis or subcostal plane is generally aligned with beam direction. Color-coded Doppler has not offered much assistance for suggesting altered pulmonary flow paths in normal flows.

PULMONARY FLOW RESULTS

Few studies have been published which relate results of Doppler and invasive pulmonary flows. The first two reports regarded pulmonary flows in chil-

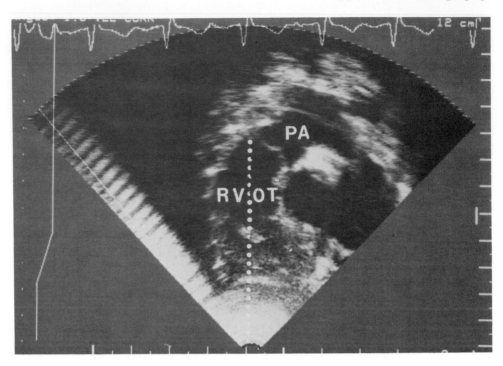

Fig. 5–13. Inverted subcostal position for right ventricular outflow tract (RVOT) imaging. Dotted line shows approximate Doppler cursor position. Pulmonary artery (PA) is not well aligned for Doppler velocities.

dren.[3,27] In one report the correlation coefficient related paired measurements was only +.72. However, when flow area was measured by angiography the correlation coefficient improved to +.94 (Fig. 5–16).[3] This difference in correlation meant that (1) mean velocities were probably accurate and (2) the earliest ultrasonic diameter measurements of the pulmonary artery were probably inaccurate. The inaccuracy arose mainly because of poor imaging of the lateral wall. It was after this finding that we began using the extreme left decubitus position and measurement of multiple diameters from videotape replay with the patient still on the examination table for possible further imaging. In the next study a high correlation was achieved between the pulmonary and aortic flow[32] (Fig. 5–17). Early results for pulmonary flows have since been reconfirmed.[18,28,34] Recently, another study[5] of simultaneous invasive (Fick) and Doppler cardiac outputs were compared and a correlation slightly weaker than that for the aorta was found. More importantly, a larger standard error of the estimate (approximately 800 ml) than reported for Doppler aortic flow measurement (approximately 500 ml) was found. The standard error of the estimate for a regression is the equivalent of a standard deviation for a mean. Accordingly, the data can be interpreted as meaning that even under quite good circumstances, more variability in paired measurements occurs for Doppler measurement of pulmonary flow as compared to aortic flow. Comparative data for reported studies of pulmonary artery flow are summarized in Table 5–2. Accurate pulmonary diameter measurement remains the key to accurate Doppler pulmonary flow measurement.

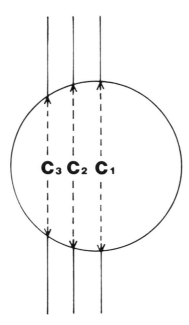

Fig. 5–14. Intercepts of a circle. Numerous chords (C) of a circle can be intercepted by a stationary beam. This figure represents a cross-sectional plane of great vessel. The transducer is stationary and placed at C1. The great vessel moves during the cardiac cycle, however, and the stationary transducer may then intercept chord 2 or chord 3. The examiner may get the impression of a large change in vessel diameter although most of the change is probably due to vessel motion to the right.

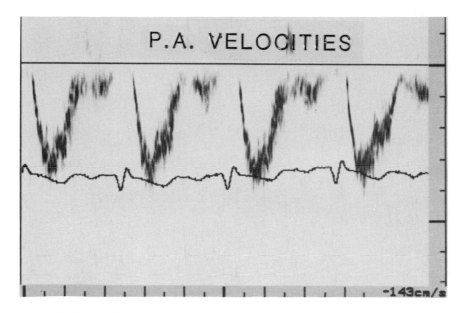

Fig. 5–15. Typical pulmonary artery velocity.

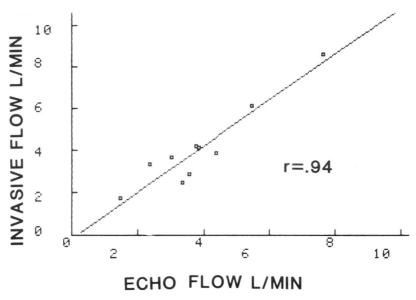

Fig. 5–16. Pulmonary flow. Comparison of invasive and Doppler echo (echo) flow measurement. These flows were performed simultaneously by indicator dilution and Doppler echocardiography.[3]

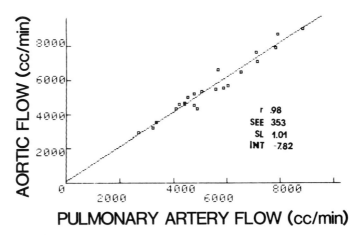

Fig. 5–17. Comparison of aortic flow and pulmonary artery flow obtained within several minutes from each individual. A high correlation is shown and slope approaches 1.0. This figure demonstrates that Doppler flow measurements in the aorta and pulmonary artery produce almost identical results.[32]

Table 5–2.   Main Pulmonary Artery Flow

First Author	r=	SEE	Slope	Y-intercept	Comparison
Sanders[18]	.88	240	1.43	370	Fick
Dickinson[5]	.94	840	0.96	730	Fick
Goldberg[3]	.72	1110	1.11	− 230	Green Dye
Goldberg[3]*	.94	510	0.79	800	Green Dye
Labovitz[28]	.81	820	NA	NA	Thermal
Lang-Jensen[34]	.80	NA	NA	NA	Thermal

Abbreviations and methods for constructing the table were similar to those cited for table 5–1. The * indicates that this set of data was computed using angiographic vessel diameter.

Tricuspid Flow

To date, only three publications document measurement of tricuspid flow.[5,32,35] Accordingly, greater experience will have to be obtained with this measurement, but initial results are extremely encouraging.

RECORDING OF TRICUSPID VELOCITIES

Imaging is performed from the apical four-chamber plane. The transducer is positioned in the short axis four chamber apical plane that allows the septum to occupy the central position of the imaging cone (Fig. 5–18). In this position, alignment of the cursor parallel to tricuspid inflow is possible. Usually, as shown by color-coded Doppler, flow passes at right angles to the plane of the annulus and generally parallel to the septum. The optimal position for the sample volume is within the right ventricle just distal to the annulus. Once the sample volume has been positioned and the signal obtained in the two visualized dimensions, small movements of the transducer can be made in the third axis (mainly a superior-inferior motion) to optimize velocity. Considerable respiratory variation is present in tricuspid velocity, and, therefore, the most reliable mean velocity can be obtained by digitizing a number of beats. Tricuspid velocity is digitized according to the same rules as used for aortic and pulmonary velocity, but digitization, in this case, is for diastolic velocity. During systole the baseline is digitized. Angle correction is not used for tricuspid velocities. Alignment from the apical plane is relatively easy.

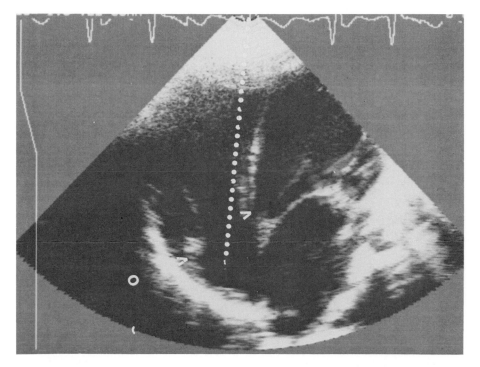

Fig. 5–18. Figure of tricuspid position with septum in mid cone. Dotted line shows best starting Doppler cursor position. < and > show points for diameter measurement.

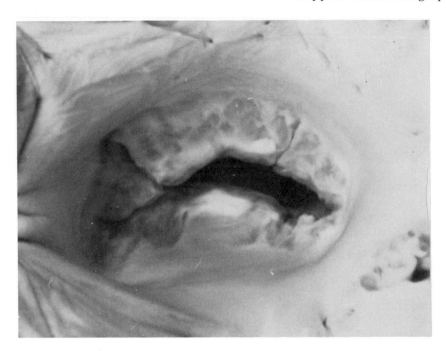

Fig. 5–19. Mitral valve photographed from the left atrium with low flow (water) passing through the leaflets. The anterior leaflet is at the top and the posterior is at the bottom. Note that the annulus is shaped like a flattened ellipse.

TRICUSPID WAVEFORMS

Waveforms are usually well demarcated except when recorded from individuals who have a large annulus. In this instance, considerable velocity spread may be encountered. If modal velocity is not well demarcated, mean velocity should not be computed. A wide velocity spread occurs relatively infrequently, but we have not yet identified a specific valve area above which identification of modal velocity is usually a problem. No angle correction appears necessary.

TRICUSPID FLOW AREA

The major assumption is that the tricuspid ring, at least during diastole, approximates a circle. Examination of the orifice visually suggests that this assumption is reasonable. Using this assumption, investigators have recommended measuring the orifice diameter at the valve ring.[5,32,35] Since tricuspid orifice diameter is imaged in lateral resolution, measurement is from endocardial surface to endocardial surface at the base of the two visualized leaflets as demonstrated in Figure 5–18. Since ring size may change or appear to change between systole and diastole, measurements are performed at maximal leaflet opening. The major problem that can occur for this measurement is imaging a foreshortened plane of the annulus. This is best avoided, in most subjects, by imaging in a plane which demonstrates that the septum is in the center of the sector, descending from the apex of the cone (Fig. 5–18).

TRICUSPID FLOW MEASUREMENT RESULTS

Three reports, to date, have compared tricuspid flows to a standard. Meijboom and co-workers[35] used the method previously outlined except that they used angle corrected velocities. They found a correlation coefficient of .98 (SEE = 430 ml) relating Doppler tricuspid and thermodilution flows. In that study, Doppler flows were measured immediately before or after thermodilution determinations. Dickenson et al.[5] used the described tricuspid Doppler flow method without angle correction and found a correlation coefficient of .96 and a standard error of the estimate of 620 ml when Doppler tricuspid flow was compared to flows measured simultaneously by the Fick technique. The only other report compared tricuspid flow to a Doppler standard.[32] They compared tricuspid flow to sequentially measured Doppler aortic flow and found a correlation coefficient of .94, SEE of 609 ml, and slope near unity and essentially no intercept. All three studies demonstrated a slope near unity and no significant Y axis intercept. Since slopes different from unity and significant intercepts suggest systematic error, it is interesting to note that tricuspid is the only post valve flow area which failed to demonstrate a systematic error of any magnitude. Although additional confirmation and investigation seems advisable, these several studies suggest that tricuspid flows measured by Doppler closely approximate flows measured by other methods.

Mitral Valve Flow

Doppler computation of mitral valve flow presents at least two aspects that are different from aortic, pulmonary or tricuspid flows. These differences include (1) inspection of the mitral valve clearly demonstrates that the annulus is more like a flattened ellipse than a circle (Fig. 5–19) and (2) imaging of the mitral valve from the four chamber plane suggests that flow might pass at an angle to the septum. However, color-coded Doppler demonstrates that mitral flow progresses generally parallel to the free wall, reaches the apex, then turns to flow in a nearly parallel stream along the septum and into the aorta.

The first technique for measuring mitral valve flow was proposed by Fisher et al.[36] They reasoned that the mitral orifice area change during the cardiac cycle was mirrored by the M-mode echogram. Accordingly an attempt was made to "adjust" annulus area by a factor determined from the average M-mode orifice. They recommended approximating mean area in the following manner: First, the maximal mitral orifice is located in the short axis plane after the technique of Henry et al.,[37] the so-called "fishmouth" plane of the mitral valve. The maximal orifice at this level was then digitized. They suggested that maximal orifice existed only for a short time during diastole, so they attempted to compute the mean orifice area. Anterior and posterior leaflets were imaged at chordal level by M-mode. Maximal leaflet separation, which should correspond to maximal mitral area observed by two-dimensional echocardiography, was measured. The area of leaflet separation on M-mode was determined, and the result was divided by the duration of leaflet separation. The quotient is the average opening of the mitral valve in millimeters. The average opening was then divided by the maximal opening to determine the percentage of the maximum that is represented by the mean. This percentage was then multiplied by the area of the two-dimensional "fishmouth" area to yield the average mitral orifice area.

This method requires a number of measurements and areas. Mitral velocity was recorded by imaging the left ventricle from the apical four chamber short axis plane. The transducer was located to image the septum as vertically as possible to allow alignment of the sample volume close to parallel with flow. If the sample volume appeared to create a beam-flow intercept angle, as judged by the septum, angular correction was performed according to the cosine of the intercept angle. Mitral flow was computed as the product of mean velocity/minute and flow area.

This method, studied mainly in dogs, provided results that were comparable to flows measured by other methods.[36] When the method was applied to humans, conflicting results were found. Although Zhang and co-workers[38] found good results, others[32] found a low correlation with aortic flow (r = .59) and a large Y axis intercept (950 ml).

The next mitral valve flow report was by Lewis and co-workers.[29] These authors used the mitral orifice size imaged in the four chamber plane as a diameter of a circle and measured velocities just distal to the mitral annulus. Doppler results were compared to thermodilution results. They found a correlation coefficient of .87 and a standard error of the estimate of 590 ml. This method had certain benefits over the earlier method. The method was simple to apply and Doppler velocity was recorded in an area close to the annular measurement. No angular corrections were made. This method, however, might overestimate mitral annulus area because the annulus is more of a flattened ellipse than a circle (Fig. 5–19). The area of a flattened ellipse is smaller than that of a circle, and flow overestimation by the circular method is due to annular overestimation. On the other hand, Lewis et al. indicated that in their population no systematic over or underestimation occurred. One other problem with the circular method is that it is not possible to be certain that the flattened ellipse is cut the same in each subject. The ratio of the minor axis to the major axis of the flattened ellipse is approximately 0.75 (Fig. 5–20).[39] Accordingly, if the minor axis was measured in the first subject, the major axis in the second, and an in-between axis in the third, little standardization would be present (Fig. 5–20). All of these axes are available for imaging from the apex.

A variation on the Lewis method was reported.[39] Velocities were measured as detailed by Lewis et al. Mitral area was determined by a different method. The mitral orifice was imaged in short axis, either at the level of the annulus or at the level of the attachment of the mitral leaflets to the annulus. The former provided a fainter image, but leaflets were not evident. Measurements in this area were performed in early diastole. The latter area provided a stronger signal,

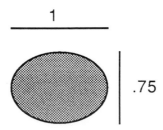

Fig. 5–20. An ellipse with a major axis of 1 unit and a minor axis of .75 units.

but area had to be measured in the first several frames following leaflet opening. Both gave similar results. Major axis was measured from leaflet junctions onto the annulus. The minor axis was measured by leading edge methodology at widest leaflet separation at annular level. Area was determined by the elliptical formula:

$$\text{area} = \text{major axis length (cm)} \times \text{minor axis length (cm)} \times \pi/4$$

Comparison of simultaneously obtained Fick outputs and Doppler mitral flows demonstrated a correlation coefficient of .93, a standard error of the estimate of 435 ml, but a slope of .81 and a Y intercept of 825 ml. The latter two data show a systematic error. When mitral Doppler flow was compared to sequentially determined Doppler aortic flow in this population, results improved to a correlation coefficient of .96, standard error of the estimate of 370 ml, slope of .93, and an intercept of 450 ml. When the Lewis method, with a modification to be mentioned, was used in this patient population and compared to Fick output, the correlation was .82, standard error of the estimate was 1024 ml, slope 1.01, and Y intercept 1656 ml. The major axis of the mitral valve was used for this computation rather than the mitral orifice measured as outlined by Lewis et al.

In summary, mitral Doppler methods are available for humans, but to date no method yields values that correlate with invasive results to the level of those obtained from the other valves.

Measurement of Flow in Other Cardiac Areas

Flow has been measured in other areas of the heart, but for these areas much less work has been accomplished and confirmatory studies are lacking in most instances.

Right ventricular outflow tract flow measurement in children was mentioned by Meijboom et al.[40] in a paper devoted to shunt measurement in dogs, and results were said to be good.

Left ventricular outflow tract flow measurement in adults was reported by Lewis et al.[29] The left ventricular outflow tract Doppler signal was interrogated in an apical short axis plane that imaged the ventricles, atria, and proximal ascending aorta. The aortic annulus was measured by M-mode echocardiography. No angle correction was used. Doppler results were compared to those of thermodilution. The correlation coefficient was .91, standard error of the estimate was 630 ml, slope was .85 and Y intercept was 1100 ml. Accordingly, this result, while useful, is not as favorable as results obtained from flow measurements of the ascending aorta from the suprasternal notch but some patients can not be studied from the suprasternal notch.

Quantitation of Semilunar Regurgitation

Direct Doppler quantitation of semilunar regurgitant flow is possible. Boughner,[41] using continuous wave echocardiography in patients with aortic regurgitation, demonstrated biphasic flow in the descending aorta. Further, he demonstrated that the integral of velocity representing retrograde flow and the integral of the velocity representing forward flow, when expressed as a regurgitant percentage, bore a strong correlation to regurgitation percentage measured by invasive means. Others later confirmed these results.[42] From this work it was but a small step to quantitation of semilunar regurgitant flow. Later investigators[43] proposed that the velocity profile in the highest portion of the ascending aorta before the curvature of the transverse aorta and in the most distal portion of the main pulmonary artery was far enough from the regurgitant valve to precede jet formation. Accordingly velocities in these areas were recorded and measured. Great vessel diameters were measured in the same location as the sample volume. Systolic velocities in the antegrade direction represented forward flow. Diastolic velocities in the great vessels were assumed to represent regurgitant flow (Fig. 5–21). Both passed through the same flow area. Accordingly, two determinations of mean velocity were required, one in systole and a second in diastole. Two immediately apparent problems remained for solution. The first was that the total velocity magnitude of systole and diastole would exceed the Nyquist limit in a number of patients with regurgitation. The second problem was to create an internal check to offer assurance that the jet created by the regurgitation was not being interrogated. The solution to the first problem is shown in Figure 5–22. The zero velocity baseline was set at the top of the tracing for pulmonary velocities and at the bottom of the tracing for aortic velocities. This action forced aliasing, which was then used to advantage. Figure 5–22 shows antegrade pulmonary velocity descending from the top baseline of the tracing and regurgitant velocity arising from the bottom baseline. Establishment of two baselines, one at the top of the tracing and one at the bottom, effectively doubles the Nyquist limit. (Suppose Nyquist limit for a given frequency and depth is + or − 100 cm/sec. Using full scale as positive only permits 200 cm/sec to be viewed without ambiguity. However,

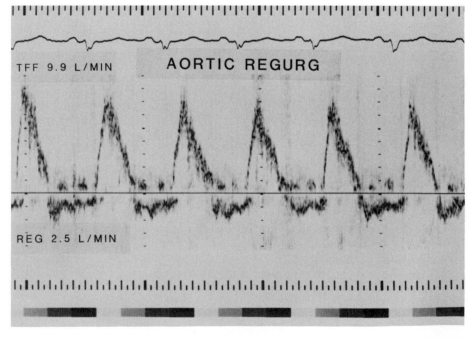

Fig. 5–21. Aortic regurgitation recorded in the mid ascending aorta distal to the position of jet formation. Note that diastolic velocity is lower than baseline, a position that indicates regurgitation (regurg). In this example total forward flow (TFF) was 9.9 L/min and regurgitation (REG) was 2.5 L/min.

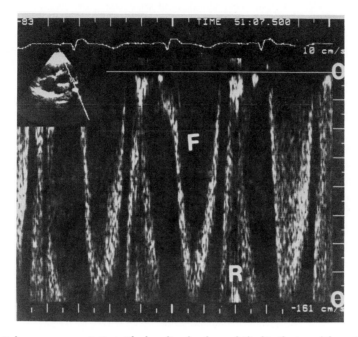

Fig. 5–22. Pulmonary regurgitation. The baseline has been shifted to the top of the velocity record. Forward flow (F) descends from the top baseline and regurgitation (R) ascends from the bottom of the velocity tracing. Note both baselines are marked zero velocity. P.A. = pulmonary artery and regurg = regurgitation. This method allows full velocity scale for both forward and regurgitant flow. (Reprinted with permission of the Am J Cardiol.[43])

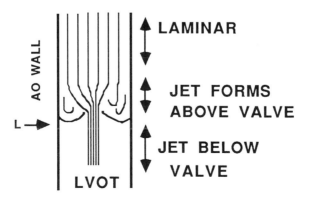

Fig. 5–23. A pictorial diagram of diastolic blood flow in the ascending aorta and left ventricular outflow tract (LVOT) in a patient with aortic valvular regurgitation (regurg). Note that well above the aortic leaflets (L) flow is laminar and without jet formation. This is the proper area for quantitative flow to be measured in a patient with aortic regurgitation. Closer to the valve, but still distal to it, jet formation is beginning. Flow measurement in this area will result in inaccuracy because the flow area is unknown. Proximal to the leaflets a typical jet is formed.

use of the described method for regurgitant velocities which go in opposite directions in systole and diastole now stretches the nonambiguous range to a total of 400 cm/sec) (200 cm/sec in each direction).

Resolution of the second problem was equally important. It seemed possible that regurgitant velocities could be recorded which would represent jet formation. In the left ventricular outflow tract, jets of the order of 5 to 6 m/sec are frequently found in patients with aortic regurgitation. Lower jet velocities are encountered in pulmonary valvular regurgitation. The jet begins to form just above the semilunar valve (Fig. 5–23), but velocities are somewhat lower than those encountered below the valve. Nonetheless, the objective is not to measure these jet velocities forming above the valve because their effective orifice would be difficult to ascertain. The objective is to measure the reversal of velocity in a portion of the great vessel which uses essentially all of the great vessel diameter as a flowpath. One useful clue during recording is that the diastolic flow velocity rarely has a peak beyond 1.5 m/sec and most regurgitant peaks do not exceed 1 m/sec. Higher velocities are probably recorded in the forming jet and the examiner is thus obligated to sample farther from the valve. However, a method which would confirm the volume of flow is desirable. If the patient has no other cardiac malformation, the volume flow past a normal valve should be equal to total forward flow minus regurgitant flow at the insufficient semilunar valve. This proved to be true in the studied population (Fig. 5–24).

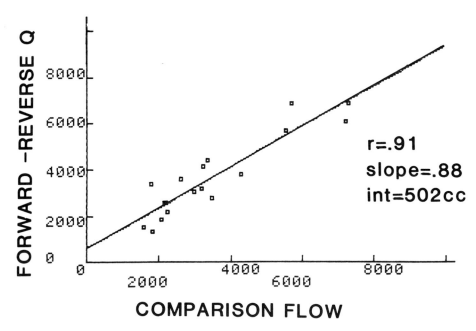

Fig. 5–24. Semilunar regurgitation. Flow on the vertical axis is the difference between forward and reverse flow. On the horizontal axis is the comparison flow (flow in another area of the heart). Each point represents one patient with semilunar insufficiency. Int = intercept. If the volume of regurgitation was precisely computed, each point on the Y-axis should match with one of similar value on the X-axis. (Reprinted with permission of the Am J Cardiol.[43])

This quantitative method has certain limitations in addition to the caveats already mentioned. One limitation is that the method requires normal flow at some point in the heart for the comparison flow. Further, shunt lesions could provide misleading information. Finally, if the affected valve is also stenotic, forward flow can not be computed unless the valve area is known.

Measurement of Mitral Regurgitation

Although qualitative methods have been reported for detecting or estimating mitral regurgitation,[44-45] few reports have had direct quantitation of regurgitation as their goal. Although no report has specifically directed attention toward mere subtraction of aortic flow (or pulmonary or tricuspid flow if they are normal) from mitral flow, this would appear to be a direct approach. Blumlein et al.[46] published a method which has some aspects of the above suggested method. The investigators report a two-dimensional echocardiographic method for computing left ventricular volume change, the value of which is equivalent to mitral inflow. Aortic flow measured by the CW Doppler technique is subtracted from this value. The authors compared this value to results of scintigraphy or cardiac catheterization. At catheterization a ventricular volume method was used to approximate mitral inflow and pulmonary thermodilution was used to approximate systemic flow. They found a correlation of .82 with catheterization measurements and a correlation of .89 with scintigraphy. The catheterization relationship had a slope of 1 and no appreciable intercept but a large SEE of 14%. The scintigraphy relationship had a 12% intercept and a slope of .7 and a lower SEE of 9%. These data suggest that the technique, while cumbersome, bears a definite relationship to mitral regurgitation measured by other techniques.

PULMONARY TO SYSTEMIC FLOW RATIOS

Pulmonary to systemic flow ratios are useful for indicating shunt flow in terms that are relative. Methodology for determining the shunt ratio reverts back to the flow methodology for each area. The questions of interest in this area are: (1) How much variability occurs between flows in individuals without shunts? (2) How often can the appropriate flows be measured? (3) What is the accuracy of the measurements compared to an invasive standard? (4) Which are the most appropriate flows for measurement in the more common lesions?

HOW MUCH VARIABILITY OCCURS BETWEEN FLOWS IN INDIVIDUALS WITHOUT SHUNTS?

Studies conducted in individuals without shunts indicate that the limits of shunt ratios under these conditions appears to be .8 to 1.2.[5] This range is not surprising since similar ranges are found during catheterization. Further, this range could be explained by considering that if each flow had an error of 10% and errors are both in the same direction, the range would be exactly that reported. Clearly, additive errors would be statistically less common than cancelling errors, so most patients will cluster closer to the center of the range.

HOW OFTEN CAN THE APPROPRIATE FLOWS BE MEASURED?

Most often this is not a problem; however, two flows, aortic and pulmonary, may present problems in some patients. Use of an off-axis transducer, in experienced hands, will allow aortic flows to be measured in at least 80% of adults and greater than 96% of children. Pulmonary flows can be measured in most children but ability to measure pulmonary flows falls off in adults, particularly older ones and those who smoke. Fortunately, pulmonary flows are not often needed in adults. Tricuspid and mitral flows can be measured in essentially all children and almost all adults.

WHAT IS THE ACCURACY OF MEASUREMENTS COMPARED TO AN INVASIVE STANDARD?

Table 5–3 contains data abstracted from reported studies of flow ratios studied by Doppler and by invasive means. These data support the proposition that flow ratios measured by Doppler and invasive means are sufficiently similar for clinical usage.

WHICH ARE THE MOST APPROPRIATE FLOWS FOR MEASUREMENT IN THE MORE COMMON LESIONS?

In the normal heart flows past the several valves must be equal. Accordingly, a set of identities can be constructed as follows:

Tricuspid Flow = Pulmonary Flow = Mitral Flow = Aortic Flow

ATRIAL SEPTAL DEFECT (ASD) QP:QS

For patients with ASD, shunted flow plus systemic flow passes through both the tricuspid and pulmonary valves. Flow through mitral and aortic valves is equal to that which leaves the left heart and is, therefore, systemic flow. Accordingly, the QP:QS can be computed as:

$$\text{ASD QP:QS} = \frac{\text{Tricuspid or Pulmonary Flow}}{\text{Aortic or Mitral Flow}}$$

Another determination would occur by measuring all four flows and making the following computation:

$$\text{ASD QP:QS} = \frac{(\text{Tricuspid + Pulmonary Flow})/2}{(\text{Aortic + Mitral Flow})/2}$$

Table 5–3.   Ratio of Pulmonary to Systemic Flow by Doppler

First Author	r =	SEE	Slope	Y-intercept	Comparison
Barron[47]	0.85	0.48	0.68	0.49	OXY, RN
Kitabatake[48]	0.92	0.28	1.11	0.30	OXY
Marx[6]	0.85	0.27	0.91	0.22	OXY
Marx[6]	0.60	0.51	0.71	0.73	RN
Meijboom[40]	0.89	0.30	NA	NA	Green Dye
Sanders[18]	0.88	NA	0.97	0.20	OXY
Valdes-Cruz[50]	0.91	0.30	0.86	0.15	Dye Curve
Dickinson[5]	0.92	0.37	0.90	0.28	OXY
Meyer[49]	0.89	0.61	0.75	0.44	OXY
Average	0.86	0.39	0.86	0.35	

Abbreviations and methods for constructing the table were similar to those cited for Table 5–1. RN = Radionuclide. The number of patients in this series was small.

VENTRICULAR SEPTAL DEFECT (VSD) QP:QS

In patients with a VSD, tricuspid and aortic flows represent systemic flow and pulmonary and mitral flows contain both systemic flow and the shunt. VSD QP:QS can be computed as follows:

$$\text{VSD QP:QS} = \frac{\text{Pulmonary or Mitral Flow}}{\text{Tricuspid or Aortic Flow}}$$

A possibly more accurate determination would occur by measuring all four flows and making the following computation:

$$\text{VSD QP:QS} = \frac{(\text{Pulmonary + Mitral Flow})/2}{(\text{Tricuspid + Aortic Flow})/2}$$

PATENT DUCTUS ARTERIOSUS (PDA) QP:QS

Estimation of the QP:QS ratio through a PDA is slightly less intuitive than the prior two flows. Systemic flow can be best measured as venous return through the tricuspid valve. Pulmonary flow in patients with this lesion is unreliable because flow here is frequently turbulent and because flow varies in different portions of the pulmonary artery. Pulmonary flow is equal to pulmonary venous return which can be measured at the mitral valve or at the aortic level. Accordingly, PDA QP:QS can be computed as:

PDA QP:QS = (Aortic or Mitral Flow)/Tricuspid Flow

A possibly more accurate determination would occur by measuring all three flows and making the following computation:

$$\text{PDA QP:QS} = \frac{(\text{Aortic + Mitral Flow})/2}{\text{Tricuspid Flow}}$$

Clearly, more complex and multiple shunts occur and principles delineated in those examples can be used to solve for shunt ratios in most cases.

CAVEATS FOR FLOW MEASUREMENT

1. Align the Doppler beam parallel to flow in three dimensions.

2. Digitize the modal velocity of curves which have the highest velocity and least velocity spread.
3. Return digitization to baseline during the part of the cardiac cycle when flow does not normally pass through the area.
4. Digitize many cycles; stroke volume varies.
5. Measure diameters at the location of the center of the sample volume, preferably with hand calipers.
6. For great vessels, measure the widest diameter.
7. Never pass the opportunity to measure several flows in the same patient.
8. If you correlate Doppler to invasive flows, remember:
   a. Invasively measured flows are not pure gold as a standard.
   b. Flows vary from time to time; compare simultaneous flows.
   c. A correspondence within 10% is all that should be expected.
9. Flow measurement requires practice and correlation.
10. Patience and experience are necessary. Better results should be expected after the first several hundred than after the first fifteen.

REFERENCES

1. Loeber, C.P., Goldberg, S.J., Marx, G.R., Carrier, M., Emery, R.W.: How much does aortic and pulmonary artery area vary during the cardiac cycle? Am Heart J *113*:95, 1987.
2. Mackenzie, J., Haiti Ne'er, Rawly, J.: Method of assessing the reproducibility of blood flow measurement: factors influencing the performance of thermal dilution cardiac output computers. Br Heart J *55*:14, 1986.
3. Goldberg, S.J., Sahn, D.J., Allen, H.D., Valdes-Cruz, L.M., Hoenecke, H., Carnahan, Y.: Evaluation of pulmonary and systemic blood flow by two-dimensional Doppler echocardiography using fast Fourier transform spectral analysis. Am J Cardiol *50*:1394, 1982.
4. Chandraratna, P.A., Nanna, M., McKay, C., Nimalasuriya, A., Swinney, R., Elkayam, U., Rahimtoola, S.H.: Determination of cardiac output by transcutaneous continuous-wave ultrasonic Doppler computer. Am J Cardiol *53*:234, 1984.
5. Dickinson, D.F., Goldberg, S.J., Wilson, N.: A comparison of information obtained by ultrasound examination and cardiac catheterization in paediatric patients with congenital heart disease. Intl J Cardiol *9*:275, 1985.
6. Marx, G.R., Allen, H.D., Goldberg, S.J., Flinn, C.J.: Transatrial septal velocity measurement by Doppler echocardiography in atrial septal defect: Correlation with QP:QS ratio. Am J Cardiol *55*:1162, 1985.
7. Gibbs, J.L., Wilson, N., Witsenburg, M., Williams, G.J., Goldberg, S.J.: Diastolic forward blood flow in the pulmonary artery detected by Doppler echocardiography. J Am Coll Cardiol *6*:1322, 1985.
8. Hatle, L., Angelsen, B.: Doppler Ultrasound in Cardiology, 2nd Ed., Philadelphia, Lea & Febiger, 1985.
9. Loeber, C.P., Goldberg, S.J., Donnerstein, R.L., Butler, M.A.: Time variability of cardiac output and stroke volume in subjects without cardiac disease. Am J Cardiol *59*:967, 1987.
10. Wilson, N., Goldberg, S.J., Allen, H.D., Marx, G.R., Loeber, C.P.: Does transducer selection affect aortic arch velocities? Am Heart J *113*:878, 1987.
11. Hegesh, J.T., Stanley, S.J., Schwartz, M.L.: Analysis of causes of velocity spread during initial deceleration in the ascending aorta in children and young adults. Am J Cardiol (in press) 1987.
12. Gardin, J.M., Iseri, L.T., Elkayam, U., Tobias, J., Childs, W., Burns, C.S., Henry, W.L.: Evaluation of dilated cardiomyopathy by pulsed Doppler echocardiography. Am Heart J *106*:1057, 1983.
13. Donnerstein, R.L., Marx, G.R.: A simplified method for determining Doppler velocity areas for cardiac output calculation. (abstr) Circulation (in press), 1987.
14. Marx, G.R., Goldberg, S.J., Allen, H.D.: Two methods for measurement of ascending aortic diameter by 2-D echocardiography as compared with cineangiography. Am Heart J *112*:172, 1986.
15. Kosturakis, D., Allen, H.D., Goldberg, S.J., Sahn, D.J., Valdes-Cruz, L.M.: Noninvasive quantification of stenotic semilunar valve areas by Doppler echocardiography. J Am Coll Cardiol *3*:1256, 1984.
16. Nishimura, R.A., Callahan, M.J., Schaff, H.V., Ilstrup, D.M., Miller, F.A., Tajik, A.J.: Noninvasive measurement of cardiac output by continuous wave Doppler echocardiography: Initial experience and review of the literature. Mayo Clin Proc *59*:484, 1984.
17. Huntsman, L.L., Stewart, D.K., Barnes, S.R., Franklin, S.B., Colocousis, J.S., Hessel, E.A.: Noninvasive Doppler determination of cardiac output in man: Clinical validation. Circulation *67*:593, 1983.

18. Sanders, S.P., Yeager, S., Williams, R.G.: Measurement of systemic and pulmonary blood flow and QP:QS ratio using Doppler and two-dimensional echocardiography. Am J Cardiol *51*:952, 1983.

19. Schwartz, M., Goldberg, S., Wilson, N., Allen, H., Marx, G.: Relation of Still's murmur, small aortic diameter and high aortic velocity. Am J Cardiol *57*:1344, 1986.

20. Sequeira, R.F., Light, L.H., Cross, G., Raftery, E.B.: Transcutaneous aortovelography. A quantitative evaluation. Br Heart J *38*:443, 1976.

21. Magnin, P.A., Stewart, J.A., Myers, S., von Ramm, O., Kisslo, J.A.: Combined Doppler and phased-array echocardiographic estimation of cardiac output. Circulation *63*:388, 1981.

22. Colocousis, J.S., Huntsman, L.L., Curreri, P.W.: Estimation of stroke volume changes by ultrasonic Doppler. Circulation *56*:914, 1977.

23. Huntsman, L.L., Gams, E., Johnson, C.C., Fairbanks, E.: Transcutaneous determination of aortic blood-flow velocities in man. Am Heart J *89*:605, 1975.

24. Light, H.: Transcutaneous aortovelography—a new window on the circulation? Br Heart J *38*:433, 1976.

25. Loeppky, J.A., Hoekenga, D.E., Greene, E.R., Luft, U.C.: Comparison of noninvasive pulsed Doppler and Fick measurements of stroke volume in cardiac patients. Am Heart J *107*:339, 1984.

26. Ihlen, H., Amlie, J.P., Dale, J., Forfang, K., Nitter-Hauge, S., Otterstad, J.E., Simonsen, S., Myhre, E.: Determination of cardiac output by Doppler echocardiography. Br Heart J *51*:54, 1984.

27. Alverson, D.C., Eldridge, M., Dillon, T., Yabek, S.M., Berman, W., Jr.: Noninvasive pulsed Doppler determination of cardiac output in neonates and children. J Pediatr *101*:46, 1982.

28. Labovitz, A.J., Buckingham, T.A., Habermehl, K., Nelson, J., Kennedy, H.L., Williams, G.: The effects of sampling site on the two-dimensional echo-Doppler determination of cardiac output. Am Heart J *109*:327, 1985.

29. Lewis, J., Kuo, L., Nelson, J., Limacher, M., Quinones, M.: Pulsed Doppler echocardiographic determination of stroke volume and cardiac output: Clinical validation of two new methods using the apical window. Circulation *70*:425, 1984.

30. Touche, T., Vervin, P., Curien, N., Merillon, J.P., Gourgon, R.: Cardiac output measurement in adult patients with combined Doppler and two-dimensional echocardiography. (abstr). Circulation *66*(II):121, 1982.

31. Goldberg, S.J., Allen, H.D., Sahn, D.J.: Pediatric and Adolescent Echocardiography. A Handbook. 1st Ed., Chicago, Yearbook Medical Publishers, Inc., 1975.

32. Loeber, C.P., Goldberg, S.J., Allen, H.D.: Doppler echocardiographic comparison of flows distal to the four cardiac valves. J Am Coll Cardiol *4*:268, 1984.

33. Williams, R.G., Bierman, F.Z., and Saunders, S.P.: Echocardiographic Diagnosis of Cardiac Malformations, Boston, Little Brown & Co., 1986.

34. Lang-Jensen, T., Berning, J., Jacobsen, E.: Stroke volume measured by pulsed ultrasound Doppler and M-mode echocardiography. Acta Anaesthesiol Scand *27*:454, 1983.

35. Meijboom, E.J., Horowitz, S., Valdes-Cruz, L.M., Sahn, D.J., Larson, D.F., Lima, C.O.: A Doppler echocardiographic method for calculating volume flow across the tricuspid valve: Correlative laboratory and clinical studies. Circulation *71*:551, 1985.

36. Fisher, D.C., Sahn, D.J., Friedman, M.J., Larson, D., Valdes-Cruz, L.M., Horowitz, S., Goldberg, S.J., Allen, H.D.: The mitral valve orifice method for noninvasive two-dimensional echo Doppler determinations of cardiac output. Circulation *67*:872, 1983.

37. Henry, W.I., Griffith Jittery, Michaelis, L.L., McIntosh, C.L., Morrow, A.G., Epstein, S.E.: Measurement of mitral valve orifice area in patients with mitral valve disease by real-time two-dimensional echocardiography. Circulation *51*:827, 1975.

38. Zhang, Y., Nitter-Hauge, S., Ihlen, H., Rootwelt, K., Myhre, E.: Measurement of aortic regurgitation by Doppler echocardiography. Br Heart J *55*:32, 1986.

39. Goldberg, S.J., Dickinson, D.F., Wilson, N.: Evaluation of an elliptical area technique for calculation of mitral flow by Doppler echocardiography. Br Heart J *54*:68, 1985.

40. Meijboom, E.J., Valdes-Cruz, L.M., Horowitz, S., Sahn, D.J., Larson, D.F., Lima, C.O., Goldberg, S.J., Allen, H.D.: A two-dimensional Doppler echocardiographic method for calculation of pulmonary and systemic blood flow in a canine model with a variable-sized left-to-right extracardiac shunt. Circulation *68*:437, 1983.

41. Boughner, D.R.: Assessment of aortic insufficiency by transcutaneous Doppler ultrasound. Circulation *52*:874, 1975.

42. Quinones, B.H.J., Quinones, M.A., Young, J.B., Waggoner, A.D., Ostojic, M.C., Ribeiro, L.G.T., Miller, L.L.: Assessment of pulsed Doppler echocardiography in detection and quantification of aortic and mitral regurgitation. Br Heart J *44*:612, 1980.

43. Goldberg, S.J., Allen, H.D.: Quantitative assessment by Doppler echocardiography of pulmonary or aortic regurgitation. Am J Cardiol *56*:131, 1985.

44. Stevenson, J.G., Kawabori, I., Guntheroth, W.G.: Differentiation of ventricular septal defect from mitral regurgitation by pulsed Doppler echocardiography. Circulation *56*:14, 1977.

45. Shah, A.A, Quinones, M.A., Waggoner, A.D., Barndt, R., Miller R.R.: Pulsed Doppler echo-cardiographic detection of mitral regurgitation in mitral valve prolapse; Correlation with cardiac arrhythmias. Cathet Cardiovasc Diagn *8*:437, 1982.
46. Blumlein, S., Bouchard, A., Schiller, N., Dae, M., Byrd, B., Ports, T., Botvinick, E.: Quantitation of mitral regurgitation by Doppler echocardiography. Circulation *74*:306, 1986.
47. Barron, J.V., Sahn, D.J., Valdes-Cruz, L.M., Lima, C.O., Grenadier, E., Allen, H.D., Goldberg, S.J.: Quantitation of the ratio by pulmonary:systemic blood flow in patients with ventricular septal defect by two-dimensional range gated Doppler echocardiography. (abstr) Circulation *66*:318, 1982.
48. Kitabatake, A., Inoue, M., Asao, M., Ito, H., Masuyama, T., Tanouchi, J., Morita, T., Hori, M, Yoshima, H.: Noninvasive evaluation of the ratio of pulmonary to systemic flow in atrial septal defect by duplex Doppler echocardiography. Circulation *69*:73, 1984.
49. Meyer, R.A., Kalavathy, A., Korfhagen, J.C., Kaplan, S.: Comparison of left-to-right shunt ratios determined by pulsed Doppler/2D-echo and Fick method. (abstr). Circulation *66*(II):232, 1982.
50. Valdes-Cruz, L.M., Horowitz, S., Mesel, E., Sahn, D.J., Fisher, D.C., Larson, D.: A pulsed Doppler echocardiographic method for calculating pulmonary and systemic blood flow in atrial level shunts: validation studies in animals and initial human experience. Circulation *69*:80, 1984.

CHAPTER **6**

CLINICAL APPLICATION OF DOPPLER DETECTED FLOW IN THE ABNORMAL CIRCULATION

The following chapter presents the Doppler echocardiographic findings in patients with abnormalities in flow direction or magnitude. These abnormalities represent altered flow states. Not all altered flow states are discussed in this chapter; however, a spectrum of defects has been chosen to demonstrate the potential of Doppler echocardiography for diagnosis and estimation of severity of disease. Many of these flow defects have an associated pressure drop that can be used to characterize the defect and estimate intracardiac pressures. Since pressure drop is discussed in detail in Chapter 4, it will not be repeated in this chapter.

Application of Doppler Cardiac Output Measurement

Doppler cardiac output measurement has extensive clinical application; it is noninvasive, can be performed expeditiously, and does not have the associated morbidity of indwelling cardiac catheters. Baseline cardiac output measurements can be obtained in the outpatient clinic, emergency room, and intensive care unit.[1-5] As an example, Figure 6–1 is the Doppler tracing obtained from a patient with a severe cardiomyopathy. Doppler velocity and aortic diameter measurements were obtained from the suprasternal notch using an off-axis transducer. Cardiac output was quickly computed using an off-line computer, digitizing pad and dedicated software program.[6] Total time for measurements and computation was approximately 5 minutes. The printout includes patient profile data, heart rate, cardiac output and stroke volume (Fig. 6–1).

Figures 6–2 and 6–3 demonstrate Doppler cardiac output determinations in two critically ill patients who presented with low cardiac output and the velocity equivalent of mechanical alternans.[4,7] Figure 6–2 shows Doppler tracings from a patient who was immediately postoperative from a Fontan operation. Peak aortic velocities and ejection times were markedly reduced in this patient (Fig. 6–2A), and Doppler calculated cardiac output was extremely low. Ascending aortic velocities were further reduced during the positive pressure phase of the ventilator. Velocities in the right atrial-to-pulmonary artery anastomosis showed low amplitude continuous velocities (Fig. 6–2B). Absence

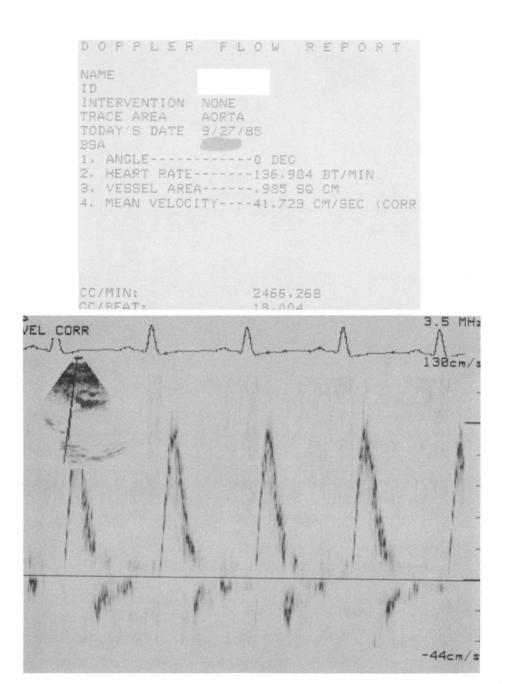

Fig. 6–1. Ascending aortic velocities from the suprasternal notch in a patient with severe cardiomyopathy. The Doppler flow report shows a cardiac output of 2.5 liters/min.

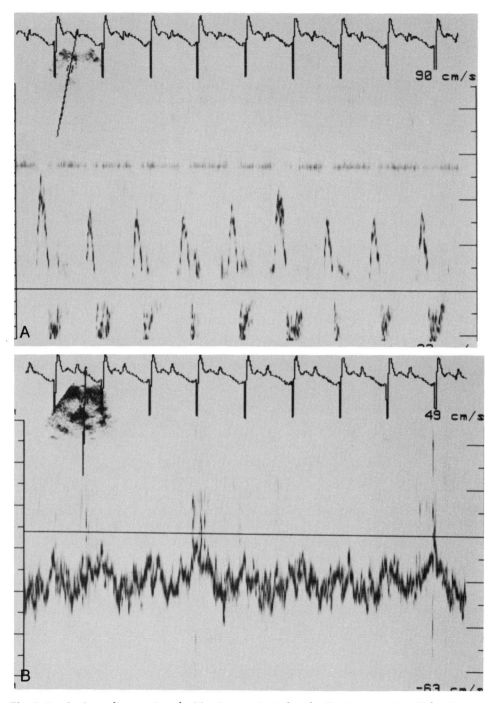

Fig. 6–2. A. Ascending aortic velocities in a patient after the Fontan operation. Velocities are decreased, and the ejection time short. Decreased peak velocities occurred during the positive pressure phase of the respirator. B. Doppler velocity tracings in the right atrial-pulmonary artery anastomosis.

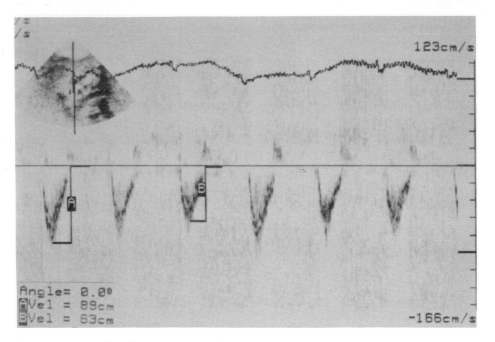

Fig. 6–3. Decreased pulmonary artery velocities in an infant with severe lung disease and low cardiac output.

of change in amplitude with respiration was indicative of abnormal flow.[8] Figure 6–3 shows pulmonary velocity tracings from an infant with severe lung disease on high pressure and high frequency ventilation. Time to peak velocity was 40 milliseconds, a value consistent with severe pulmonary artery hypertension.[9] Decreased flow velocities occurred on alternating beats during the positive pressure ventilator phase.

Doppler echocardiography can provide noninvasive assessment of response to drug therapy.[10–13] Figure 6–4A and B shows velocity tracings in two patients with mitral regurgitation, poor left ventricular function, and low cardiac output despite a dobutamine infusion. The clinical question was whether the patients would benefit from afterload reduction by an increase in cardiac output. The patient, whose tracing is shown in Figure 6–4A had no significant change in cardiac output during a nitroprusside infusion dose of 3.0 mcg/kg/min. However, the other patient (Fig. 6–4B) increased cardiac output during an infusion dose of 2.5 mcg/kg/min.

Doppler is also useful for evaluating patients with dysrhythmias.[14] Figure 6–5 shows pulmonary velocity tracings from a patient with atrial bigeminy. Atrial premature beats were associated with reduced stroke volume, shown as reduced area under the time velocity curve. Figure 6–6A shows pulmonary velocity tracings from a patient with supraventricular tachycardia (heart rate 260 beats per minute), and low cardiac output. Velocity alternans was present with a peak velocity of 25 to 30 cm/s. After conversion to normal sinus rhythm, heart rate decreased to 165 beats per minute and peak aortic Doppler velocities increased to 65 cm/s (Fig. 6–6B). The alternans pattern disappeared.

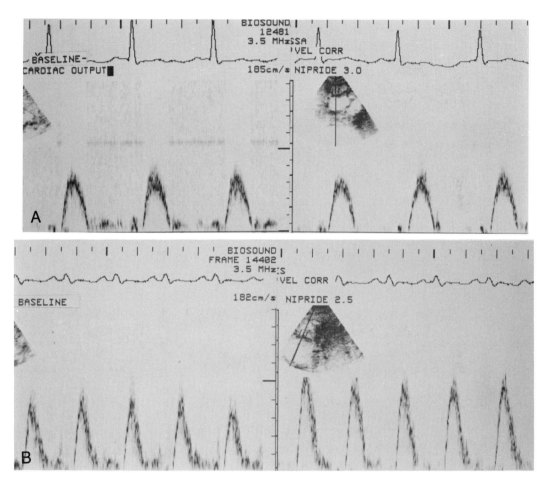

Fig. 6–4.   A. Ascending aortic velocities at baseline (left panel) and after nitroprusside infusion (right panel). Cardiac output showed no increase even at a nitroprusside dose of 3.0 mcg/Kg/min. B. Ascending aortic velocities at baseline (left panel) and after nitroprusside infusion dose of 2.5 mcg/Kg/min. Doppler measured cardiac output increased 60% from baseline.

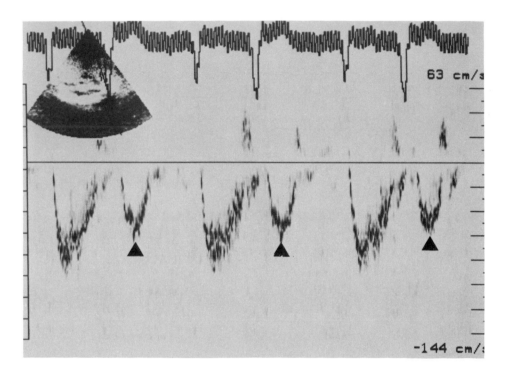

Fig. 6–5. Pulmonary velocity tracings in a patient with atrial bigeminy. Atrial premature beats (arrow) had decreased stroke volume as indicated by decreased area under the time velocity curve.

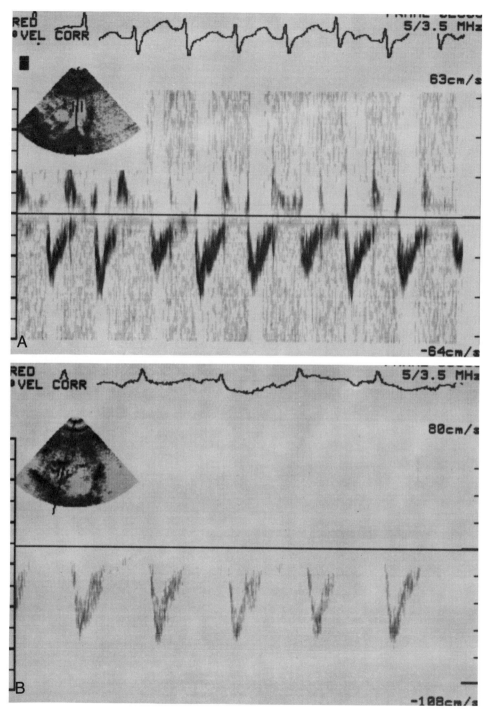

Fig. 6–6.   A. Pulmonary artery velocities in a patient with supraventricular tachycardia, from a short axis parasternal plane. Velocity alternans was present with peak velocities of 25–30 cm/s. B. Ascending aortic tracings from an apex five chamber plane after conversion to normal sinus rhythm. Peak velocities increased to 65 cm/s.

VALVE INSUFFICIENCIES

Mitral Valve Regurgitation

DIAGNOSTIC DOPPLER FINDINGS

Doppler findings of mitral regurgitation are systolic retrograde velocities within the left atrium near the level of the mitral valve (Fig. 6–7).[7,15–21] Doppler interrogation for mitral regurgitation is best accomplished from an apical four chamber plane using pulsed (Fig. 6–7A) (including color-coded Doppler) or continuous wave Doppler (Fig. 6–8). Velocities in this plane are negative in polarity. Positive systolic velocities can be interrogated from the suprasternal notch in small babies and young infants, and in some older patients with severe regurgitation. Jet direction in mitral regurgitation may be in a different alignment than forward flow. Jet orientation has been reported to occur in different directions, depending on the type of regurgitant lesion.[22] Direction is probably best determined by color-coded Doppler. The timing of mitral regurgitation is important; mitral regurgitation jets begin at mitral valve closure and continue past the second heart sound until the mitral valve opens (Fig. 6–8).[7]

In patients with mitral valve prolapse the systolic regurgitation jet is usually mid-systolic (Fig. 6–9).[7] This Doppler finding is easily differentiated from holosystolic mitral regurgitation.

Color-coded Doppler demonstrates mitral regurgitation from both the long axis parasternal (Plate 16A) and apical four chamber planes (Plate 16B). In both planes, blue systolic velocities (away from the transducer) are seen in the left atrium.[23–26] Color-coded Doppler demonstrates that mitral regurgitant jets are often directed toward the lateral wall of the left atrium (Plate 16B).

ASSOCIATED DOPPLER FEATURES

Mitral velocities are increased in amplitude when regurgitation is significant (Fig. 6–10A and B). In particular, the area beneath the rapid filling phase, and peak "E" wave velocities are increased.[7] In mitral regurgitation the E wave deceleration is shortened, whereas with mitral stenosis the E wave deceleration phase is prolonged.

DOPPLER DIFFERENTIATION FROM OTHER LESIONS

Systolic jets of aortic stenosis can be mistaken for mitral regurgitation. In the apex five chamber plane both are negative in polarity, whereas from a suprasternal notch plane both are positive in polarity. Magnitude of peak jets velocities may be similar, depending on severity of disease. Hatle has exquisitely described jet timing and morphology including the differentiation of mitral regurgitation from aortic stenosis.[7] Aortic stenosis jets begin after termination of isovolumetric contraction, whereas mitral regurgitation jets begin immediately after mitral valve closure (Fig. 6–8). Mitral regurgitation jets occur during both the isovolumetric contraction and relaxation phases, and therefore are longer in duration than aortic stenosis.

Antegrade mitral velocities are increased when mitral regurgitation is significant due to increased forward flow across the mitral valve (Fig. 6–10). Measurement of mitral velocities proximal and distal to the valve, within the same flow area, is necessary to determine presence of a pressure gradient. In the absence of a pressure gradient, the velocity differential before and after the

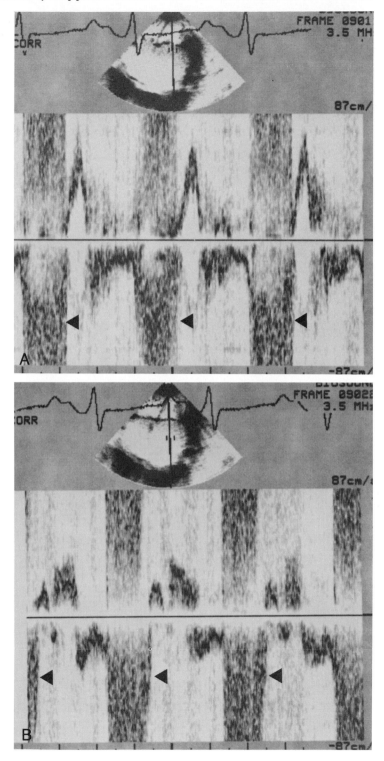

Fig. 6–7. Pulsed wave Doppler interrogation proximal to the mitral valve within the left atrium from an apical four chamber view. Dense systolic negative jets of mitral regurgitation (arrows) are shown just proximal to the mitral valve (A) and mid left atrium (B). (Figure 6–7 is continued on the following page.)

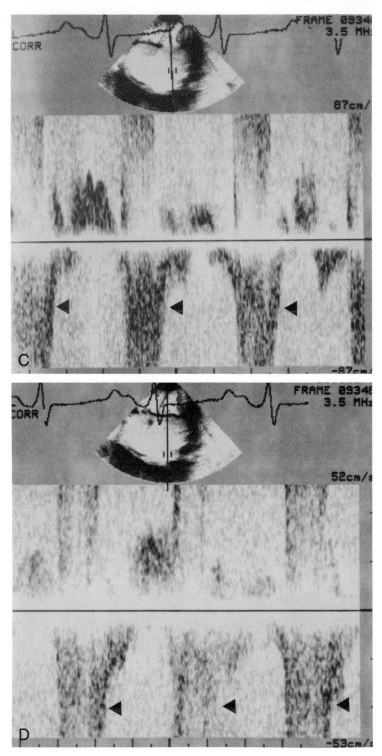

Fig. 6–7 (continued). Dense systolic negative jets of mitral regurgitation (arrows) are also seen in the posterior third of the left atrium (C), and near the entrance of the pulmonary veins (D).

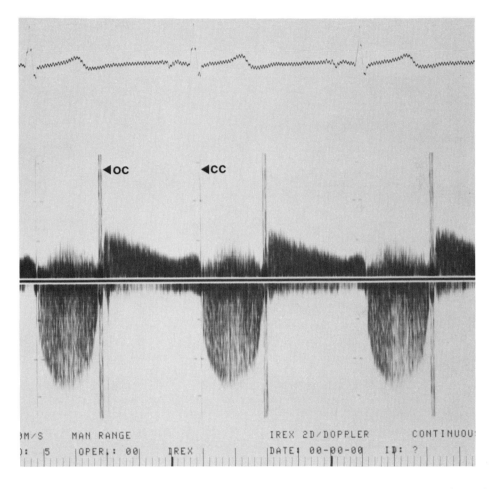

Fig. 6–8. Continuous wave Doppler interrogation showing a dense negative systolic jet of mitral regurgitation. Opening (oc) and closing clicks (cc) of the mitral valve are shown by the arrows.

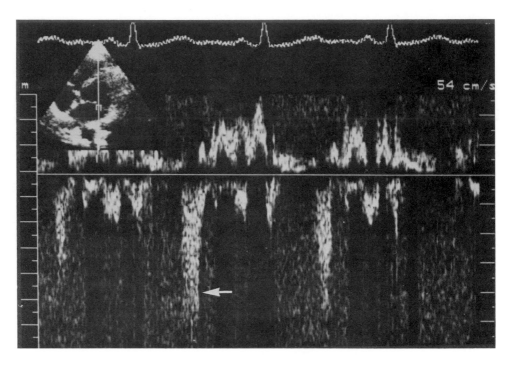

Fig. 6–9. Mid-systolic regurgitant jet (arrow) in a patient with mitral valve prolapse. The jet is directed toward the posterior lateral wall of the left atrium.

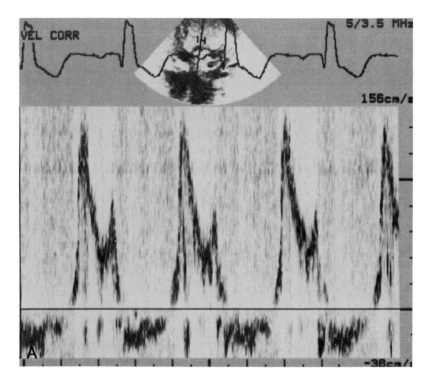

Fig. 6–10. Mitral velocities in a patient with severe regurgitation (A). Peak early filling phase "E wave" velocities are significantly increased as compared to the "A" wave velocities.

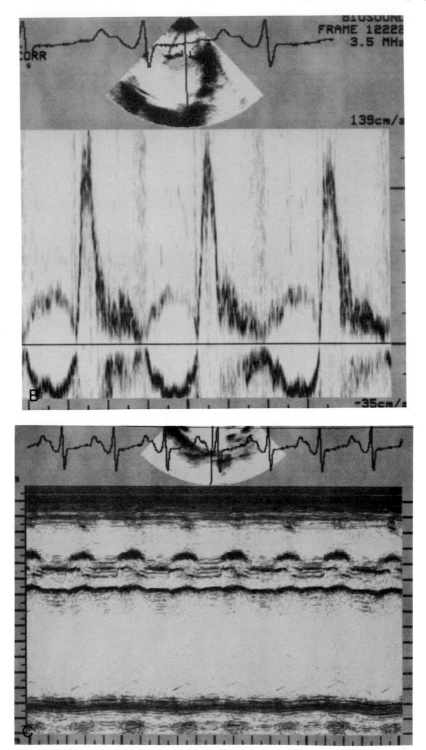

Fig. 6–10 (continued).   Panels B and C show peak mitral velocities (B) and M-mode echocardiogram (C) from another patient with critical mitral regurgitation, low cardiac output, and massively dilated left atrium. The peak amplitude "E" wave velocities are increased, and the "A" wave velocities reduced (B). The left atrium is significantly dilated, and the aortic tracing shows a markedly shortened ejection time (C).

valve does not exceed 20 to 30 cm/s.[27] Measurement of mitral pressure half time,[7] and effective orifice area (Chapter 7) can assist in differentiation of flow related gradients and anatomic mitral stenosis.

Other cardiac lesions which result in increased flow will also cause elevated peak mitral velocities. These lesions include large left to right shunts from patent ductus arterioses, surgically placed aortic-pulmonary shunts, and ventricular septal defects.[27]

DOPPLER ESTIMATION OF SEVERITY OF DISEASE

Intensity of the Doppler signal, and peak amplitude of antegrade velocities increase with severity of disease.[7] Regurgitant fractions can be calculated by comparison of regurgitant to forward mean velocities (Fig. 6–11). This assumes that mitral flow area remains constant during systole and diastole (Chapter 5), which probably is not true. In mitral valve disease, regurgitant velocities close to the mitral orifice form a high velocity jet. Formation of a jet suggests orifice constriction and precludes flow measurement unless flow area is known. Regurgitant flow can, however, be calculated as total forward flow across the mitral valve, minus net forward flow across either the aortic, pulmonary or tricuspid valve (assuming no stenosis or insufficiency of these valves).

Abassi and co-workers introduced the concept of "mapping" the mitral regurgitant jet in the left atrium as an indicator of severity of disease.[15] A jet that can be interrogated farther posteriorly and in a larger area was equated with more significant disease.[15,28] Figure 6–7A–D shows an example of severe mitral regurgitation in which a dense systolic negative jet was mapped into the posterior left atrium and entrance of the pulmonary veins.

Reports have shown a good correlation between the area of regurgitation defined by color coding, to the area of regurgitation found by angiography.[24–26,29] Weak signals in the posterior left atrium, problems with signal to noise ratio, and improper gain setting may prevent accurate determination of velocities far from the transducer.

Tricuspid Regurgitation

DIAGNOSTIC DOPPLER FINDINGS

Doppler findings of tricuspid regurgitation are systolic retrograde velocities within the right atrium at the tricuspid valve level (Fig. 6–12).[7,30,31] Similar to mitral regurgitation, Doppler interrogation for tricuspid regurgitation is best accomplished from the apical four chamber plane. Jet direction in tricuspid regurgitation may be in a different alignment than forward flow, requiring interrogation for the regurgitant jet in several planes. Negative systolic jets of tricuspid regurgitation are usually directed along the atrial septal surface as shown by standard pulsed[30] (Fig. 6–13) and color-coded Doppler (Plate 17).[23,25,26]

Timing of tricuspid regurgitation shows that velocities begin at tricuspid valve closure and continue past the second heart sound until the tricuspid valve opens (Fig. 6–12).

Color-coded Doppler demonstrates tricuspid regurgitation from the short axis parasternal (Plate 18A) and apical four chamber planes (Plate 18B). In both planes, blue systolic velocities (away from the transducer) are seen within the right atrium.[23,25,26]

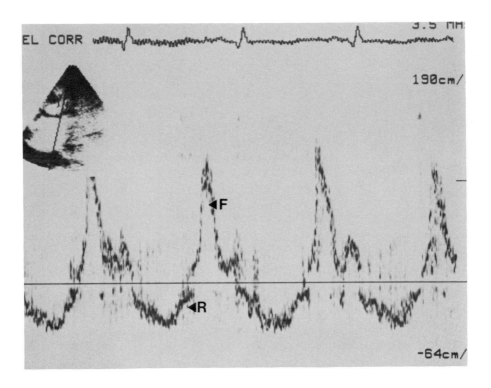

Fig. 6–11. Mitral velocities in a patient with significant regurgitation. R = regurgitant velocities. F = forward velocities.

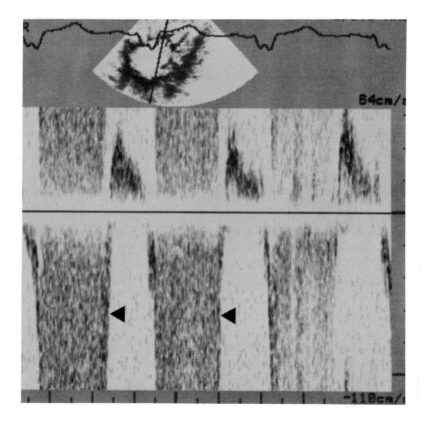

Fig. 6–12.   Negative systolic velocities (arrow) of tricuspid regurgitation with the sample volume within the right atrium proximal to the tricuspid valve.

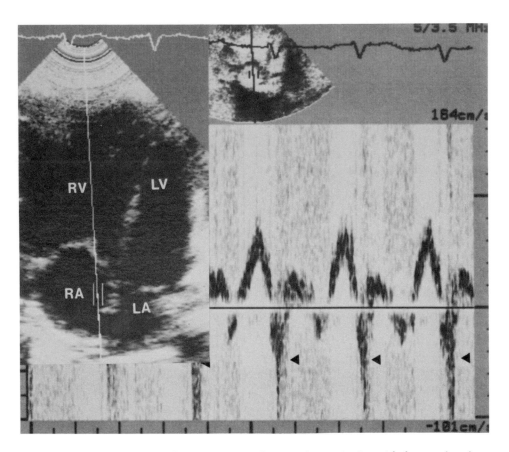

Fig. 6–13.   Negative systolic velocities (arrows) of tricuspid regurgitation with the sample volume placed along the right atrial septal surface (insert).

Doppler echocardiography is a sensitive test for the detection of tricuspid regurgitation. A tricuspid jet can be found in patients with negative auscultatory findings.[32] Tricuspid regurgitation is a common Doppler finding in patients of all ages with either heart or lung disease, especially in those patients with right ventricular hypertension (Fig. 6–14).[7]

Negative systolic velocities can usually be found in the right atrium of normal individuals.[7,33,34] We prefer to use the term "tricuspid backflow" for this entity. These velocities are interrogated only a short distance from the tricuspid valve (Fig. 6–15), as opposed to more severe tricuspid regurgitation where the velocities can be tracked further posteriorly into the right atrium (Fig. 6–16).

ASSOCIATED DOPPLER FEATURES

Increased tricuspid velocity amplitudes are seen in patients with significant tricuspid regurgitation secondary to increased flow across the tricuspid valve. Tricuspid velocities are measured proximal and distal to the valve, within the same flow area, to determine presence of a velocity gradient.[27] Increased velocities resulting from increased tricuspid flow can also occur as the result of atrial septal defects, left ventricular to right atrial shunts, and anomalous pulmonary venous drainage.[27]

DOPPLER DIFFERENTIATION FROM OTHER LESIONS

Left ventricular to right atrial shunts associated with membranous and endocardial cushion defects may produce systolic jet lesions within the right atrium originating near the tricuspid valve. These jets are differentiated from other types of tricuspid regurgitation since their direction is frequently diagonal across the right atrium. In contrast, tricuspid regurgitation jets are usually directed medially along the atrial septal surface. Jets across restrictive atrial septal defects may also be seen within the right atrium. These jets are best interrogated from the subcostal plane from which atrial septal interrogation can be performed nearly perpendicular to the septum. Jet velocities across atrial septal defects are usually of short duration, and peak amplitude rarely exceeds 2 m/s. On the other hand, even the lowest tricuspid regurgitation jets approximate 2.5 m/s, and may be much higher depending on magnitude of peak right ventricular systolic pressure.

DOPPLER ESTIMATION OF SEVERITY OF DISEASE

Severity of tricuspid regurgitation can be estimated in a manner similar to that used for study of mitral regurgitation: (1) calculation of regurgitant fraction, and (2) Doppler mapping of the regurgitant velocities.[30] Regurgitant fraction can be calculated by comparison of regurgitant to forward mean velocities (Chapter 5). Similar to mitral regurgitation, retrograde velocities form a high velocity jet close to the tricuspid orifice, suggesting orifice constriction. Regurgitant flow can be calculated as total forward flow across the tricuspid valve, minus net forward flow across either the aortic, pulmonary or mitral valve.

Mapping negative systolic velocities in the right atrium by pulsed Doppler[30] (Fig. 6–16) and color-coded Doppler (Plate 19)[23,25,26,35] can estimate severity of tricuspid regurgitation. In general, tricuspid regurgitation is considered more severe the larger the area, and the further from the valve that jet velocities can be interrogated. Positive systolic velocities can be interrogated in the inferior

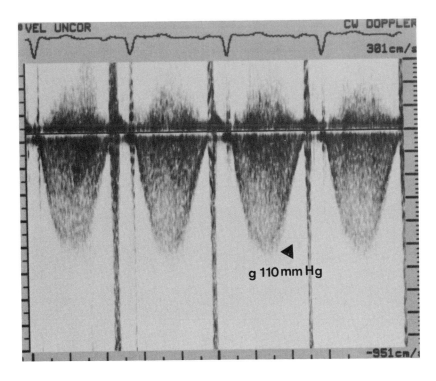

Fig. 6–14. Continuous wave Doppler tracings of tricuspid regurgitation in a patient with severe lung disease. Peak systolic velocity gradient (g) was 110 mm Hg, consistent with suprasystemic right ventricular pressure.

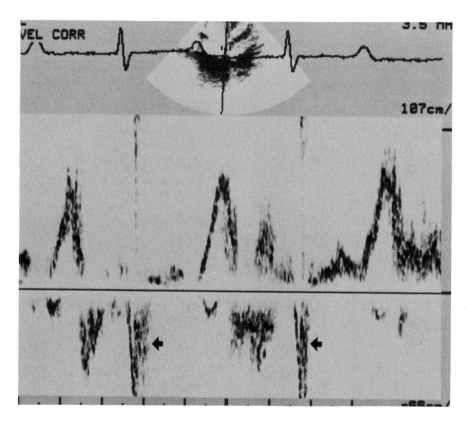

Fig. 6–15. Pulsed wave negative systolic jet (arrow) of tricuspid regurgitation with the sample volume placed along the atrial septal surface near the tricuspid valve.

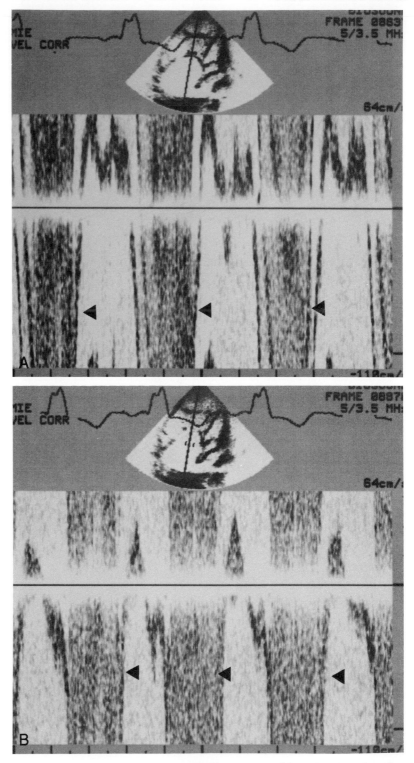

Fig. 6–16. (A–D) Pulsed Doppler interrogation from an apical four chamber plane in a patient with severe tricuspid regurgitation. Negative systolic velocities (arrows) were sequentially mapped posteriorly from immediately proximal to the valve (A); proximal third (B); middle third (C) and distal portion of the right atrium (D).

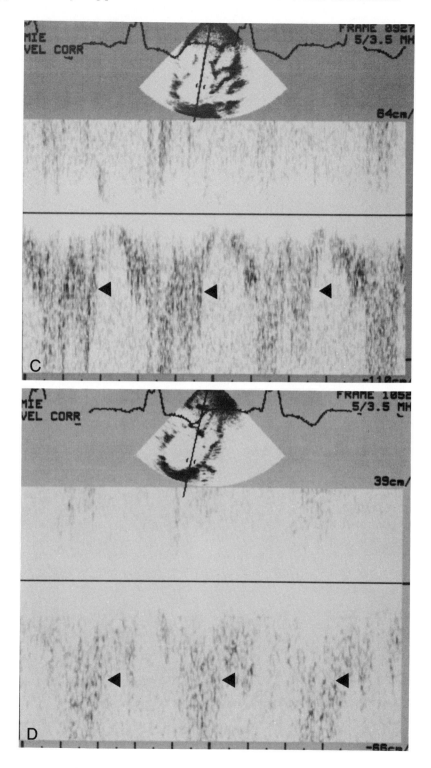

Fig. 6–16 (continued).

and superior vena cava in patients with severe tricuspid regurgitation (Fig. 6–17).[36] Ratio of systolic to diastolic velocities in the hepatic veins,[37,38] and inferior vena cava[39] have also been related to severity of disease.

Aortic Regurgitation

DIAGNOSTIC DOPPLER FINDINGS

Doppler features of aortic regurgitation are diastolic retrograde velocities in the aorta and left ventricular outflow tract.[7,40–42] These velocities are positive from an apical five chamber plane with the Doppler sample volume placed proximal to the valve (Fig. 6–18), and negative when interrogated from the suprasternal notch (Fig. 6–19). In infants and small children the subcostal approach can also be used to demonstrate aortic regurgitation.

Aortic regurgitation velocities almost always alias when using pulsed Doppler. Accordingly, continuous wave Doppler is also used to detect the regurgitant jet (Fig. 6–19). Doppler is a sensitive modality for detection of aortic regurgitation, which can be present in patients without a murmur.[41,43]

On color-coded exams from the apical plane, aortic regurgitation is detected as red diastolic velocities in the aortic outflow tract (Plate 20).[23,25,26]

ASSOCIATED DOPPLER FEATURES

Systolic forward velocities are increased in patients with significant aortic regurgitation, commensurate with increased total forward flow. Since antegrade velocities are increased, Doppler interrogation both proximal and distal to the valve, within the same flow area, must be done to rule out a significant pressure drop (Fig. 6–20).[27]

DOPPLER DIFFERENTIATION FROM OTHER LESIONS

Increased velocities across the non-stenotic aortic valve can also occur as the result of increased pulmonary venous return. These lesions include patent ductus arterioses and surgically placed aortic to pulmonary artery shunts.

The diastolic jet of aortic regurgitation can be mistaken for mitral stenosis.[7] Aortic regurgitation starts earlier at aortic valve closure and continues throughout diastole (Fig. 6–21).[7,42] Doppler velocity tracings in mitral stenosis begin at mitral valve opening and continue until mitral valve closure. Mitral stenosis jet peak velocity amplitude rarely exceeds 2.5 m/s, whereas aortic regurgitant jets generally are greater than 2.5 m/s.

DOPPLER ESTIMATION OF SEVERITY OF DISEASE

Severity of aortic regurgitation can be estimated by (1) calculation of regurgitant fraction,[44–47] and (2) Doppler mapping of the regurgitant velocities.[23,25,40,48] Regurgitant fraction can be calculated by comparison of regurgitant to forward mean velocities[45,47] (Chapter 5). Mean aortic regurgitant velocities can usually be directly quantitated from diastolic reversal of flow in the ascending aorta. In this region retrograde velocities rarely exceed 1.5 m/s. Retrograde and forward velocities have the same flow area, allowing for calculation of regurgitant fraction. Jet velocities occur more proximal to the valve, precluding flow computation. Regurgitant flow can be quantitated by measurement of total forward flow across the aortic outflow tract, minus net forward flow across the mitral, tricuspid or pulmonary valve.[45,49]

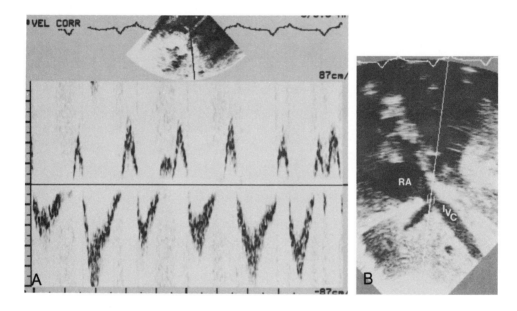

Fig. 6–17.　Positive systolic velocities (A) of severe tricuspid regurgitation from a subcostal short axis plane with the Doppler sample volume placed in the inferior vena cava-right atrial junction (B).

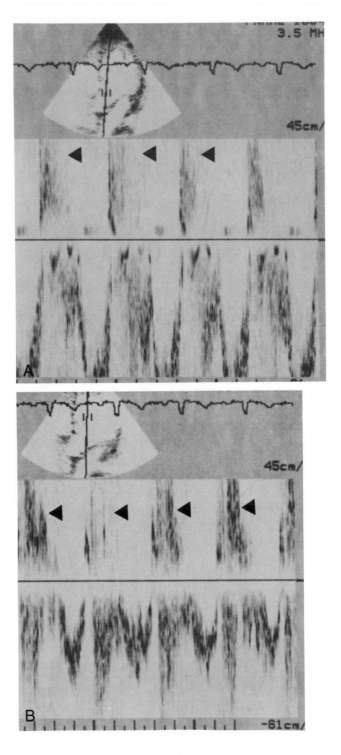

Fig. 6–18. Pulsed Doppler aortic outflow tract velocity tracings from an apical five chamber plane. Positive diastolic velocities of aortic regurgitation (arrows) were mapped from immediately below the aortic valve (A); middle third (B); and distal third of the left ventricle (C).

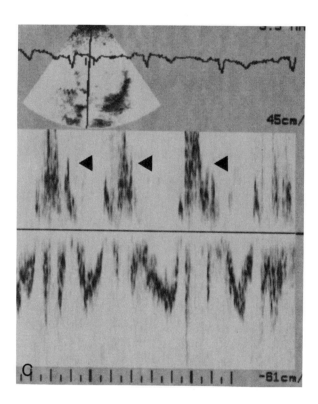

Fig. 6–18 (continued).

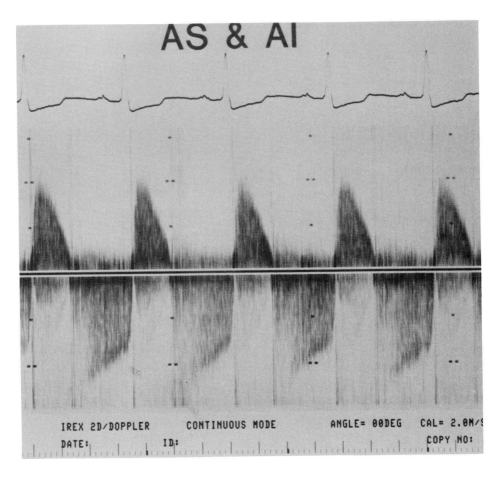

Fig. 6–19. Continuous wave Doppler ascending aortic velocities from the suprasternal notch demonstrating negative diastolic velocities of aortic regurgitation.

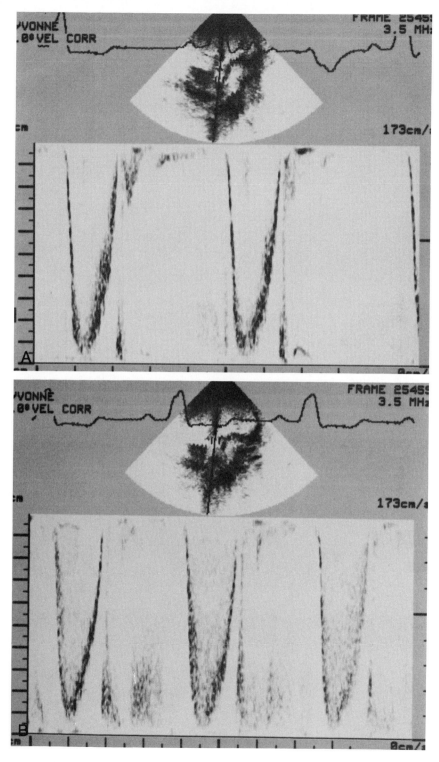

Fig. 6–20.   Pulsed Doppler aortic outflow tract velocities distal (A) and proximal (B) to the aortic valve in a patient with aortic regurgitation. Although the distal peak velocities are 1.8 m/s, no valve gradient exists since the proximal peak velocities are also 1.8 m/s.

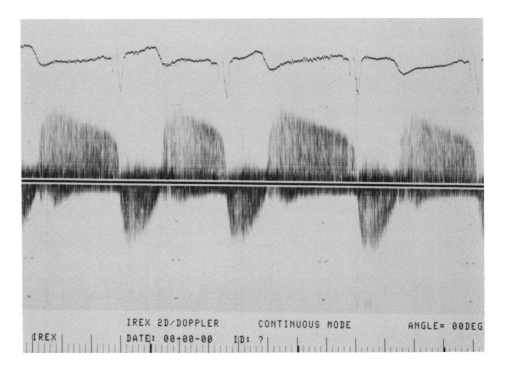

Fig. 6–21. Continuous wave Doppler tracings of aortic regurgitation demonstrating positive diastolic velocities starting with aortic valve closure and continuing throughout diastole until aortic valve opening.

Retrograde diastolic velocities occur in the transverse and descending aorta[50–53] in patients with severe regurgitation. This pattern is found most often in patients with severe disease (Fig. 6–22). Other lesions such as patent ductus arterioses and surgically created aortic-pulmonary shunts can create generally similar velocity patterns in the transverse aortic arch and descending aorta (Fig. 6–23).[7,51] Some investigators have found a good correlation between ratio of forward to retrograde velocities in this area, and magnitude of regurgitation.[50,52]

Intensity of the Doppler regurgitant signal is related to the severity of disease.[7] Further, the Doppler pattern in severe aortic regurgitation is associated with a rapid slope following peak velocity, and a minimal velocity gradient at end diastole (Fig. 6–24).[7] This pattern indicates reduced diastolic aortic pressure and elevated left ventricular end-diastolic pressure.

Aortic regurgitation may be assessed qualitatively by both standard pulsed[40,42,48] and color coded Doppler mapping techniques.[23,25,26,54] Regurgitant jets can be mapped further posteriorly towards the apex of the left ventricle (Figs. 6–18 and 6–25), and in a larger area of the left ventricle in patients with severe disease (Plate 21). Veyrat and co-workers caution that increased accuracy is obtained when the regurgitant area is mapped in two planes.[46] As in other regurgitation forms, weak signals far from the transducer may prevent accurate determination of the most distal velocities.

Pulmonary Regurgitation
DIAGNOSTIC DOPPLER FINDINGS

The diagnostic feature of pulmonary regurgitation is retrograde diastolic velocities detected in the right ventricular outflow tract (Fig. 6–26).[7,55,56] Pulmonary regurgitant velocities can also be interrogated in the main pulmonary artery, right ventricular outflow tract, or conduit following repair of complex congenital heart defects. Diastolic velocities of pulmonary regurgitation are optimally obtained in the short axis parasternal plane. In infants and small children the subcostal short axis and coronal planes can also be used to detect pulmonary regurgitation velocities. In these planes pulmonary regurgitant velocities are positive in direction, begin at pulmonic valve closure, and are continuous throughout diastole (Fig. 6–26).[7,55,56] Pulmonary regurgitant velocities can be detected in the absence of auscultatory findings of disease.[57]

In normal subjects, positive diastolic velocities can be seen proximal to the pulmonary valve (Fig. 6–27).[33,34] These velocities are usually low in magnitude (less than 2 m/s) and can be detected only in a small area close to the pulmonary valve. These velocities are sometimes recorded in mid-diastole and not immediately after valve closure,[7,33] perhaps because of poor alignment with the small jet. This normal pulmonary velocity pattern cannot be distinguished from mild pulmonic regurgitation following pulmonary valvotomies, or balloon dilation angioplasty. We prefer to use the term "pulmonary backflow" for minimal regurgitation velocities occurring in individuals with no underlying cardiovascular or pulmonary disease.

Color-coded Doppler will show diastolic red velocities proximal to the pulmonary valve in patients with pulmonary regurgitation (Plate 22).[23]

ASSOCIATED DOPPLER FINDINGS

When pulmonary regurgitation is significant, a large regurgitant volume will result in increased total forward flow and peak systolic velocities (Fig. 6–28).

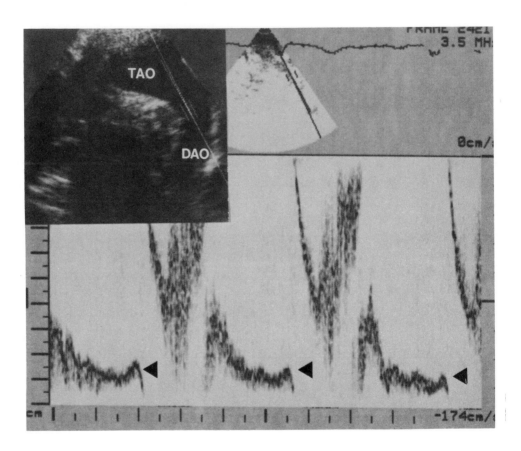

Fig. 6–22.   Aortic velocity tracings with the Doppler sample volume (insert) placed within the transverse aortic arch (TAO), descending aorta (DAO) junction. Positive diastolic velocities (arrows) found at this site indicate significant regurgitation.

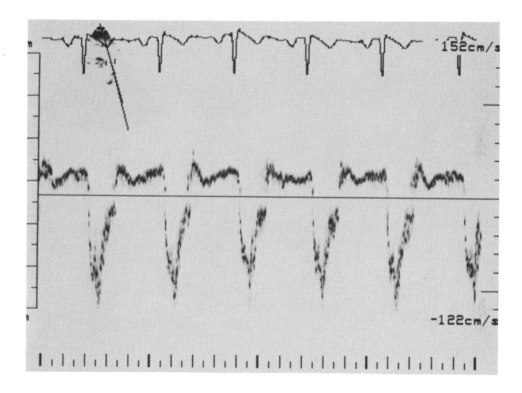

Fig. 6–23. Aortic velocity tracings with the Doppler sample volume placed in the transverse arch from a patient with a Blalock-Taussig shunt. Note positive diastolic velocities indicating run-off into the pulmonary arteries.

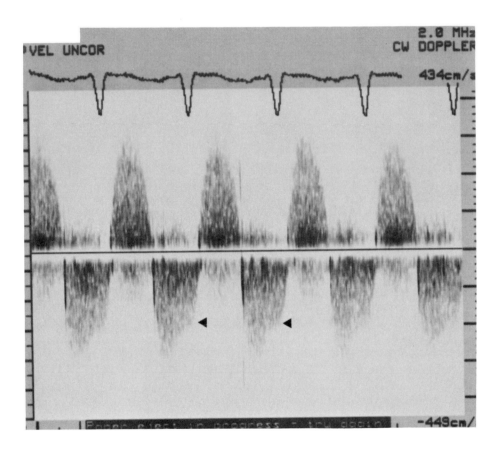

Fig. 6–24. Continuous wave Doppler tracings form the suprasternal notch in a patient with severe aortic insufficiency. Negative velocities show a rapid slope with an end diastolic velocity gradient (arrows) of only 16 mm Hg. Peak velocities may have been missed in order to demonstrate the end diastolic velocity gradient.

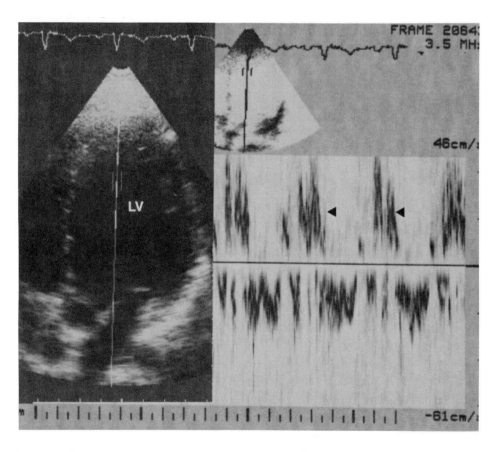

Fig. 6–25. Positive diastolic velocities (arrows) interrogated near the apex of the left ventricle in a patient with severe aortic regurgitation.

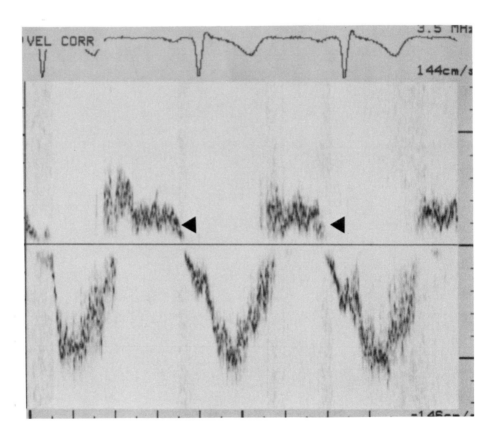

Fig. 6–26. Positive diastolic velocities of pulmonary regurgitation (arrow) with the pulsed wave Doppler sample volume in the main pulmonary artery.

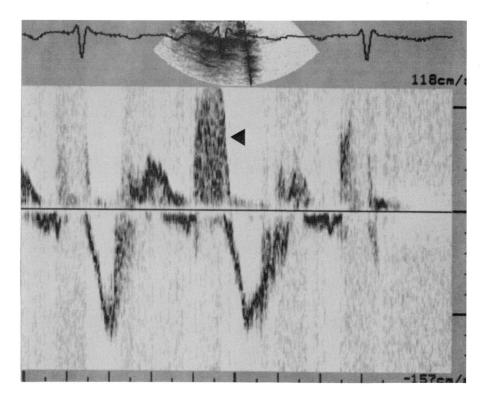

Fig. 6–27. Positive diastolic velocities with the sample volume in the main pulmonary artery close to the pulmonary valve in a normal subject. The jet (arrow) was recorded in this example in mid-diastole.

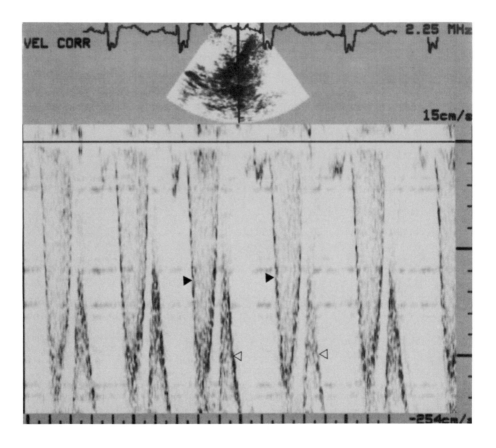

Fig. 6–28. Increased antegrade velocities (black arrows) and retrograde pulmonary velocities (white arrows) from a patient with pulmonary regurgitation with the sample volume placed within a nonvalved right ventricular-to-pulmonary artery conduit.

A pressure drop can be determined by comparing velocities proximal and distal to the pulmonic valve in the same flow area.[27] Significant, pulmonary regurgitation, however, as well as large left-to-right shunts, may be associated with a flow related gradient.

DOPPLER DIFFERENTIATION FROM OTHER LESIONS

Increased systolic velocities from increased pulmonary flow can also be found in patients with atrial septal defects, ventricular septal defects, and anomalous pulmonary venous return.[27]

Diastolic retrograde velocities can also be detected in the main pulmonary artery in patients with a patent ductus arteriosus (Fig. 6–29), surgical aortic-pulmonary artery shunts, and rarely aorticopulmonary windows (Fig. 6–30). However, unless pulmonary regurgitation co-exists, diastolic velocities from these diseases are not interrogated in the right ventricular outflow tract.

DOPPLER ESTIMATION OF SEVERITY OF DISEASE

Intensity of the Doppler regurgitant signal is generally related to severity of disease.[7] Patients with severe pulmonary regurgitation have a rapid slope following peak velocity, and minimal velocity gradient at end diastole.[7,56] This velocity pattern indicates equilibration of low pulmonary artery diastolic pressure, and elevated right ventricular end diastolic pressure. Peak diastolic velocities will be significantly increased when pulmonary artery hypertension coexists.

Regurgitant fraction can also provide an estimate of the severity of disease. The sample volume is placed in the mid pulmonary artery proximal to the bifurcation. A time velocity envelope with minimal velocity spread can be seen during both systole and diastole (Fig. 6–31). Total forward (negative) and regurgitant mean velocities (positive) can be measured, allowing for calculation of regurgitant fraction.[45] A diastolic jet will be interrogated if the Doppler sample volume is placed too inferiorly in the pulmonary outflow tract, or near the pulmonary valve. Regurgitant volume can also be quantitated by measurement of total forward flow across the pulmonary valve, minus net forward flow across the mitral, tricuspid or aortic valve.

Severity of pulmonary regurgitation can also be assessed by pulsed Doppler, including color coded Doppler (Plate 23). The area and distance that diastolic velocities can be visualized into the right ventricle relate to severity of disease.[23]

SHUNT LESIONS

Atrial Septal Communications

DIAGNOSTIC DOPPLER FEATURES

Two-dimensional echocardiography is extremely useful for visualizing atrial septal communications. However, Doppler provides important additional information concerning magnitude and direction of flow across these defects.[58–63]

When the Doppler sample volume is placed along the right atrial septal surface in patients with left to right atrial shunts, the Doppler velocity pattern is positive, nearly continuous, and has two to three peaks (Fig. 6–32).[59,61,62] The first peak is broadest with highest velocities, and occurs during late systole. The second velocity peak occurs during mid-diastole and has less breadth and

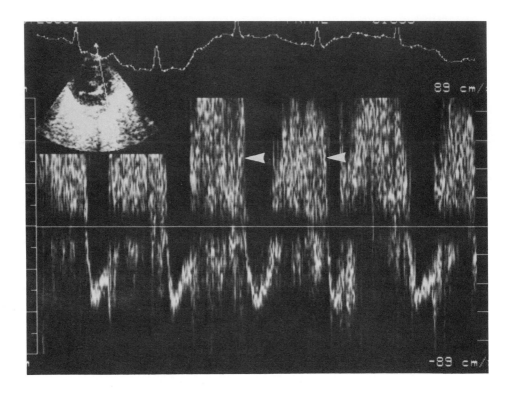

Fig. 6–29. Positive diastolic velocities in the main pulmonary artery from a patient with a patent ductus arteriosus. These velocities were not present within the right ventricular outflow tract, proximal to the pulmonary valve.

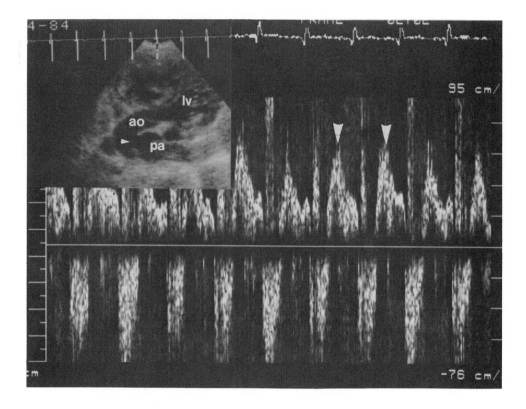

Fig. 6–30. Positive diastolic velocities (arrows) from the main pulmonary artery in a patient with an aorticopulmonary window (insert).

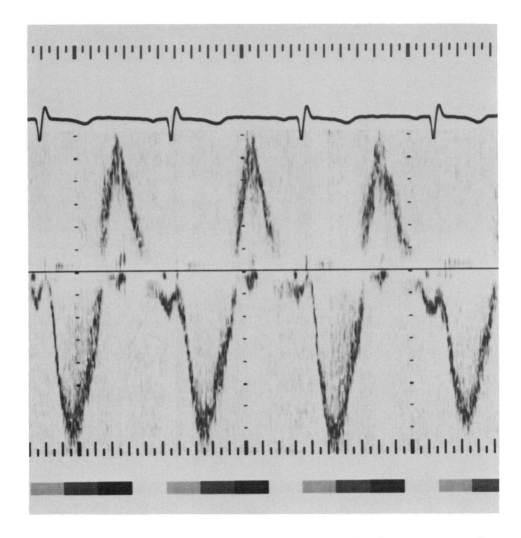

Fig. 6–31. Negative systolic (total forward flow) and positive diastolic velocities (regurgitant flow) in a patient with significant pulmonary regurgitation. The sample volume was placed in the midportion of the main pulmonary artery.

height than the first. These two waveforms usually return to baseline and then a third peak occurs during atrial systole. Velocity amplitude rarely exceeds 1.5 m/s (Fig. 6–32) when atrial septal defects are large. Doppler velocities are negative in patients with right to left atrial shunts when the Doppler sample volume is placed along the right atrial septal surface (Fig. 6–33).[7,61]

Alignment with flow across atrial defects is best obtained from subcostal long and short axis planes with the transducer aligned nearly perpendicular to the septum. The entire length of the septum should be interrogated for the highest velocities with simultaneous movement of the transducer in the non-visualized or azimuthal plane.

Color-coded Doppler provides rapid visualization of flow direction.[23,25] Although color-coded Doppler patterns of the atrial shunt can be seen from an apical four chamber plane (Plate 24), the preferred planes are subcostal (Plate 25). Left to right atrial shunts appear as a red/orange pattern within the right atrium (Plates 24, 25, 26). Right to left atrial shunts appear as a blue pattern within the left atrium (Plate 27).

ASSOCIATED DOPPLER FEATURES

Patients with significant atrial septal defects and large left to right shunts have increased velocities across the tricuspid and pulmonary valves.[27]

DOPPLER DIFFERENTIATION FROM OTHER LESIONS

Tricuspid regurgitation, and left ventricular to right atrial shunts can produce increased systolic velocities along the right atrial septal surface. Peak velocity amplitude is generally higher in tricuspid regurgitation than velocities which occur across atrial septal communications.

DOPPLER ESTIMATION OF SEVERITY OF DISEASE

Pulmonary-to-systemic flow ratio can be accurately estimated in patients with an atrial septal defect.[60,62,64–68] Figure 6–34 schematically shows possible flow measurement sites for patients with an atrial septal defect. Systemic flow can be calculated from the aorta, and pulmonary flow from the tricuspid valve, right ventricular outflow tract or pulmonary artery. Flow related gradients may occur in patients with significant shunts. In these patients pulmonary flow is calculated across the tricuspid valve.

Mean shunt velocity across atrial defects can be determined by digitizing the outer envelope of the velocity tracings.[61,62] Mean velocity provides an estimate of pulmonary to systemic flow ratio. However, if the atrial septal defect is restrictive (Fig. 6–35), i.e. peak velocities exceed 1.5 m/s, mean velocities have less predictive value. Doppler mean velocity calculation can be helpful when the atrial septal defects are difficult to image, or when the atrial septum has multiple fenestrations.

Combined two-dimensional and Doppler echocardiography can be used to demonstrate efficacy of atrial septostomy. Figure 6–36A shows transatrial septal velocities in a patient with hypoplastic left heart syndrome. Velocities approached 2.5 m/s for an estimated pressure drop of 25 mm Hg. At catheterization the mean left atrial pressure was 30 mm Hg, and the right atrial pressure was 5 mm Hg. A balloon septostomy was performed for stabilization for a palliative operation. Figure 6–36B shows reduction of the atrial septal velocities to

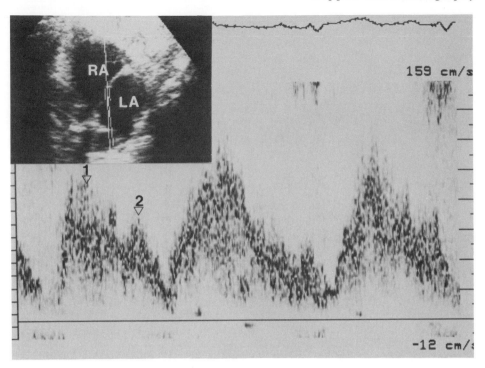

Fig. 6–32. Continuous turbulent velocities with two merging peaks (1 and 2) obtained from a patient with a non-restrictive secundum atrial septal defect. The sample volume was placed across the defect from a subcostal short axis plane (insert).

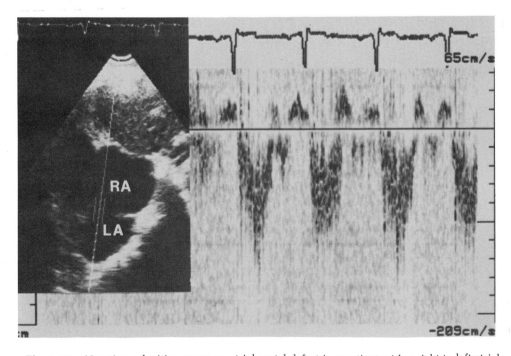

Fig. 6–33. Negative velocities across an atrial septal defect in a patient with a right to left atrial shunt. The sample volume was placed perpendicular to flow across the defect from a subcostal short axis plane.

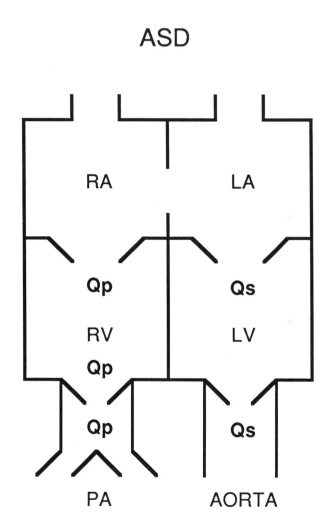

Fig. 6–34. Schematic drawing showing possible sample sites for the measurement of pulmonary (Qp) and systemic (Qs) flow in a patient with an atrial septal defect.

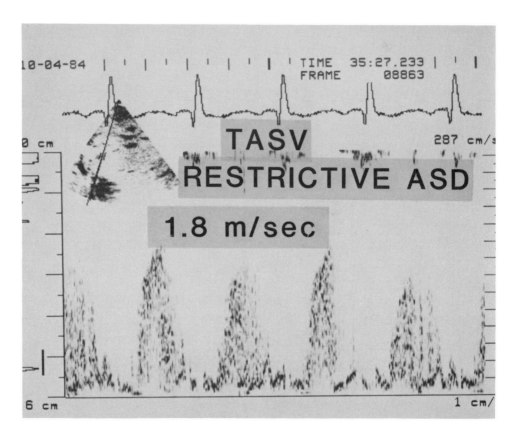

Fig. 6–35. High velocity jets (1.8 m/s) across the atrial septum from a patient with a restrictive atrial septal communication. (Reprinted with permission, American Journal of Cardiology.[62])

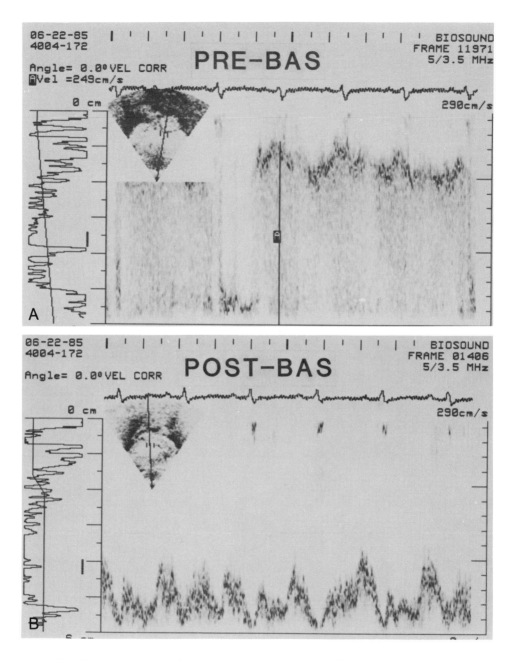

Fig. 6–36.   Transatrial septal velocities prior (A) and following (B) a balloon atrial septostomy in a patient with hypoplastic left heart syndrome. Note the marked reduction in peak velocities from 250 cm/s to 100 cm/s.

1.0 m/s after septostomy. No gradient was found by pressure manometry at catheterization.

Figure 6–37 demonstrates pulsed Doppler velocities across a patent foramen ovale before and after balloon atrial septostomy in a baby with transposition of the great arteries, intact ventricular septum. Note the significant increase in the mean transatrial septal velocities after the atrial septal communication was enlarged.

Ventricular Septal Defects

DIAGNOSTIC DOPPLER FINDINGS

Multiple investigators have documented the utility of Doppler echocardiography for detection of ventricular septal defects.[69–73] If the defect is imaged, the pulsed Doppler sample volume may be placed along the ventricular septum to verify its existence. If the pressure difference between the ventricles is high, the signal will alias (Fig. 6–38).

When the defect is difficult to image, pulsed Doppler can be used in multiple planes to scan the right ventricular surface of the septum. For example, a membranous VSD is usually found by interrogating the ventricular septum in the parasternal long axis (Fig. 6–38) or apical four chamber planes (Fig. 6–39). Muscular defects can be detected in the parasternal long axis or short axis views. In infants and children, the subcostal imaging planes are also useful for the Doppler evaluation of ventricular septal defects (Fig. 6–40). In many adults, imaging in this plane is difficult.

A high velocity jet will not be detected if right and left ventricular pressures are comparable. Situations which cause similar right and left ventricular pressures in the presence of a VSD include, among others, large, unrestrictive ventricular septal defects (Fig. 6–41), right ventricular outflow obstruction, and elevated pulmonary vascular resistance. Velocity polarity may indicate right to left shunts in these patients (Fig. 6–41 and Plate 28).

On occasion, even after a careful conventional pulsed Doppler examination, the jet associated with a small, restrictive ventricular septal defect may not be detected. Frequently, even these small defects can be found after a thorough examination wth continuous wave Doppler (Fig. 6–42). The jet associated with a ventricular septal defect usually lasts throughout systole. However, particularly in the presence of a small muscular defect, the duration of the jet may be abbreviated because the jet moves out of the sample volume or the defect functionally closes later in systole.

Color-coded Doppler is highly sensitive and specific for identification of the presence of ventricular septal defects (Plate 29).[74] Signal aliasing, as shown by the mosaic pattern in this patient, is found on the right side of the ventricular septum. Color-coded images of ventricular septal defects can be obtained from the long axis and short axis parasternal, apical and subcostal planes. Very small defects may pose problems even for color-coded Doppler. Color-coded Doppler is reported to be more sensitive than conventional Doppler and two-dimensional imaging for detection of multiple ventricular septal defects.[74] However, even color-coded Doppler failed to identify multiple defects in some cases.[74]

ASSOCIATED DOPPLER FEATURES

In the presence of a significant ventricular septal defect, increased peak velocities can be detected across the pulmonary and mitral valves. Occasion-

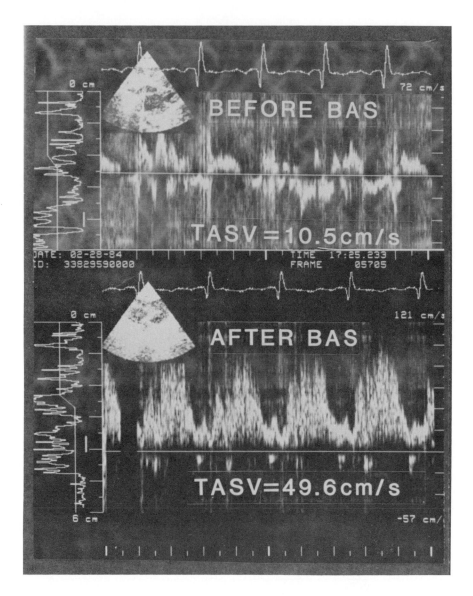

Fig. 6–37. Transatrial septal velocities prior (top panel) and following (bottom panel) balloon atrial septostomy in an infant with transposition of the great arteries, intact ventricular septum. Note the marked increase in velocities after the septostomy was performed.

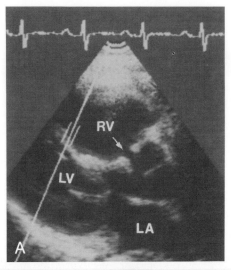

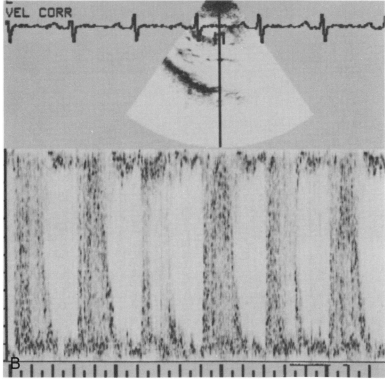

Fig. 6–38. Two-dimensional image (A) and pulsed Doppler velocities (B and C) obtained from the parasternal view from a patient with a membranous ventricular septal defect (arrow). High jet velocities result in signal aliasing (B and C).

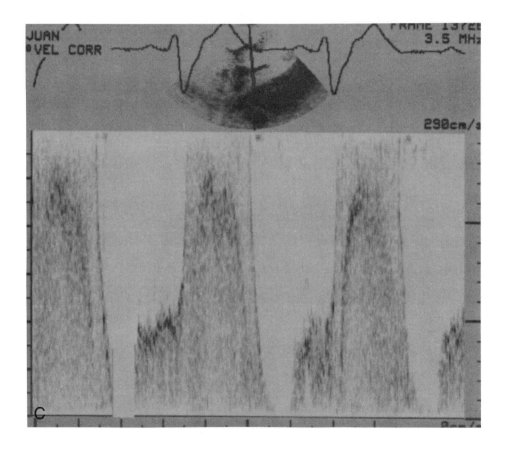

Fig. 6–38 (continued). The jet envelope can be seen within the aliased signal in Panel C.

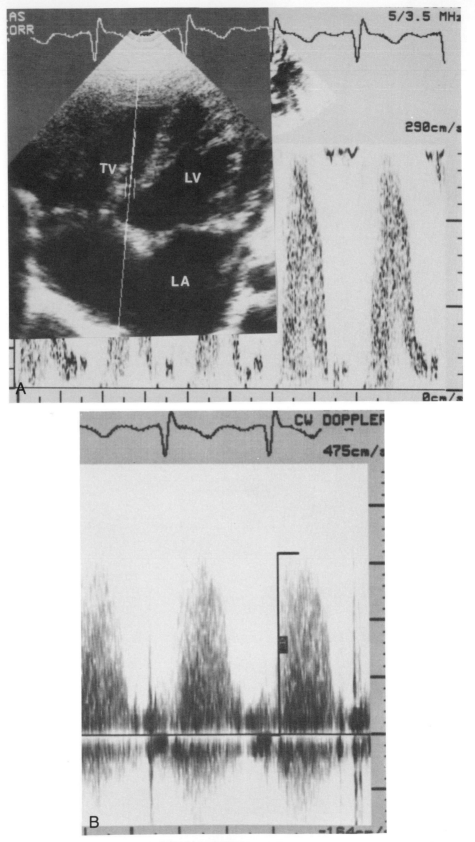

Fig. 6–39. Two-dimensional image and pulsed Doppler velocities (A) obtained from the apical four chamber view from a patient with a membranous ventricular septal defect. The defect is seen near the septal leaflet of the tricuspid valve (TV). The pulsed Doppler study shows signal aliasing. The continuous wave velocities (B) demonstrate a 40 mm Hg pressure drop between the left and right ventricles.

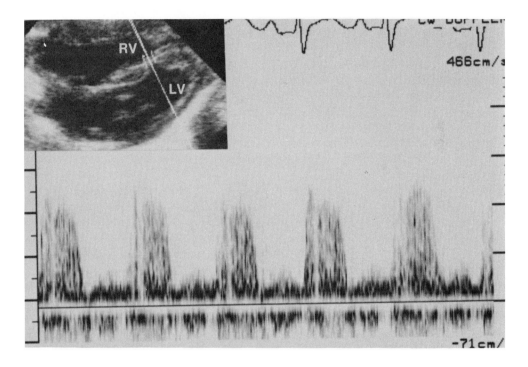

Fig. 6–40. Two-dimensional subcostal image and continuous wave Doppler velocity tracings from a patient with a small muscular ventricular septal defect. The pulsed Doppler sample volume is placed on the right ventricular side of the defect.

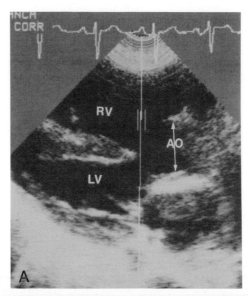

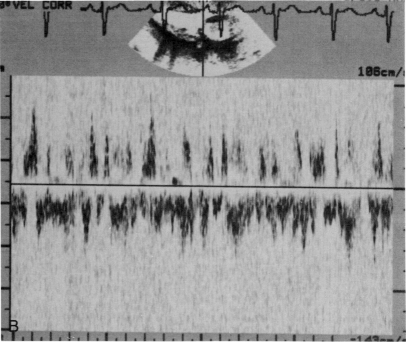

Fig. 6–41. Two-dimensional long axis parasternal image (A) and pulsed Doppler velocities (B) obtained from a patient with a large malalignment ventricular septal defect. The pulsed Doppler waveform shows low amplitude bidirectional velocities.

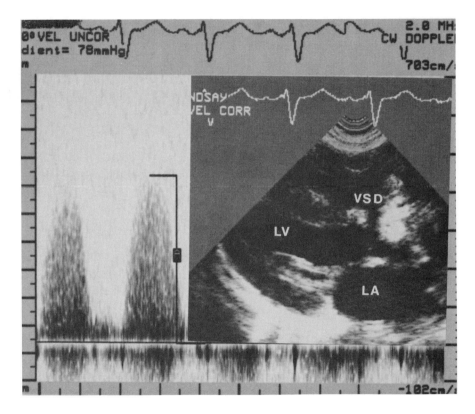

Fig. 6–42. Two-dimensional parasternal long axis image and continuous wave Doppler velocities obtained from a patient with a restrictive membranous ventricular septal defect.

ally, increased peak flow velocities will result in a flow related gradient. Because of a series effect, the flow disturbance associated with a ventricular septal defect may also be detected in the pulmonary artery (Chapter 4). Pulsed Doppler detection of a flow disturbance proximal to the pulmonary valve suggests that the disturbance originated within the right ventricle. Differentiating an associated pulmonary stenosis from a series effect may occasionally be difficult.

DOPPLER DIFFERENTIATION FROM OTHER LESIONS

Other lesions that may cause a flow disturbance within the right ventricle include tricuspid stenosis, pulmonary regurgitation, and subvalvar pulmonic stenosis or anomalous right ventricular muscle bundles. Tricuspid stenosis and pulmonary regurgitation cause diastolic flow disturbances and are therefore easily differentiated from the systolic disturbance resulting from a ventricular septal defect. However, subvalvar pulmonic stenosis and right ventricular muscle bundles can cause flow disturbances within the right ventricle which appear similar to those resulting from a restrictive ventricular septal defect. Generally, pulsed Doppler combined with two-dimensional imaging will differentiate these lesions.

DOPPLER ESTIMATION OF SEVERITY OF DISEASE

Pulmonary-to-systemic flow ratio can be estimated for patients with a ventricular septal defect.[64–67,75] Potential sites for evaluating pulmonary and systemic flows are shown in Figure 6–43. Systemic flow is usually determined in the ascending aorta but may also be measured across the tricuspid valve. Pulmonary flow should be evaluated in the main pulmonary artery whenever possible. However, abnormal velocity patterns in the pulmonary artery may result from systolic flow through the ventricular defect, associated pulmonary stenosis or a flow related gradient. In these situations pulmonary flow can be measured as pulmonary venous return across the mitral valve.

Doppler can accurately assess right ventricular pressure for patients with a VSD. Techniques for performing these calculations are discussed in detail in Chapter 4.

Patent Ductus Arteriosus

DIAGNOSTIC DOPPLER FINDINGS

Detection of a patent ductus was an important early application of pulsed Doppler.[76] Doppler evidence of a patent ductus can be found even in the absence of a heart murmur.[77,78] After imaging the pulmonary artery in the short axis precordial plane, the Doppler sample volume is placed in the distal main pulmonary artery to detect a diastolic positive jet (Fig. 6–44). A narrow patent ductus may direct flow in other directions and the entire main pulmonary artery must be scanned to detect the jet.[79] The pulmonary artery can be well visualized from the subcostal window in infants and many children and the jet associated with a PDA can also be detected from this view. A patent ductus and its origin from the distal aortic arch may also be imaged from the high right parasternal region or the suprasternal notch.[80,81] The Doppler sample volume can be placed within the PDA and velocity patterns traced from this aortic origin to the pulmonary artery. Even when the PDA is not visualized in the two-dimensional image, a jet may be detected. However, since the Doppler

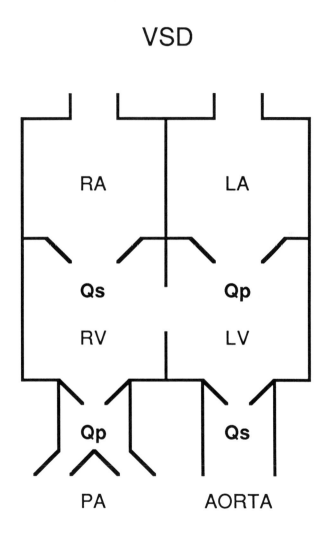

Fig. 6–43.   Schematic drawing showing possible sample sites for the measurement of pulmonary (Qp) and systemic (Qs) flow in a patient with a ventricular septal defect.

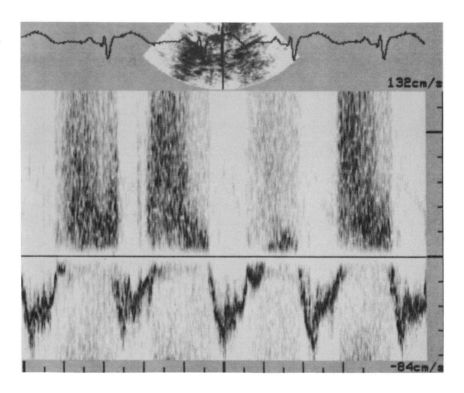

Fig. 6–44. Pulsed Doppler velocities obtained in the main pulmonary artery from the parasternal short axis view in a patient with a restrictive patent ductus arteriosus. The sample volume is within the jet and aliased retrograde velocities are present throughout diastole.

beam will not usually be aligned with flow in this plane, this procedure only confirms the presence of a patent ductus and may not provide quantitative information regarding pressure drop.

The presence of a patent ductus may also be inferred indirectly by demonstrating abnormal velocity patterns in other areas. The connection to the usually lower resistance pulmonary bed will result in a diastolic runoff from the aorta into the pulmonary artery.[7] Depending upon the size of the ductus and the balance of systemic and pulmonary vascular resistance, reversal of diastolic flow may be noted in the descending aorta distal to the patent ductus or may extend into other arch vessels.[51,82] These regions are best visualized and interrogated from the suprasternal notch (Fig. 6–45). Diastolic flow in the aortic arch proximal to the patent ductus arteriosus should be in the forward direction. Presence of antegrade diastolic flow in the main pulmonary artery is highly sensitive and specific for detection of a patent ductus arteriosus (Fig. 6–46).[83] This is felt to represent diastolic ductal flow reversing at the closed pulmonary valve and then flowing in a forward direction out of the pulmonary artery. This finding is present even in patients in whom the jet disturbance from the patent ductus can not be identified. Therefore, the flow disturbance associated with a patent ductus arteriosus will depend upon the location of the sample volume. If the sample volume is within the main pulmonary artery and not within the jet, antegrade flow will be present both during systole and diastole (Fig. 6–46). If the sample volume is placed within the jet of a restrictive patent ductus arteriosus, retrograde velocities will be seen throughout diastole (Fig. 6–44).

Interrogation from the parasternal region with continuous wave Doppler will demonstrate continuous retrograde pulmonary artery velocities in the presence of a restrictive PDA (Fig. 6–47). Velocities will follow the aortic to pulmonary artery pressure difference and will therefore rise to a peak during late systole and fall during diastole.

Color-coded Doppler will demonstrate systemic to pulmonary velocity patterns associated with a patent ductus in the precordial short axis plane (Plate 30). Signal aliasing is seen when a large pressure drop is encountered between the aorta and pulmonary artery. Although slow videotape playback will usually define the direction of the jet, the examiner should verify that flow occurs during diastole and does not continue in significant amounts retrograde through the pulmonary valve. Ductal flow can also be visualized in the high right parasternal,[79] suprasternal and subcostal image planes. Right-to-left ductal shunting secondary to pulmonary hypertension may also be visualized with color-coded Doppler.[79]

ASSOCIATED DOPPLER FEATURES

A patent ductus with a significant left to right shunt will cause increased peak velocities at the mitral and aortic levels.[27]

DOPPLER DIFFERENTIATION FROM OTHER LESIONS

A ventricular septal defect, pulmonic stenosis, peripheral pulmonic stenosis, pulmonary regurgitation, and other great artery level shunts may also cause abnormal velocities in the pulmonary arteries. Both a ventricular septal defect and valvar pulmonic stenosis will cause antegrade systolic jet velocities in the main pulmonary artery. These should not be confused with the retrograde jet

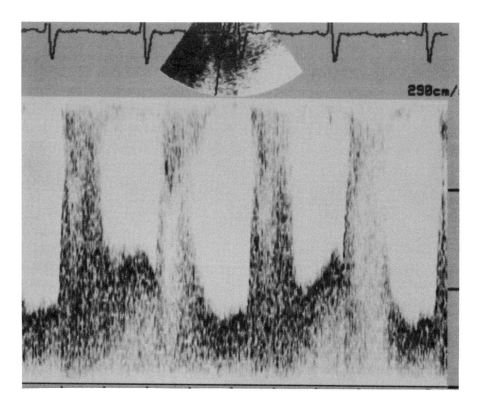

Fig. 6–45. Aliased pulsed Doppler velocities in a patient with a patent ductus arteriosus obtained from the suprasternal notch in the region of the PDA.

COLOR PLATES

Plate 16A. Color-coded Doppler long axis parasternal view from a patient with severe mitral regurgitation. Negative systolic regurgitant velocities within the left atrium are encoded as blue.

Plate 16B. Color-coded Doppler apical four chamber view showing a large left atrium with systolic velocities of mitral regurgitation encoded as blue. Panel to the left is early systole, and to the right is mid to late systole.

Plate 17. Color-coded Doppler apical four chamber view from a patient with mild tricuspid regurgitation showing systolic velocities (blue) along the right atrial septal surface (double arrows).

Plate 18A. Color-coded Doppler parasternal short axis view demonstrates blue velocities (arrow) of tricuspid regurgitation within the right atrium.

Plate 18B. Color-coded Doppler apical four chamber view shows blue velocities (arrow) of tricuspid regurgitation within the right atrium.

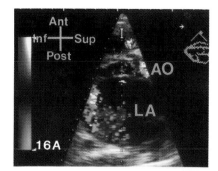

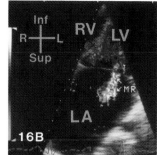

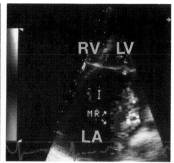

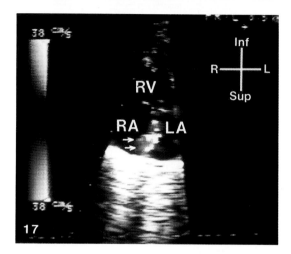

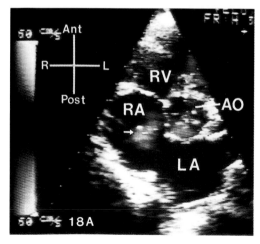

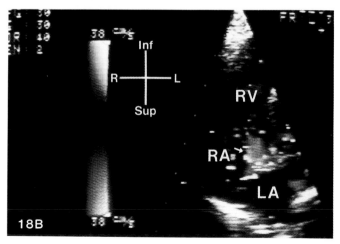

Plate 19A.   Apical four chamber view in a patient with severe tricuspid regurgitation demonstrates marked dilation of the pulmonary venous atrium (PVA), and incomplete apposition of the tricuspid valve leaflets. The patient had a Senning procedure for transposition of the great arteries. (SVA = systemic venous atrium.)

Plate 19B.   Color-coded Doppler apical four chamber view from the same patient shown in Plate 19A. Blue mosaic systolic velocities (double arrows) are seen far posteriorly and in a large area within the pulmonary venous atrium.

Plate 20.   Color-coded Doppler velocities from an apex five chamber plane. Red diastolic velocities of aortic regurgitation visualized proximal to the aortic valve (arrow) allowed easier alignment of the continuous wave Doppler cursor and recording of regurgitant jet velocities.

Plate 21.   Color-coded Doppler velocities from an apex five chamber plane from a patient with severe aortic regurgitation. Diastolic red mosaic pattern is traced inferiorly from the aortic valve to the apex of the left ventricle.

Plate 22.   Color-coded Doppler velocities from a high short axis parasternal plane. Diastolic red velocities of pulmonary regurgitation are visualized within the right ventricular outflow tract (RVOT) proximal to the pulmonary valve.

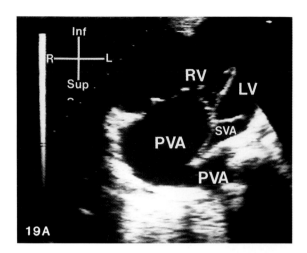

19A

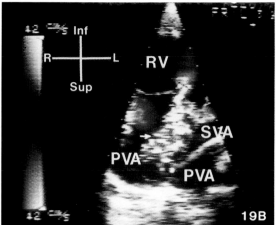

19B

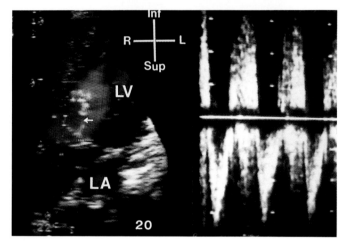

20

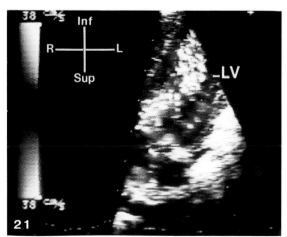

21

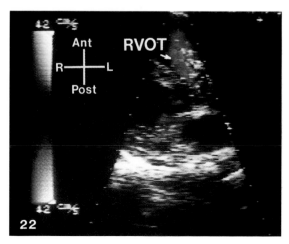

22

Plate 23. Short axis subcostal plane with right ventricle anterior and left ventricle posterior. Diastolic red velocities of pulmonary regurgitation are seen within a large area of the right ventricle.

Plate 24. Apical four chamber plane with red-orange pattern (double arrows) at the atrial septum indicating a left to right atrial shunt.

Plate 25A. Subcostal long axis view of a secundum atrial septal defect (arrow).

Plate 25B. Color-coded Doppler velocities from the same patient in Plate 25A. Red-orange velocity pattern demonstrates left to right atrial shunt.

Plate 26. Subcostal short axis view demonstrates red velocity pattern of left to right atrial shunt.

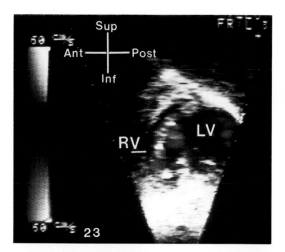

23

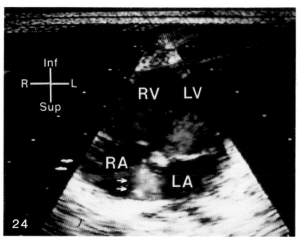

24

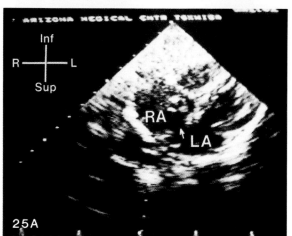

25A

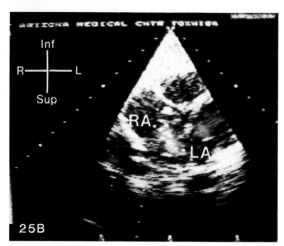

25B

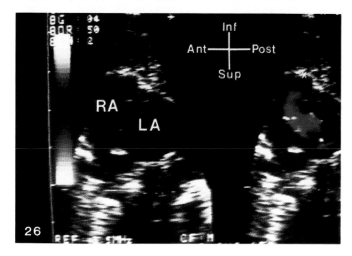

26

Plate 27.   Subcostal long axis plane demonstrates right to left bowing (double arrows) of the interatrial septum in a patient with tricuspid atresia (A). Blue velocities within the right and left atria demonstrate the right to left atrial shunt (B).

Plate 28.   Color-coded Doppler velocities obtained from the parasternal long axis view from a patient with a large malalignment ventricular septal defect. The blue and red-orange velocities within the defect indicate bidirectional shunting.

Plate 29.   Color-coded Doppler velocities obtained from a patient with a restrictive membranous ventricular septal defect. High velocities across the defect result in signal aliasing (mosaic pattern) in the long-axis parasternal view.

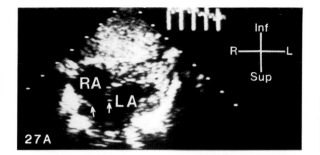

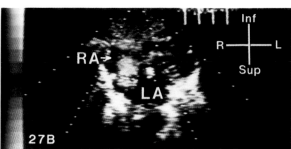

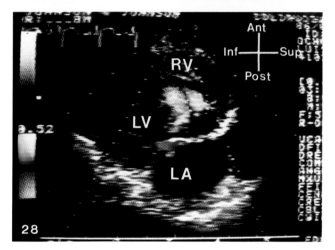

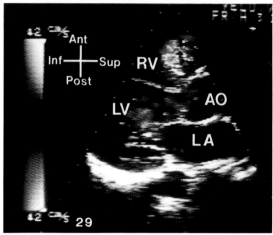

Plate 30. Color-coded Doppler velocities demonstrate a patent ductus arteriosus with red diastolic velocities (arrow) directed toward the left lateral wall of the pulmonary artery.

Plate 31. Subcostal color-coded Doppler velocities in a patient after a Senning operation. (A) Normal systemic inflow velocities (red) (arrow) course through the systemic venous atrium (SVA) toward the mitral valve. (B) Normal pulmonary venous inflow velocities (arrow) are directed from the posterior to anterior pulmonary venous atrium (PVA).

Plate 32. Color-coded Doppler velocities from an apical four chamber plane in a patient after a Senning operation. Severe tricuspid regurgitation is shown as a systolic blue mosaic pattern within the pulmonary venous atrium (PVA).

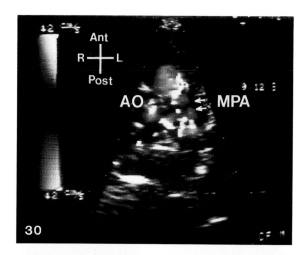

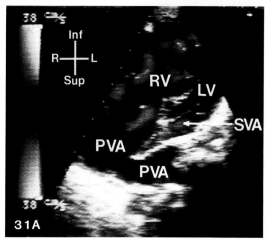

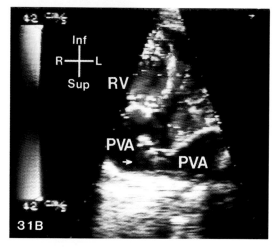

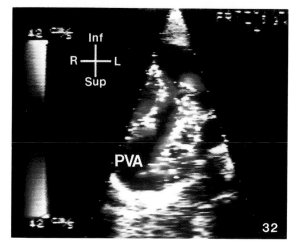

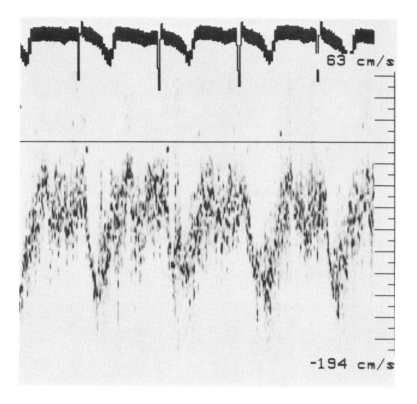

Fig. 6–46. Pulsed Doppler velocities obtained in the main pulmonary artery from the parasternal short axis view in a patient with a patent ductus arteriosus. Antegrade velocities are present during systole and diastole.

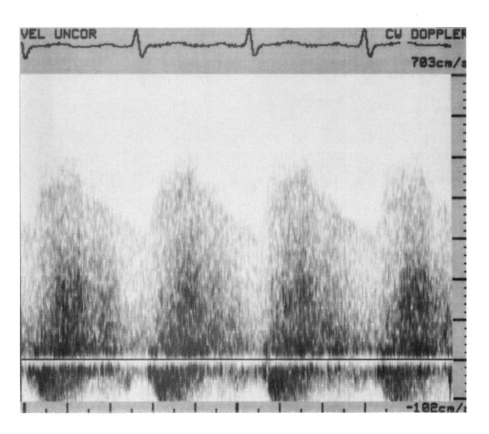

Fig. 6–47. Continuous wave Doppler velocities obtained from the parasternal region in a patient with a restrictive patent ductus arteriosus. Positive velocities are present throughout the cardiac cycle.

from a PDA. Similar to a patent ductus arteriosus, peripheral pulmonic stenosis can also be associated with continuous velocities. However, from the parasternal region, these velocities are directed away from the transducer and will therefore be in a different direction than those associated with the jet of a patent ductus arteriosus. Pulsed Doppler can verify increased velocity in the pulmonary artery branches when the stenosis is near the pulmonary bifurcation.

Pulmonary regurgitation causes retrograde diastolic flow in the main pulmonary artery. However, velocities in this region are generally not as high as those found within the jet of a PDA. Retrograde diastolic velocities proximal to the pulmonary valve are not found with a ductus arteriosus unless associated with pulmonary regurgitation.

Difficulty may arise in differentiating a PDA from other great artery level shunts such as an aorticopulmonary artery window, pulmonary origin of the left coronary artery or a surgically created systemic to pulmonary artery shunt. An anomalous left coronary artery can usually be imaged with two-dimensional echocardiography. If retrograde coronary flow exists, pulsed Doppler can be used to detect the abnormal velocities at the origin of the coronary artery into the proximal main pulmonary artery. Surgically created systemic to pulmonary artery shunts are discussed later.

Color-coded Doppler can be helpful in differentiating a patent ductus from the above lesions. The origin of the flow disturbance within the pulmonary artery can be ascertained relatively quickly with this modality.

DOPPLER ESTIMATION OF SEVERITY OF DISEASE

Pulmonary-to-systemic flow ratio can be estimated for a patent ductus arteriosus.[64–66] Pulmonary flow in a patient with a patent ductus or other great artery shunt is calculated as pulmonary venous return at the mitral or aortic levels (Fig. 6–48). Although good quality Doppler signals can usually be obtained from either site, measurements are usually made most easily in the ascending aorta. Systemic flow should be calculated as systemic venous return through the tricuspid valve or right ventricular outflow tract. Theoretically, flow in the proximal pulmonary artery may represent systemic venous return. However, in the presence of a significant shunt, flows in this location are usually too abnormal to permit accurate measurement. Additionally, the sample site which represents forward flow is speculative.

Several studies have shown that Doppler can accurately estimate pulmonary artery pressures for patients with a PDA. Aorta to pulmonary artery pressure difference was calculated from the peak pulmonary artery jet velocity. Techniques for performing these calculations are discussed in detail in Chapter 4.

Operative Aorticopulmonary Shunts

DIAGNOSTIC DOPPLER FINDINGS

The main diagnostic Doppler finding in patients with aortico-pulmonary shunts is continuous velocities in the pulmonary artery (Fig. 6–49).[7,84,85] Doppler interrogation of shunt velocities is achieved by placement of the Doppler sample volume in the corresponding pulmonary artery from the short axis parasternal, subcostal, or suprasternal notch planes (Fig. 6–49).

Continuous wave Doppler interrogation is best achieved by aiming the transducer in the direction of anticipated shunt flow. Alignment with velocities in

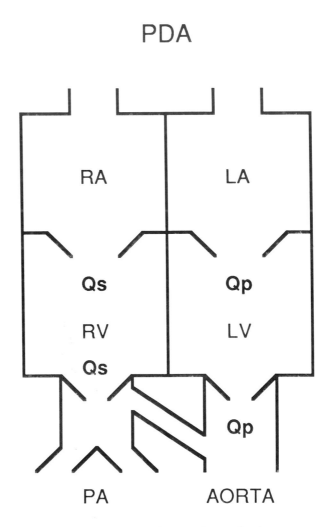

PDA

Fig. 6–48. Schematic drawing showing possible sample sites for the measurement of pulmonary (Qp) and systemic (Qs) flow in a patient with a patent ductus arteriosus.

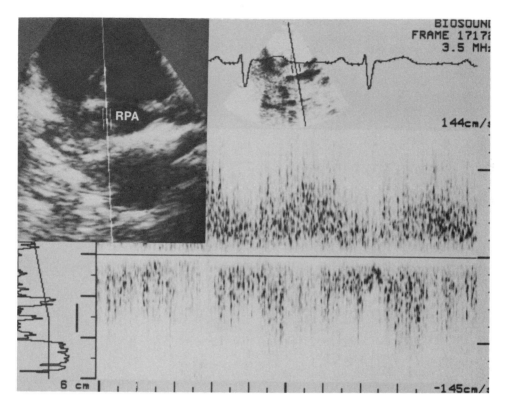

Fig. 6–49. Pulsed Doppler interrogation from the suprasternal notch with the sample volume in the right pulmonary artery (insert) in a patient with a Blalock-Taussig Shunt. Turbulent continuous velocities confirm patency of the shunt.

patients with right Blalock-Taussig shunts can best be achieved from the suprasternal notch or right supraclavicular area.[85] The transducer is aimed inferiorly, in all directions, until optimal Doppler waveforms are achieved. Shunt velocities are continuous, and do not return to baseline (Fig. 6–50), indicating a pressure drop at end diastole. Alignment with the jet occurs when the peak velocities are concentrated on the perimeter of the time velocity envelope (Fig. 6–50). Systolic pulmonary artery pressure can be estimated by subtracting the peak pressure drop from systolic systemic arterial pressure (Chapter 4).

Doppler alignment with flow in a patient with a Waterston shunt is best achieved by placement of the sample volume in the right or left parasternal border and aiming the transducer toward the patient's right side. The waveform will be similar to that in a Blalock-Taussig shunt.

DOPPLER DIFFERENTIATION FROM OTHER LESIONS

Retrograde diastolic velocities can be found in the transverse aortic arch and descending aorta in patients with left to right aorticopulmonary shunts (Fig. 6–23). This pattern is similar to that which occurs in patients with aortic regurgitation. Doppler interrogation in the aortic outflow tract in a patient with aortic regurgitation will show a jet, whereas patients with an aortic-pulmonary shunt alone will have no diastolic jet in this area.

Truncus arteriosus may provide a diagnostic dilemma. Patients with this lesion also have negative diastolic velocities in the transverse arch secondary to run-off flow into the pulmonary artery (Fig. 6–51). These patients may also have a jet of truncal regurgitation within the left ventricular outflow tract (Fig. 6–52).

Total Anomalous Pulmonary Venous Drainage

DIAGNOSTIC DOPPLER FEATURES

Total anomalous pulmonary venous drainage is difficult to diagnose despite advances in imaging echocardiography.[86–90] Visualization of pulmonary veins, and detection of pulmonary venous velocities entering the posterior left atrium precludes the diagnosis of this disease. Confirmation of anomalous pulmonary venous drainage occurs when the confluence of the pulmonary veins to the anomalous drainage site is shown. Pulsed Doppler can be extremely useful in demonstrating the anomalous drainage.[91–93]

Anomalous pulmonary venous drainage to the vertical vein, innominate, and superior vena cava can be mapped by pulsed Doppler from either a subcostal or suprasternal notch plane (Fig. 6–53).[93] First, the pulmonary vein confluence behind the left atrium is visualized. The Doppler sample volume is placed in the superior aspect of the confluence, at the entrance of the vertical vein. From the suprasternal notch positive continuous velocities, indicating pulmonary venous flow in a cephalad direction, are traced superiorly into the vertical vein (Fig. 6–53A,B). These velocities can be sequentially mapped into the left innominate. Doppler interrogation in the right superior vena cava demonstrates significantly increased amplitude negative velocities (Fig. 6–53C) into the right atrium.

Anomalous pulmonary venous return to the coronary sinus can also be diagnosed by a combination of two-dimensional imaging and pulsed Doppler[93] (Fig. 6–54A). From a subcostal short axis plane, pulmonary veins can be seen

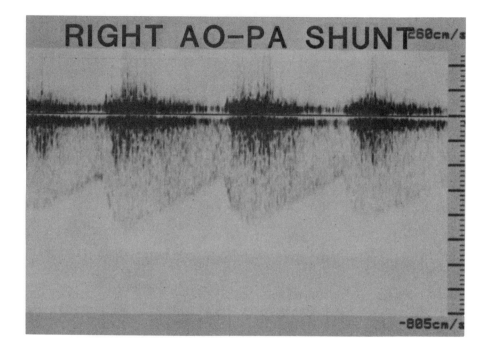

Fig. 6–50. Continuous wave Doppler tracings from a patient with a central Gortex® shunt. Concentration of peak velocities on the perimeter indicates alignment with the jet.

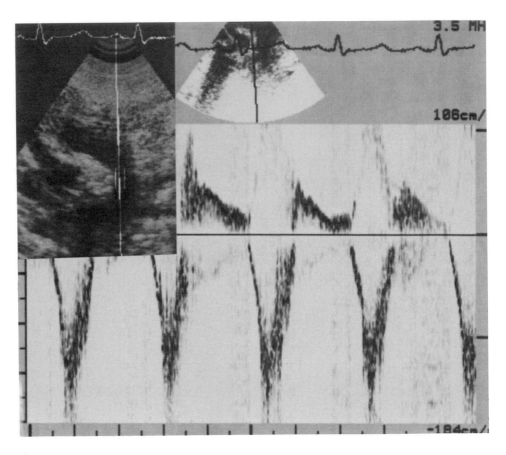

Fig. 6–51. Pulsed wave Doppler tracings in the transverse aortic arch (insert) from a patient with truncus arteriosus. Positive diastolic velocities of flow into the pulmonary arteries are seen.

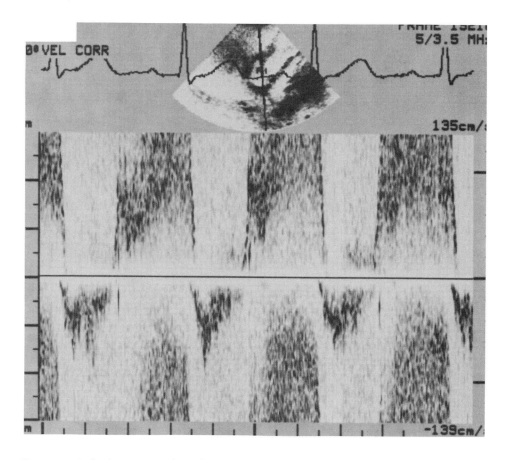

Fig. 6–52. Pulsed wave Doppler velocities from an apex four chamber plane with the sample volume proximal to the truncal valve in a patient with truncus arteriosus. High velocity, positive diastolic jets of severe truncal regurgitation are shown.

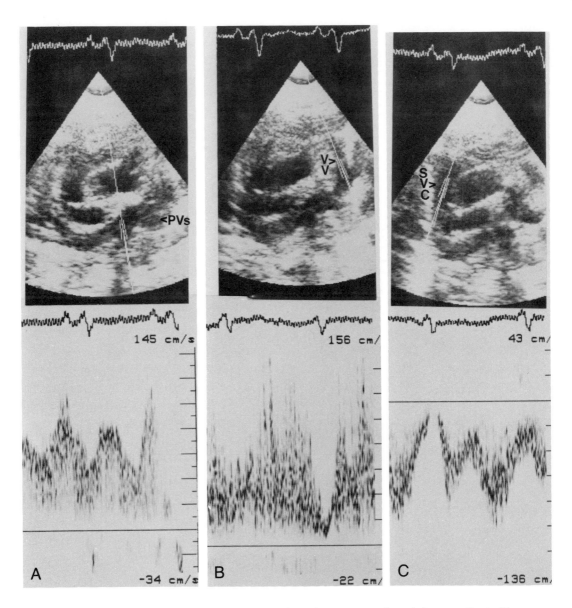

Fig. 6–53. Pulsed wave Doppler velocities from the suprasternal notch from a patient with anomalous pulmonary venous drainage to the superior vena cava. Positive continuous velocities, with the sample volume within the pulmonary veins (PV) confluence (A), can be traced superiorly into the vertical vein (VV) (B). Increased negative velocities are interrogated in the right superior vena cava-right atrial junction (C).

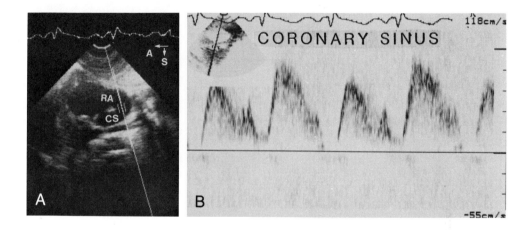

Fig. 6–54. Subcostal (A and B) and suprasternal (C and D) Doppler echo interrogation from a patient with mixed total anomalous pulmonary venous drainage. Increased positive biphasic pulmonary velocity tracings (B) are seen with the sample volume within the coronary sinus (A).

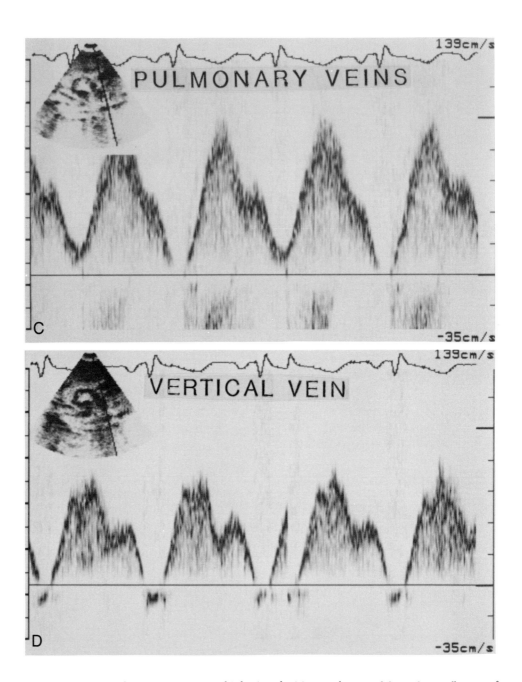

Fig. 6–54 (continued). Positive venous biphasic velocities can be traced from the confluence of the pulmonary veins (C) to the vertical vein (D).

entering a dilated vertical chamber that empties into the right atrium. Positive continuous velocities of pulmonary venous inflow can be mapped posteriorly from the entrance of the pulmonary veins, through the coronary sinus and into the entrance of the right atrium (Fig. 6–54B). Pulmonary venous velocities may appear to be entering the left atrium if the Doppler transducer is inadvertently aimed anteriorly.

Occasionally, as shown in Figure 6–54C and D, anomalous drainage can be mixed. In addition to anomalous pulmonary venous drainage to the coronary sinus, standard interrogation from the suprasternal notch demonstrated a confluence of pulmonary veins draining into a vertical vein. Velocities were sequentially mapped (Fig. 6–54C and D) demonstrating anomalous pulmonary venous drainage to the superior vena cava.

Anomalous pulmonary venous drainage below the diaphragm can also be accurately imaged by two-dimensional echocardiography, and velocities mapped by pulsed Doppler technique (Fig. 6–55).[91] Three vessels are visualized, from a subcostal short axis view, as they traverse posteriorly across the diaphragm. Rightward orientation demonstrates the inferior vena cava entering the right atrium. Doppler velocities are negative, biphasic, and low amplitude. Leftward orientation of the transducer demonstrates the vertical vein posterior to the left atrium, and anterior to the aorta (Fig. 6–55A). Velocity tracings in the vertical vein are also low amplitude and continuous, but are positive in direction (Fig. 6–55B). Aortic velocities have characteristic positive, high velocity systolic envelopes.

ASSOCIATED DOPPLER FEATURES

Anomalous pulmonary venous drainage is associated with right to left atrial shunting. Tricuspid and pulmonary valve velocities are significantly higher than normal due to increased flow. One major exception occurs in patients with obstructed anomalous pulmonary venous drainage in whom all velocities may be decreased as the result of low cardiac output.

DOPPLER DIFFERENTIATION FROM OTHER LESIONS

Increased superior vena caval velocities can also occur in patients with cerebral or upper extremity arterial-venous malformations. Increased inferior vena caval velocities occur in patients with hepatic arterial-venous malformations. Both result in increased intracardiac and great vessel velocities.

Persistence of a left superior vena cava to the coronary sinus can result in increased velocities at the entrance of the coronary sinus to right atrium. A dilated vertical vein can be seen entering the coronary sinus from either a subcostal or suprasternal notch plane (Fig. 6–56). Doppler interrogation in this vessel shows negative, continuous low amplitude velocities that can be mapped to the level of the coronary sinus.

Partial Anomalous Pulmonary Venous Return

DIAGNOSTIC DOPPLER FINDINGS

Partial anomalous pulmonary venous return can have a myriad of possible anatomic locations. Precise anatomic delineation of the anomalous return by two-dimensional echocardiography is best accomplished from complimentary orthogonal subcostal planes (Fig. 6–57A). Doppler interrogation in these anom-

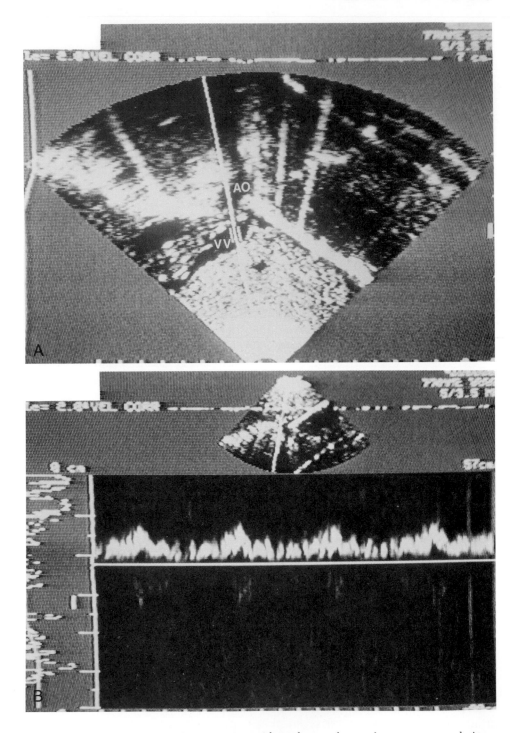

Fig. 6–55. Subcostal view (A) from a patient with total anomalous pulmonary venous drainage below the diaphragm with the Doppler sample volume placed within the vertical vein (vv). Low amplitude, continuous, positive pulsed Doppler velocities are found within the vertical vein (B).

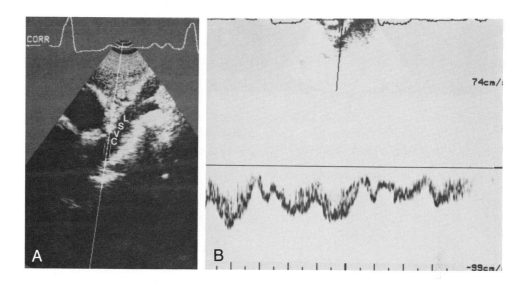

Fig. 6–56. Doppler sample volume placed in a persistent left superior vena cava (LSVC), as imaged from the suprasternal notch (A). Negative, low amplitude, biphasic tracings of systemic venous return are seen (B).

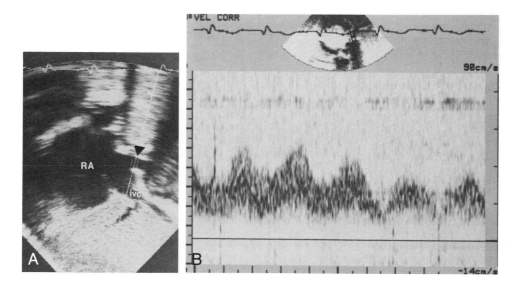

Fig. 6–57. Short axis subcostal plane demonstrating the Doppler sample volume within a pulmonary vein (arrow) draining to the right atrium (A). Velocities are turbulent, continuous and low amplitude (B). Amplitude is low because of the intercept angle.

alous vessels demonstrates turbulent, continuous, low amplitude velocities (Fig. 6–57B). Decreased velocities are, in part, related to inability to interrogate parallel to flow in these vessels.

ASSOCIATED DOPPLER FEATURES

Partial anomalous pulmonary venous return may be associated with increased velocities across the tricuspid and pulmonary valves.

DOPPLER DIFFERENTIATION FROM OTHER LESIONS

Increased tricuspid and pulmonary velocities are also seen in patients with atrial septal defects which often occur with partial anomalous pulmonary venous return (see prior for diagnosis of atrial septal defects).

Hypoplastic Left Heart Syndrome

DIAGNOSTIC DOPPLER FINDINGS

Although two-dimensional echocardiography can accurately diagnose hypoplastic left heart syndrome, Doppler can confirm the physiologic parameters associated with this disease.[94] Hypoplastic left heart syndrome is most often associated with aortic and or mitral atresia. In some cases, however, both the aortic and mitral valves appear anatomically normal but are severely hypoplastic. Hence, no diagnostic Doppler velocity patterns exist for all forms of this disease.

In cases of hypoplastic left heart syndrome with mitral atresia, Doppler confirms absence of flow across the mitral valve (Fig. 6–58A). Absence of antegrade systolic velocities in the ascending aorta confirms aortic atresia (Fig. 6–58B). Retrograde velocities from a patent ductus arteriosus can be detected traversing around the transverse aortic arch into the ascending aorta to provide coronary perfusion[94] (Fig. 6–58B). Tricuspid inflow velocities can be used to assess right ventricular function, and extent of tricuspid regurgitation. Patients with significant tricuspid regurgitation, as detected by Doppler, are reported to have a worse outcome for the first stage of the Norwood procedure.[95]

DOPPLER DIFFERENTIATION FROM OTHER LESIONS

Critical aortic stenosis of the newborn period can also present with hypoplasia of the left ventricle, mitral valve apparatus and aortic outflow tract. Those patients with critical aortic stenosis, severe ventricular dysfunction, and low cardiac output may be difficult to differentiate from those with hypoplastic left heart syndrome. In general, those patients with critical aortic stenosis still have an aortic jet, but peak velocity may approach only 2 m/s because of low cardiac output.

Pulmonic Valve Atresia

DIAGNOSTIC DOPPLER FINDINGS

Diagnostic features of pulmonary valve atresia are absence of antegrade velocities in the main pulmonary artery, and turbulent retrograde velocities from a patent ductus arteriosus or aortic pulmonary collaterals (Fig. 6–59). Right-to-left shunting at the atrial level can be demonstrated in patients with pulmonary atresia and intact ventricular septum (Fig. 6–60).[88] These patients often have either tricuspid atresia or tricuspid stenosis. Either lesion can be visu-

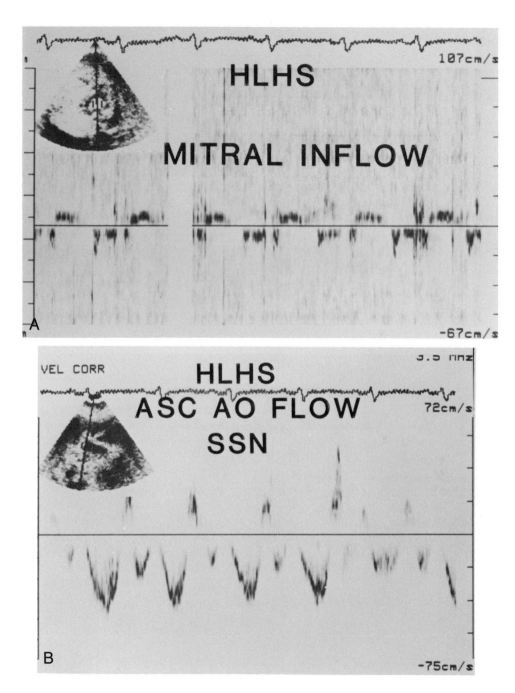

Fig. 6–58.   Absence of antegrade mitral velocities from an apical four chamber plane from a patient with hypoplastic left heart syndrome (A). Ascending aorta Doppler interrogation from the suprasternal notch shows absence of antegrade velocities confirming aortic atresia (B). Negative systolic retrograde velocities (below baseline) represent ductal flow to provide perfusion of the coronary arteries.

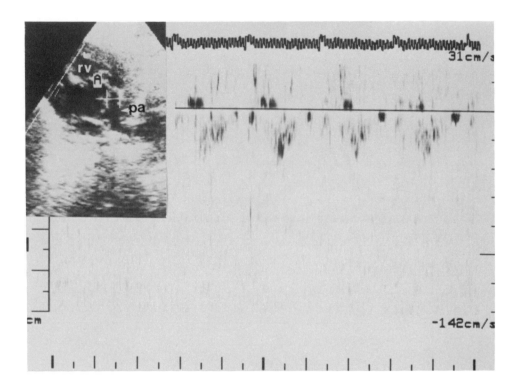

Fig. 6–59. Absence of antegrade pulmonary velocities in a patient with pulmonary atresia (insert).

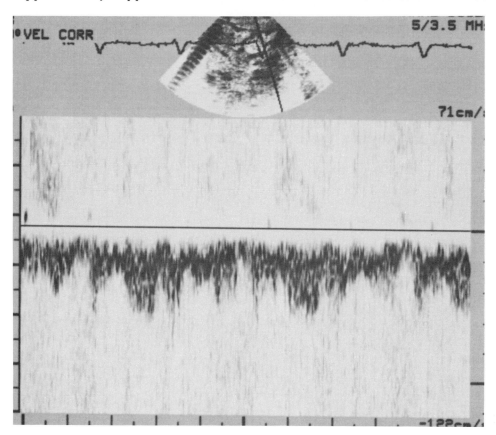

Fig. 6–60. Negative pulsed Doppler velocities demonstrating right to left atrial shunt in an infant with pulmonary atresia and intact ventricular septum. The sample volume was placed in the left atrium.

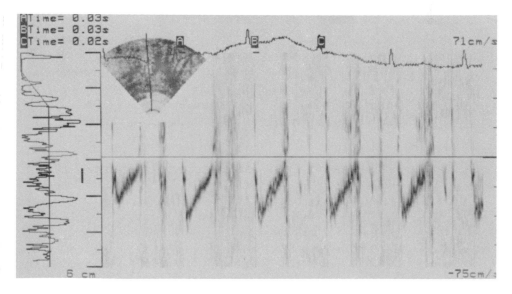

Fig. 6–61. Pulmonary velocity tracings from an infant with persistent fetal circulation. Time to peak velocity was 30 m/sec consistent with severe pulmonary artery hypertension.

alized by two-dimensional echocardiography with Doppler demonstrating absence of velocities in tricuspid atresia, or increased velocities in stenosis.

DOPPLER DIFFERENTIATION FROM OTHER LESIONS

Differentiation of persistent fetal circulation from valvar pulmonary atresia can be difficult to assess in critically ill newborn infants. In both lesions the right atrium and ventricle can be significantly enlarged, with right to left shunting at the atrial or ductal level. Infants with severe persistent fetal circulation and elevated pulmonary resistance, have minimal systolic excursion of the pulmonary valve leaflets. The leaflets may appear thickened, simulating valvar pulmonary atresia. Valvar atresia is characterized by absence of forward velocities (Fig. 6–59), while persistent fetal circulation is characterized by low amplitude antegrade pulmonary velocities with decreased acceleration times (Fig. 6–61). In persistent fetal circulation, Doppler may detect pulmonic regurgitation, which would be absent in pulmonary valve atresia. Patients with critical pulmonic stenosis will demonstrate a systolic jet, which may be low amplitude if right ventricular dysfunction co-exists.

Transposition of the Great Arteries

DIAGNOSTIC DOPPLER FINDINGS

Two-dimensional echocardiography provides precise anatomic diagnosis of d-transposition of the great arteries (Fig. 6–62)[88,89,96,97] including visualization of associated ventricular septal defects,[98,99] abnormal attachment of the tricuspid valve apparatus,[98,99] and left ventricular outflow tract obstruction.[88,97,100] Doppler provides additional important information concerning preoperative tricuspid regurgitation, and magnitude and site of left ventricular outflow tract obstruction (Fig. 6–63).[100,101] Both potential lesions have implications for an atrial baffle or vessel switch operation.

Doppler Assessment of Baffle Obstruction after Mustard or Senning Repair

DIAGNOSTIC DOPPLER FINDINGS

Pulmonary and systemic venous obstruction, and tricuspid regurgitation are known complications after both the Mustard and Senning operation for transposition of the great arteries. Pulmonary venous obstruction can be insidious and life threatening. Several investigators have demonstrated the accurate two-dimensional echocardiographic diagnosis of systemic and pulmonary venous obstruction following the Mustard and Senning operations.[88,97,102] However, two-dimensional imaging may not be diagnostic in older patients in whom subcostal imaging is not possible, or in patients with lung disease or chest wall abnormalities in whom imaging from the apex plane is difficult.

Detection of pulmonary venous inflow velocities (Fig. 6–64) is best achieved from the subcostal plane where interrogation can be done in two orthogonal views. In older patients Doppler interrogation can be accomplished from the apex four chamber plane. After a baffle operation pulmonary venous inflow velocities are usually bi-phasic with reversal of flow during atrial systole (Fig. 6–64).[103]

Doppler interrogation of systemic venous inflow velocities is difficult following both the Senning (Fig. 6–65) and Mustard operation. After surgery,

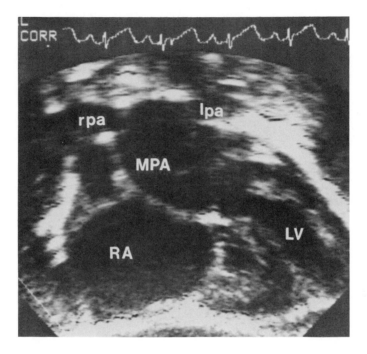

Fig. 6–62.   Subcostal long axis plane in d-transposition of the great arteries demonstrating origination of the main pulmonary artery from the left ventricle.

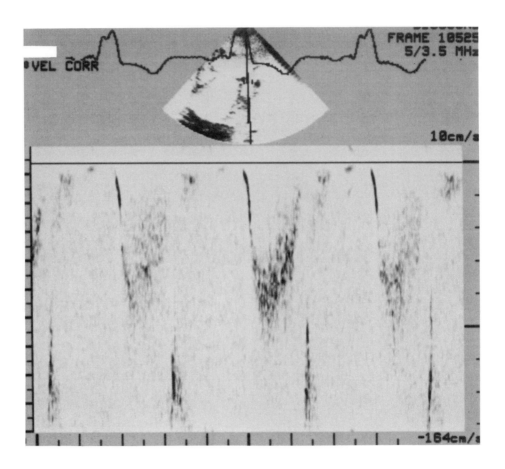

Fig. 6–63. Left ventricular outflow tract velocities in a patient with transposition of the great vessels with the sample volume placed directly underneath the pulmonary valve. A turbulent velocity pattern is seen; the patient had mild subpulmonary valve obstruction.

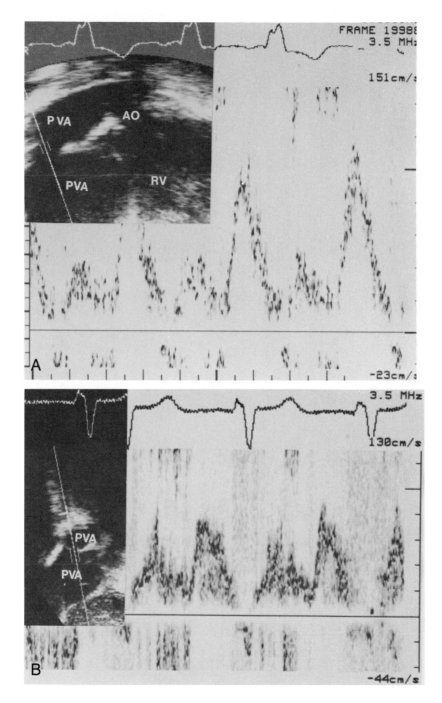

Fig. 6–64. Subcostal long (A) and short axis (B) Doppler echocardiographic tracings from a patient after a Senning operation. The Doppler sample volume is at the usual area of obstruction of the pulmonary venous atrium (PVA). Positive biphasic velocities are seen, with the highest peak preceding the QRS complex.

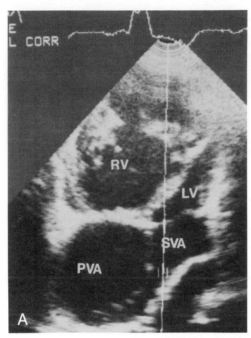

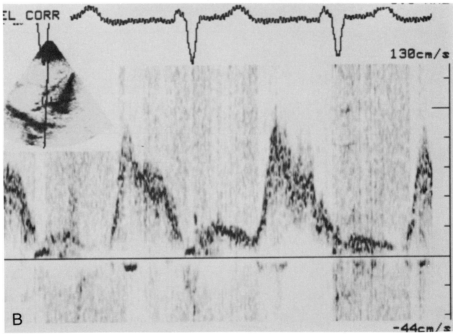

Fig. 6–65. Doppler velocities in the systemic venous atrium (SVA) from an apex four chamber plane in a patient after a Senning operation (A). The velocities are biphasic and positive with lower amplitude and greater velocity spread than found in normal patients (B).

systemic venous inflow pathways are directed at an angle away from the vertical plane. This orientation makes parallel alignment with flow entering the heart from both the inferior and superior vena cava difficult. A nonturbulent biphasic pattern can be seen in the systemic venous atrium in the absence of a gradient.[104] Superior vena caval velocities are lower and have increased velocity spread after an atrial baffle operation (Fig. 6–65B). Color-coded Doppler usually provides an expedient view of pulmonary and systemic inflow velocities (Plate 31).

Interrogation for pulmonary venous obstruction after the Senning operation requires visualization of the narrowed pulmonary venous pathway coursing from dilated pulmonary veins, through the pulmonary venous atrium towards the tricuspid valve.[88,102] The site of obstruction can be visualized, and the pulsed wave Doppler sample volume moved proximal and distal to the expected area of obstruction (Fig. 6–66). After the Mustard operation the obstruction is usually at the entrance of the pulmonary veins to the pulmonary venous atrium. When significant obstruction is present, velocities distal to the obstruction also form a continuous jet (Fig. 6–67).[103]

An example of superior vena caval obstruction after a Mustard operation is shown in Figure 6–68. The Doppler sample volume was placed at the mitral valve annulus from an apical four chamber plane. A turbulent jet of systemic venous obstruction can be seen adjacent to the mitral valve inflow velocities.

DOPPLER DIFFERENTIATION FROM OTHER LESIONS

Dilated pulmonary venous atrium and pulmonary veins can also be secondary to significant tricuspid regurgitation after an atrial baffle procedure. This entity can be differentiated by standard pulsed or color-coded imaging (Plate 32).

Intracardiac Masses

Doppler interrogation can provide important information about intracardiac masses that cannot be gleaned from an imaging study alone.[105,106] The following two cases will illustrate this point.

Figure 6–69 shows a large mass in the aortic outflow tract in an infant with tuberous sclerosis and multiple intracardiac rhabdomyomas. Despite what appeared to be nearly complete anatomic obstruction, continuous wave Doppler interrogation showed only a mild gradient (Fig. 6–69D). Doppler cardiac output calculated across the pulmonary valve was normal at 3.5 liters/min/m^2. Since this patient had no significant dysrhythmias or obstruction, intervention was postponed. Serial two-dimensional Doppler echocardiograms have shown regression of the tumors.

The second case was a young infant with a single large tumor occluding the left ventricular outflow tract (Fig. 6–70A). Continuous wave Doppler interrogation showed an aortic outflow tract gradient of 58 mm Hg (Fig. 6–70B). Surgical intervention successfully removed the tumor.

These two cases illustrate the use of Doppler echocardiography in the management of patients with intracardiac masses. In such patients cardiac catheterization is hazardous, and masses are demonstrated only as filling defects at angiography. Combined two-dimensional Doppler studies not only directly visualize the masses, but also provide physiologic information to determine necessity for surgical intervention.

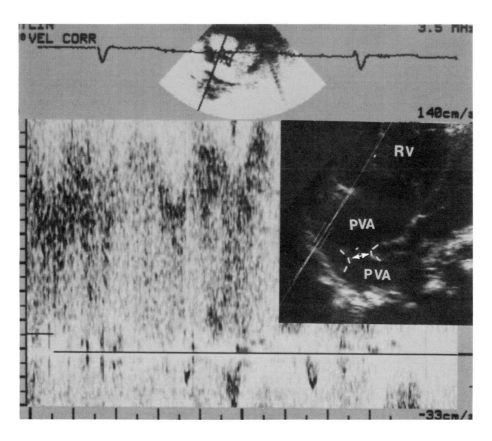

Fig. 6–66. Pulsed Doppler velocities distal to site of pulmonary venous obstruction (insert, arrows) after a Senning operation. Turbulent, continuous high velocities confirm obstruction. PVA = pulmonary venous atrium.

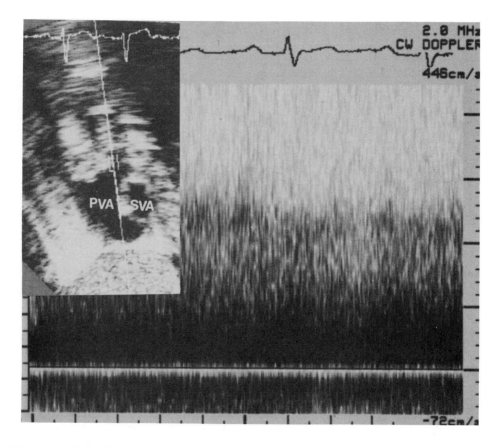

Fig. 6–67.   High velocity (2.6 m/s) continuous wave Doppler tracing across obstructed pulmonary veins in a patient after the Mustard operation. The velocities are dense and occur throughout the cardiac cycle. In the subcostal long axis view (insert), the sample volume is seen at the entrance of the pulmonary veins into the superior portion of the pulmonary venous atrium (PVA).

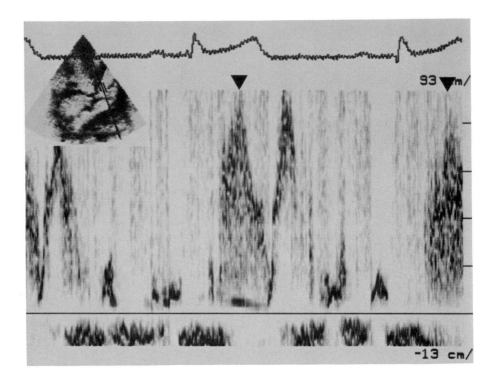

Fig. 6–68. Pulsed Doppler velocities at the mitral valve orifice in a patient after a Mustard operation. Turbulent systolic velocities (arrows) due to systemic venous obstruction are seen adjacent to mitral inflow velocities.

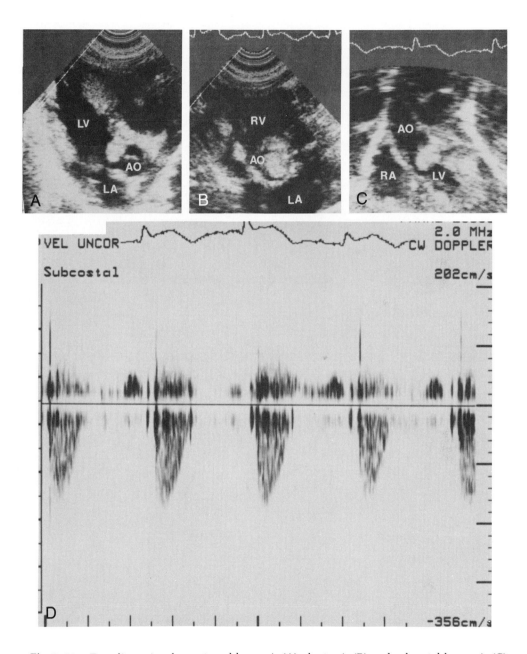

Fig. 6–69. Two-dimensional parasternal long axis (A), short axis (B), and subcostal long axis (C) planes showing a large mass apparently nearly occluding the left ventricular outflow tract. Continuous wave Doppler interrogation across the outflow tract showed minimal obstruction (D).

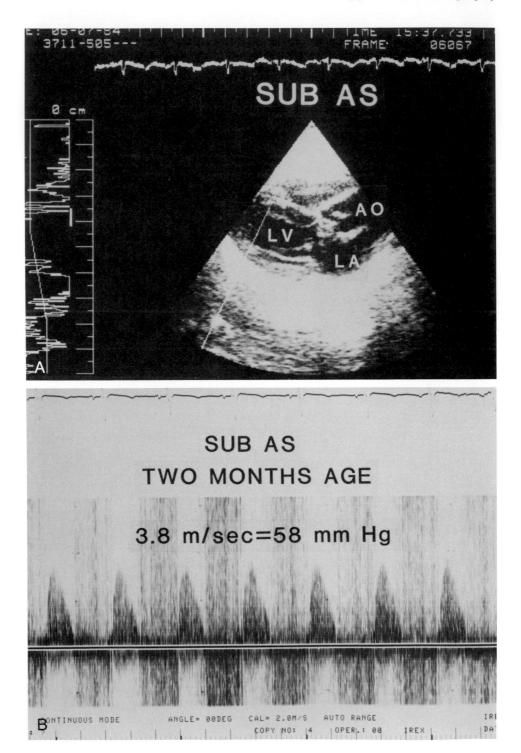

Fig. 6–70. Long axis parasternal image demonstrating a large tumor mass occluding the left ventricular outflow tract (A). Continuous wave Doppler velocities showed a gradient of 58 mm Hg (B).

Cardiac Function

SYSTOLIC FUNCTION

Many parameters of ventricular ejection have been used to assess ventricular performance. Most of these indices do not assess contractility independently since they are influenced by preload, afterload, and heart rate. The most commonly used measurements include cardiac output, stroke volume, ejection fraction and the rate of left ventricular pressure rise, LVdP/dt.

Various measurements of the aortic velocity curve have been studied to see how they correlate with ventricular performance. As shown in Figure 6–71 these include:

1. Peak Velocity (PV)—the maximal modal velocity obtained in the aorta during left ventricular ejection. The units are cm/s.

2. Systolic Velocity Integral (SVI)—The area under the systolic aortic velocity curve. The units are cm.

3. Acceleration Time (AT)—the time from onset of aortic flow to attainment of peak velocity. The units are ms.

Average and peak accelerations can be calculated from the systolic aortic velocity curve. The average acceleration during the rise in aortic velocity is computed by dividing peak velocity by acceleration time and multiplying by 1000 (to convert acceleration time from ms to seconds). The units are cm/s^2. Peak acceleration is the maximal slope of the aortic velocity curve during the early systolic rise in aortic velocity. The units are cm/s^2.

Animal studies have demonstrated a good correlation between Doppler peak velocity and invasively measured peak value of LVdp/dt.[107,108] This correlation is relatively insensitive to changes in heart rate and preload but is affected by afterload.[107] Human investigations have demonstrated a good relationship between Doppler peak aortic velocity and angiographically determined ejection fraction in patients without mitral or aortic disease.[109] Inducing myocardial ischemia in animals results in decreased aortic peak velocity which is related to the amount of ischemic left ventricular myocardium.[110] Decreased peak velocities may also be predictive of three vessel disease in patients with a previous myocardial infarction.[111]

Peak velocities have also been demonstrated to decrease with increasing systemic vascular resistance.[13] Since aortic area is not considered in this relationship, the correlation is stronger for changes in these parameters than for the absolute values themselves. Figure 6–4B shows an increase in aortic peak velocities after starting afterload reduction in a patient with a dilated cardiomyopathy. Peak velocities have been shown to be decreased in dilated cardiomyopathy[112] (Fig. 6–72) and increased in hypertrophic cardiomyopathy.[113] Peak velocities decrease significantly with age.[114,115] This finding is due, in part, to an age related increase in aortic diameter.[114]

Stroke volume may be calculated by multiplying the systolic velocity integral by the aortic cross-sectional area (Chapter 5). Factors affecting stroke volume would, therefore, be expected to influence SVI. SVI has been shown to decrease with myocardial ischemia[109–111] and dilated cardiomyopathy[112] and to vary inversely with systemic vascular resistance.[13] When compared to other Doppler indices, SVI is more sensitive to loading conditions and not as sensitive to the inotropic state.[108,109,116] Since stroke volume is a function of both SVI and the

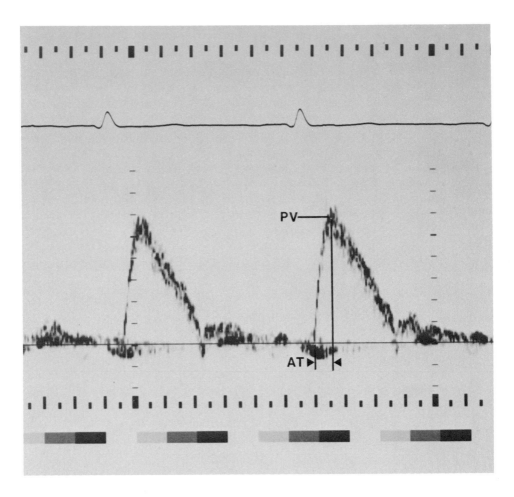

Fig. 6–71. Ascending aortic velocity curve showing Peak Velocity (PV) and Acceleration Time (AT). See text for details.

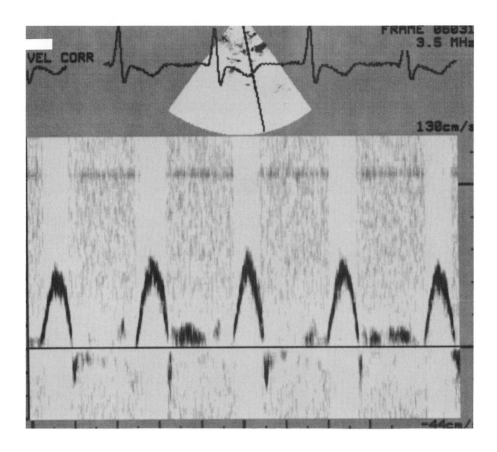

Fig. 6–72. Ascending aortic velocities from a patient with a severe dilated cardiomyopathy. Note the decreased peak velocities and abnormal upstroke velocities.

aortic cross-sectional area, changes in SVI correlate better with ventricular performance than do the absolute values.[13] Similar to peak velocity, SVI has been shown to decrease with age.[114,115]

Animal studies have shown a decrease in Doppler aortic acceleration time with an increase in inotropic state.[108] This parameter has not been studied as well as other Doppler indices of left ventricular function or pulmonary acceleration time. In addition to left ventricular function, the shape of the aortic velocity curve is affected by several factors including systemic impedance, preload, and aortic size.[7] Clinical studies have shown no significant change in AT in patients with nonobstructive hypertrophic cardiomyopathy[113] and a decrease in AT in patients with dilated cardiomyopathy.[112] Acceleration time does not significantly change with age.[114]

In theory, aortic peak acceleration should be related to the maximal force attained by the left ventricle in early systole.[109] It will also be influenced by other factors such as mass of blood ejected, opposing forces or afterload, and viscous factors. Peak acceleration has been shown to increase with increases in left ventricular dp/dt in animals and is relatively insensitive to alterations in heart rate or preload.[107] In these studies, increased afterload caused a decrease in peak acceleration and a rise in LV dp/dt. Human investigations have also demonstrated that peak acceleration correlates with the inotropic state.[109,116] In both animals[110] and humans,[111] an increase in left ventricular ischemic mass has been associated with decreased peak acceleration.

Average acceleration is influenced by those factors that affect peak velocity and acceleration time and has been shown to correlate with LV dp/dt.[108] Average acceleration is decreased in patients with dilated cardiomyopathy.[112] Like peak velocity, average acceleration decreases with age.[114]

DIASTOLIC FUNCTION

Numerous methods have been proposed to assess cardiac function with Doppler. Early signs of cardiac dysfunction in many patients are impaired diastolic relaxation or ventricular compliance.[117–121] Abnormal diastolic function may be detected by Doppler as alterations in ventricular filling. Instantaneous left ventricular filling rate (mitral flow) can be computed as the product of transmitral instantaneous velocity and mitral orifice cross-sectional area. Most Doppler studies of left ventricular diastolic function have investigated mitral velocities rather than left ventricular filling rates. It should be kept in mind that although these values may correlate, they are not equivalent.

As described in Chapter 3, the normal mitral velocity waveform is composed of two diastolic peaks. The amplitude of the first peak (E wave) is generally the greater and occurs during early diastolic filling. The second filling peak (A wave) represents atrial contraction. It is postulated that left ventricular dysfunction results in impairment of early diastolic filling,[122–125] represented in the Doppler waveform as a lower peak velocity of the E wave and prolongation of this portion of diastole. Compensatory mechanisms should result in increased filling during atrial systole with higher A wave velocities.

Many parameters of mitral velocities have been proposed to assess diastolic function. These may be subdivided into those that measure peak filling velocities,[123–132] fractional filling,[125,129,133] and acceleration or deceleration rates or times.[123–127,129–131]

Figure 6–73 schematically shows a waveform demonstrating the most common measurements including the peak velocities of the E and A waves and their ratio, A/E. Closely related measurements include the areas under these curves and the ratio of these areas. Diastolic dysfunction would be expected to result in:

1. decreased E wave peak velocity
2. decreased area under the E wave
3. increased A wave peak velocity
4. increased area under the A wave
5. increased A/E peak velocity ratio
6. increased ratio of A wave area to E wave area

Figure 6–74 shows an abnormal A/E ratio in a patent with myocardial tumors.

Left ventricular "filling fractions,"[125,129,133] shown in Figure 6–75, are also used to assess diastolic function. To obtain true "filling fractions," instantaneous velocities should be multiplied by instantaneous mitral valve cross-sectional area (Chapter 5). Computations are greatly simplified, however, by ignoring changes in mitral valve cross-section and making calculations solely on the basis of areas under the velocity curve. Filling fractions are calculated by dividing the area under a selected portion of the transmitral velocity waveform by the area under the entire waveform. The selected area is generally the first 50% or first 33% of total diastolic flow time. The method for calculating the 50% fraction is shown schematically in Figure 6–75. The area under the cross-hatched portion of the curve, representing the first half of diastole, is divided by the area under the entire curve. As noted, diastolic dysfunction should cause a shift of left ventricular filling from early to late diastole. This in turn should result in a decrease in the 50% and 33% fractions.

Various measurements of E wave velocity acceleration or deceleration are also used to assess diastolic function.[123–127,129–132] These are shown schematically in Figure 6–76. The most commonly used measurements and their units are:

1. Acceleration Time (ms) (AT)—time interval from the onset of diastolic filling to the peak of the E wave.

2. Acceleration Half Time (ms) (AHT)—time interval from the point when the E wave reaches half peak velocity to the point when it reaches peak velocity.

3. Deceleration Time (ms) (DT)—time interval from the peak of the E wave to the point when the extrapolated downslope of the E wave crosses the baseline.

4. Deceleration Half Time (ms) (DHT)—time interval from peak of the E wave to the point when the E wave reaches half peak velocity.

5. Average Acceleration (cm/s^2)—Peak E wave velocity divided by acceleration time (AT) or one half peak E wave velocity divided by acceleration half time (AHT).

6. Average Deceleration (cm/s^2)—Peak E wave velocity divided by deceleration time (DT) or one half peak E wave velocity divided by deceleration half time (DHT).

Impaired left ventricular relaxation or compliance may result in increased acceleration and deceleration times and decreased average acceleration and deceleration.[122 124,127]

Early studies used cineangiography[117,118] and radionuclide angiography[120,121]

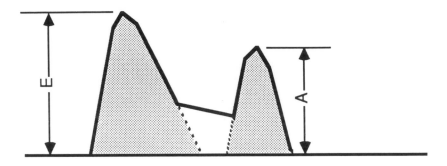

Fig. 6–73. Schematic drawing of a normal Doppler mitral velocity curve showing the peak velocity during diastolic filling (E wave) and the peak velocity during atrial systole (A wave). The areas under the E and A waves are shaded.

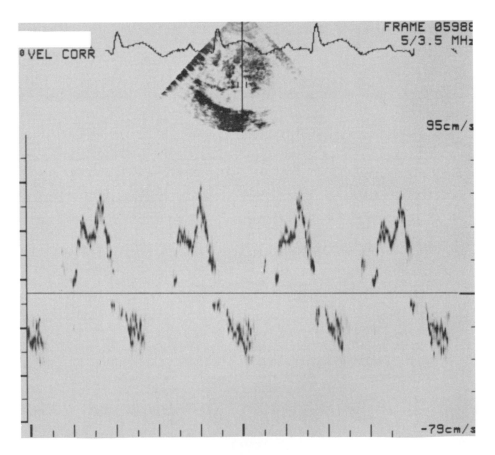

Fig. 6–74. Mitral valve velocities from a patient with myocardial tumors. The A/E ratio is abnormally increased.

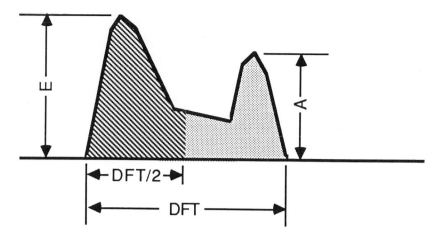

Fig. 6–75. Schematic drawing of a normal Doppler mitral velocity waveform showing the 50% filling fraction. E and A waves are shown. The entire shaded area represents the area under the velocity curve during the total diastolic filling time (DFT). The cross-hatched area represents the area under the velocity curve during the first half of diastole (DFT/2).

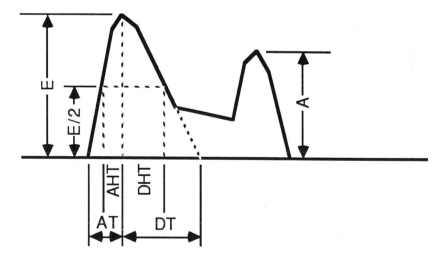

Fig. 6–76. Schematic drawing of a normal Doppler mitral velocity waveform showing various measurements of E wave acceleration and deceleration. E = peak E wave velocity; A = peak A wave velocity; AHT = acceleration half time; AT = acceleration time; DHT = deceleration half time; DT = deceleration time. See text for details.

to assess left ventricular filling parameters. Rokey et al.[133] compared Doppler peak filling rates and filling fractions with similar data obtained by cineangiography and found generally good correlations. Spirito et al.[126] did a similar study comparing Doppler measurements of diastolic velocity with volumetric measurements of left ventricular filling obtained by radionuclide angiography and found that Doppler results compared well with those of radionuclide angiography for assessing left ventricular function.

Patients with myocardial infarction have been found to have increased A/E ratios,[123,124] decreased average deceleration[124] and increased acceleration and deceleration half times.[123] The later investigation by Fujii et al. demonstrated more significant increases in deceleration half times than in acceleration half times. They postulated that one of the causes of significant prolongation of the deceleration phase in these patients was presence of fibrotic tissue, which would be expected to influence left ventricular filling throughout diastole. Impaired biochemical relaxation might also affect diastolic filling but these effects would be expected to predominate during early diastole and therefore should significantly affect acceleration phase.

Takenaka et al.[130] demonstrated that patients with dilated cardiomyopathy without mitral regurgitation have decreased E wave velocities and increased A/E ratios. Mitral regurgitation resulted in normalization of the peak E and A wave velocities and the A/E ratio. They suggested that this was because mitral regurgitation led to increased early diastolic left atrial pressures which in turn resulted in increased flow and increased E wave velocities.

Patients with hypertrophic cardiomyopathy[124,129] have shown a decrease in peak E wave velocity without a compensatory increase in A wave peak velocity. Kitabatake et al.[124] noted significant decreases in average deceleration rates in adults with hypertrophic cardiomyopathy, while significant increases in acceleration times were not found in children.[129] Although changes in the deceleration phase may be a more sensitive indicator of diastolic dysfunction than the acceleration phase, at least part of the above discrepancy can be explained by the incorporation of peak E wave velocity into computation of average acceleration and deceleration rates. A significant decrease in the 33% filling fraction has been demonstrated in children with hypertrophic cardiomyopathy.[129]

Adults with systemic hypertension have been found to have decreased E waves,[124,127] increased A waves,[124] and increased A/E ratios.[124,127,134] In children with systemic hypertension, Snider et al.[125] found increased A wave peak velocities and mildly increased A/E ratios, but did not note any significant difference in E wave peak velocities when compared to normal subjects. Similar to hypertrophic cardiomyopathy, decreased average E wave deceleration was seen in hypertensive adults,[124] while children did not have significant prolongation of acceleration time.[125]

Pearson et al.[132] investigated Doppler filling rates in weight lifters with left ventricular hypertrophy. Although they noted that both the E and A peak filling rates were higher than those of normal control subjects, no significant differences were found in the A/E ratios. They concluded that in the presence of an otherwise normal heart, left ventricular hypertrophy resulting from isometric exercises does not result in diastolic dysfunction as assessed by these criteria.

Several precautions are in order when using Doppler to assess left ventricular diastolic function. Several studies have demonstrated significant changes in mitral velocity with age.[128,131] E wave peak velocity has been shown to decrease with age, while A wave peak velocity and A/E ratio have been found to increase.[128,131] Gardin et al.[131] also demonstrated a significant age related increase in the E wave deceleration time and decrease in the average deceleration. None of these parameters were significantly influenced by heart rate. Therefore, until the relationship between age alone and ventricular function is clarified, patient age must be considered when using mitral velocity measurements to assess left ventricular function.

Ishida et al.[135] demonstrated that peak E wave velocity correlated strongly with the peak pressure difference between the left atrium and left ventricle during early diastole. They did not find a good correlation between the peak E wave velocity and left ventricular relaxation and postulated that this is because left ventricular relaxation is only one determinant of transmitral pressure difference. Other factors which must be considered are left ventricular and atrial compliance, left ventricular end-systolic volume, and left atrial early diastolic pressure. Leeman et al.[136] demonstrated that changes in preload will significantly alter Doppler indices of mitral velocity including the A/E ratio. Several other recent studies have also noted that that these indices must be used with caution when assessing left ventricular diastolic function.[137–139]

Although diastolic filling characteristics have been shown to change in various disease states, the majority of studies investigated Doppler mitral velocities in the presence of known pathologic conditions. Therefore, while these measurements may confirm already suspected cardiac dysfunction, it has not as yet been clearly demonstrated that they can provide independent information.

REFERENCES

1. Huntsman, L.L., Stewart, D.K., Barnes, S.R., Franklin, S.B., Colocousis, J.S., Hessel, E.A.: Noninvasive Doppler determination of cardiac output in man: Clinical validation. Circulation *67*:593, 1983.
2. Labovitz, A.J., Buckingham, T.A. Habermehl, K., Nelson, J., Kennedy, H.L., Williams, G.: The effects of sampling site on the two-dimensional echo-Doppler determination of cardiac output. Am Heart J *109*:327, 1985.
3. Lewis, J., Kuo, L., Nelson, J., Limacher, M., Quinones, M.: Pulsed Doppler echocardiographic determination of stroke volume and cardiac output: Clinical validation of two new methods using the apical window. Circulation *70*:425, 1984.
4. Schuster, A.H., Nanda, N.C.: Doppler echocardiographic features of mechanical alternans. Am Heart J *107*:580, 1984.
5. Rein, A.J., Hsieh, K.S., Elixson, M., Colan, S.D., Lang, P., Sanders, S.P., Castaneda, A.R.: Cardiac output estimates in the pediatric intensive care unit using a continuous-wave Doppler computer Validation and limitations of the technique. Am Heart J *112*:97, 1986.
6. Goldberg, S.J., Sahn, D.J., Allen, H.D., Valdes-Cruz, L.M., Hoenecke, H., Carnahan, Y.: Evaluation of pulmonary and systemic blood flow by two-dimensional Doppler echocardiography using fast Fourier transform spectral analysis. Am J Cardiol *50*:1394, 1982.
7. Hatle, L., Angelsen, B.: Doppler Ultrasound in Cardiology. Physical Principles and Clinical Applications. 2nd Ed., Philadelphia, Lea & Febiger, 1985.
8. Hagler, D.J. Seward, J.B., Tajik, A.J., Ritter, D.G.: Functional assessment of the Fontan operation: Combined M-mode, two-dimensional and Doppler echocardiographic studies. J Am Coll Cardiol *4*:756, 1984.
9. Kosturakis, D., Goldberg, S.J., Allen, H.D., Loeber, C.: Doppler echocardiographic prediction of pulmonary arterial hypertension in congenital heart disease. Am J Cardiol *53*:1110, 1984.
10. FitzGerald, D.E., Harry, J.D.: The use of Doppler ultrasound techniques to study the effects of isoprenaline and beta-adrenoceptor blocking drugs on peripheral blood vessels in man. Br J Clin Pharmacol *17*:773, 1984.
11. Ihlen, H., Amlie, J.P., Dale, J., Forfang, K., Nitter-Hauge, S., Otterstad, J.E., Simonsen, S.,

Myhre, E.: Determination of cardiac output by Doppler echocardiography. Br Heart J *51*:54, 1984.

12. Matsuda, M., Sekiguchi, T., Sugishita, Y., Ito, I.: Adverse effect of nifedipine on left ventricular obstruction detected by pulsed Doppler echocardiography. Jpn Heart J *25*:1081, 1984.

13. Elkayam, U., Gardin, J.M., Berkley, R., Hughes, C., Henry, W.: The use of Doppler flow velocity measurement to assess the hemodynamic response to vasodilators in patients with heart failure. Circulation *67*:377, 1983.

14. Rosenbloom, M., Saksena, S., Nanda, N.C., Rogal, G., Werres, R.: Two-dimensional echocardiographic studies during sustained ventricular tachycardia. PACE *7*:136, 1984.

15. Abbasi, A.S., Allen, M.W., DeCristofaro, D., Ungar, I.: Detection and estimation of the degree of mitral regurgitation by range gated pulsed Doppler echocardiography. Circulation *61*:143, 1980.

16. Diebold, B., Theroux, P., Bourassa, M.G., Thuillez, C., Peronneau, P., Guermonprez, J.L., Xhaard, M., Waters, D.D.: Noninvasive pulsed Doppler study of mitral stenosis and mitral regurgitation. Preliminary study. Br Heart J *42*:168, 1979.

17. Keren, G., LeJemtel, T., Zelcer, A., Meisner, J.S., Bier, A., Yellin, E.: Time variation of mitral regurgitant flow in patients with dilated cardiomyopathy. Circulation *74*:684, 1986.

18. Kalmanson, D., Veyrat C., Bernier, A., Savier, C.H., Chiche, P., Witchitz, S.: Diagnosis and evaluation of mitral valve disease using transseptal ultrasound catheterization. Br Heart J *37*:257, 1975.

19. Miyatake, K., Kinoshita, N., Nagata, S., Beppu, S., Park, Y., Sakakibara, H., Nimura, Y.: Intracardiac flow pattern in mitral regurgitation studied with combined use of the ultrasonic pulsed Doppler technique and cross-sectional echocardiography. Am J Cardiol *45*:155, 1980.

20. Johnson, S.L., Baker, D.W., Lute, R.A., Murray, J.A.: Detection of mitral regurgitation by Doppler echocardiography. (abstr) Am J Cardiol *33*:146, 1974.

21. Goldberg, S.J., Allen, H.D., Marx, G.R., Flinn, C.F.: Doppler Echocardiography. Philadelphia, Lea & Febiger, 1985.

22. Miyatake, K., Nimura, Y., Sakakibara, H., Kinoshita, N., Okamoto, M., Nagata, S., Kawazoe, K., Fujita, T.: Localization and direction of mitral regurgitant flow in mitral orifice studied with combined use of ultrasonic pulsed Doppler technique and two-dimensional echocardiography. Br Heart J *48*:449, 1982.

23. Miyatake, K., Okamoto, M., Kinoshita, N., Izumi, S., Owa, M., Takao, S., Sakakibara, H., Nimura, Y.: Clinical applications of a new type of real-time two-dimensional Doppler flow imaging system. Am J Cardiol *54*:857, 1984.

24. Miyatake, K., Izumi, S., Okamoto, M., Kinoshita, N., Asonuma, H., Nakagawa, H., Yamamoto, K., Takamiya, M., Sakakibara, H., Nimura, Y.: Semiquantitative grading of severity of mitral regurgitation by real-time two-dimensional Doppler flow imaging technique. J Am Coll Cardiol *7*:82, 1986.

25. Omoto, R.: Color Atlas of Real-Time Two-Dimensional Doppler Echocardiography. 2nd Ed., Tokyo, Shindan-To-Chiryo Co., Ltd., 1987.

26. Omoto, R., Yokote, Y., Takamoto, S., Kyo, S., Ueda, K., Asano, H., Namekawa, K., Kasai, C., Kondo, Y.: The development of real-time two-dimensional Doppler echocardiography and its clinical significance in acquired valvular diseases. With special reference to the evaluation of valvular regurgitaiton. Jpn Heart J *25*:325, 1984.

27. Goldberg, S.J., Wilson, N., Dickinson, D.F.: Increased blood velocities in the heart and great vessels of patients with congenital heart disease. An assessment of their significance in the absence of valvar stenosis. Br Heart J *53*:640, 1985.

28. Houda, N., Takeuchi, M., Morita, N., Nakano, T., Takezawa, H.: Diagnosis and estimation of mitral regurgitation by two dimensional pulsed echocardiography. J Cardiogr *15*:449, 1985.

29. Helmcke, F., Nanda, N.C., Hsiung, M.C., Soto, B., Adey, C.K., Goyal, R.G., Gatewood, R.P., Jr.: Color Doppler assessment of mitral regurgitation with orthogonal planes. Circulation *75*:175, 1985.

30. Miyatake, K., Okamoto, M., Kinoshita, N., Ohta, M., Kozuka, T., Sakakibara, H., Nimura, Y.: Evaluation of tricuspid regurgitation by pulsed Doppler and two-dimensional echocardiography. Circulation *66*:777, 1982.

31. Veyrat, C., Kalmanson, D., Farjon, M., Manin, J.P, Abitbol, G.: Noninvasive diagnosis and assessment of tricuspid regurgitation and stenosis using one and two-dimensional echo pulsed Doppler. Br Heart J *47*:596, 1982.

32. Nimura, Y., Miyatake, K. Okamoto, M., Beppu, S., Kinoshita, N., Sakakibara, H.: Pulsed Doppler echocardiography in the assessment of tricuspid regurgitation. Ultrasound Med Biol *10*:239, 1984.

33. Kostucki, W., Vandenbossche, J., Friart, A., Engert, M.: Pulsed Doppler regurgitant flow patterns of normal valves. Am J Cardiol *58*:309, 1986.

34. Yock, P.G., Naasz, C., Schnittger, I., Popp, R.L.: Doppler tricuspid and pulmonic regurgitation in normals: Is it real? Circulation (abstr) *70*(II):40, 1984.

35. Suzuki, Y., Kambara, H., Kadota, K., Tamaki, S., Yamazato, A., Nohara, R. Osakada, G., Kawai, C.: Detection and evaluation of tricuspid regurgitation using a real-time, two-dimensional, color-coded Doppler flow imaging system: Comparison with contrast two-dimensional echocardiography and right ventriculography. Am J Cardiol *57*:811, 1986.
36. Garcia-Dorado, D., Falzgraf, S., Almazan, A., Delcan, J., Lopez-Bescos, L., Menarguez, L.: Diagnosis of functional tricuspid insufficiency by pulsed wave Doppler ultrasound. Circulation *66*:1315, 1982.
37. Pennestri, F., Loperfido, F., Salvatori, M.P., Mongiardo, R., Ferrazza, A., Guccione, P., Manzoli, U.: Assessment of tricuspid regurgitation by pulsed Doppler ultrasonography of the hepatic vein. Am J Cardiol *54*:363, 1984.
38. Sakai, K., Nakamura, K., Satomi, G., Kondo, M., Hirosawa, K.: Evaluation of tricuspid regurgitation by blood flow pattern in the hepatic vein using pulsed Doppler technique. Am Heart J *108*:516, 1984.
39. Diebold, B., Touati, R., Blanchard, D., Colonna, G., Guermonprez, J.L., Peronneau, R., Forman, J., Maurice, P.: Quantitative assessment of tricuspid regurgitation using pulsed Doppler echocardiography. Br Heart J *50*:443, 1983.
40. Giobanu, M., Abbasi, A.S., Allen, M., Hermer, A., Spellberg, R.: Pulsed Doppler echocardiography in the diagnosis and estimation of severity of aortic insufficiency. Am J Cardiol *49*:339, 1982.
41. Takahashi, H., Sakamoto, T., Hada, Y., Amano, K., Yamaguchi, T., Ishimitsu, T., Takikawa, R., Hasegawa, I., Takahashi, T.: Pulsed Doppler echocardiography and pharmacodynamic phonocardiography in the diagnosis of silent aortic regurgitation: A correlative study. J Cardiogr *15*:495, 1986.
42. Toguchi, M., Ichimiya, S., Yokoi, K., Hibi, N., Kambe, T.: Clinical investigation of aortic insufficiency by means of pulsed Doppler echocardiography. Jpn Heart J *22*:537, 1981.
43. Esper, R.J.: Detection of mild aortic regurgitation by range gated pulsed Doppler echocardiography. Am J Cardiol *50*:1037, 1982.
44. Fukushima, M., Hiramatsu, M., Yoshima, H., Yamada, M., Ohkubo, N., Matsuwaka, R., Yoshii, Y., Ohgidani, N., Hoki, N., Hata, S., Onishi, K., Kobayashi, H.: Quantitative assessment of regurgitant fraction in aortic regurgitation: Comparison of two-dimensional Doppler echocardiography with other methods. J Cardiogr *15*:483, 1985.
45. Goldberg, S.J., Allen, H.D.: Quantitative assessment by Doppler echocardiography of pulmonary or aortic regurgitation. Am J Cardiol *56*:131, 1985.
46. Veyrat, C., Ameur, A., Gourtchiglouan, C., Lessana, A., Abitbol, G., Kalmanson, D.: Calculation of pulsed Doppler left ventricular outflow tract regurgitant index for grading the severity of aortic regurgitation. Am Heart J *108*:507, 1984.
47. Quinones, M.A., Young, J.B., Waggoner, A.D., Ostojic, M.C., Ribeiro, L.G.T., Miller, L.L.: Assessment of pulsed Doppler echocardiography in detection and quantification of aortic and mitral regurgitation. Br Heart J *44*:612, 1980.
48. Bommer, W.J., Mapes, R., Miller, L. Mason, D.T., DeMaria, A.N.: Quantitation of aortic regurgitation with two-dimensional Doppler echocardiography. (abstr) Am J Cardiol *47*:412, 1981.
49. Kitabatake, A., Ito, H., Inoue, M., Tanouchi, J., Isihara, K., Morita, T., Fuijii, K., Yoshida, Y., Masayama, T., Yoshima, H., Hori, M., Kamada, T.: A new approach to noninvasive evaluation of aortic regurgitant fraction by two-dimensional Doppler echocardiography. Circulation *72*:523, 1985.
50. Boughner, D.R.: Assessment of aortic insufficiency by transcutaneous Doppler ultrasound. Circulation *52*:874, 1975.
51. Serwer, G.A., Armstrong, B.E., Anderson, P.A.W.: Noninvasive detection of retrograde descending aortic flow in infants using continuous wave Doppler ultrasonography. J Pediatr *97*:394, 1980.
52. Nakayama, N., Yoshimura, S., Hara, M., Teruya, H., Nakatsuka, T., Furuhata, H.: Noninvasive quantitative evaluation of aortic regurgitation using an ultrasonic pulsed Doppler flowmeter. Jpn Circ J *47*:641, 1983.
53. Takenaka, K., Dabestani, A., Gardin, J., Russell, D., Clark, S., Allfie, A., Henry, W.: A simple Doppler echocardiographic method for estimating severity of aortic regurgitation. Am J Cardiol *57*:1340, 1986.
54. Sahn, D.J., Valdes-Cruz, L., Scagnelli, S., Tomizuka, F., Elias, W., Covell, J.: Two-dimensional Doppler color flow mapping for spatial localization and quantitation of aortic insufficiency: Validation of a new diagnostic modality using an open chest dog model. (abstr) Circulation *70*:38, 1984.
55. Masuyama, T., Kodama, K., Kitabatake, A., Sato, H., Nanto, S., Inoue, M.: Continuous-wave Doppler echocardiographic detection of pulmonary regurgitation and its application to noninvasive estimation of pulmonary artery pressure. Circulation *74*:484, 1986.
56. Miyatake, K., Okamoto, M., Kinoshita, N., Matsuhisa, M., Nagata, S., Beppu, S., Park, Y.,

Sakakibara, H., Nimura, Y.: Pulmonary regurgitation studied with the ultrasonic pulsed Doppler technique. Circulation *65*:969, 1982.

57. Waggoner, A.D., Quinones, M.A., Young, J.B., Brandon, T.A., Shah, A.A., Verani, M.S., Miller, R.R.: Pulsed Doppler echocardiographic detection of right-sided valve regurgitation. Experimental results and clinical significance. Am J Cardiol *47*:279, 1981.

58. Goldberg, S.J., Areias, J.C., Spitaels, S.E.C., de Villeneuve, V.H.: Use of time interval histographic output from echo Doppler to detect left-to-right atrial shunts. Circulation *58*:147, 1978.

59. Kalmanson, D., Veyrat, C., Derai, C., Savier, C., Berkman, M., Chiche, P.: Non-invasive technique for diagnosing atrial septal defect and assessing shunt volume using directional Doppler ultrasound. Correlations with phasic flow velocity patterns of the shunt. Br Heart J *34*:981, 1972.

60. Kitabatake, A., Inoue, M., Asao, M., Ito, H., Masuyama, T., Tanouchi, J., Morita, T., Hori, M., Yoshima, H.: Noninvasive evaluation of the ratio of pulmonary to systemic flow in atrial septal defect by duplex Doppler echocardiography. Circulation *69*:73, 1984.

61. Minagoe, S., Tei, C., Kisanuki, A., Arikawa, K., Nakazono, Y., Yoshimura, H., Kashima, T., Tanaka, H.: Noninvasive pulsed Doppler echocardiographic detection of the direction of shunt flow in patients with atrial septal defect: usefulness of the right parasternal approach. Circulation *71*:745, 1985.

62. Marx, G.R., Allen, H.D., Goldberg, S.J., Flinn, C.J.: Transatrial septal velocity measurement by Doppler echocardiography in atrial septal defect: Correlation with QP:QS ratio. Am J Cardiol *55*:1162, 1985.

63. Stevenson, G.J.: Experience with qualitative and quantitative applications of Doppler echocardiography in congenital heart disease. Ultrasound Med Biol *10*:771, 1984.

64. Barron, J.V., Sahn, D.J., Valdes-Cruz, L.M., Lima, C.O., Goldberg, S.J., Grenadier, E., Allen, H.D.: Clinical utility of two-dimensional Doppler echocardiographic techniques for estimating pulmonary to systemic blood flow ratios in children with left-to-right shunting atrial septal defect, ventricular septal defect or patent ductus arteriosus. J Am Coll Cardiol *3*:169, 1984.

65. Dickinson, D.F., Goldberg, S.J., Wilson, N.: A comparison of information obtained by ultrasound examination and cardiac catheterization in paediatric patients with congenital heart disease. Int J Cardiol *9*:275, 1985.

66. Meyer, R.A., Kalavathy, A., Korfhagen, J.C., Kaplan, S.: Comparison of left-to-right shunt ratios determined by pulsed Doppler/2D-echo and Fick method. (abstr). Circulation *66*(II):232, 1982.

67. Sanders, S.P., Yeager, S., Williams, R.G.: Measurement of systemic and pulmonary blood flow and QP:QS ratio using Doppler and two-dimensional echocardiography. Am J Cardiol *51*:952, 1983.

68. Valdes-Cruz, L.M., Horowitz, S., Mesel, E., Sahn, D.J., Fisher, D.C., Larson, D.: A pulsed Doppler echocardiographic method for calculating pulmonary and systemic blood flow in atrial level shunts: validation studies in animals and initial human experience. Circulation *69*:80, 1984.

69. Stevenson, J.G., Kawabori, I., Dooley, T., Guntheroth, W.G.: Diagnosis of ventricular septal defect by pulsed Doppler echocardiography: sensitivity, specificity and limitations. Circulation *58*:322, 1978.

70. Magherini, A., Azzolina, G., Wiechman, V., Fantini, F.: Pulsed Doppler echocardiography for diagnosis of ventricular septal defects. Br Heart J *43*:143, 1980.

71. Johnson, S.L., Baker, D.W., Lute, R.A., Kawabori, I.: Detection of small ventricular septal defects by Doppler flowmeter. (abstr) Circulation *50*(III): 142, 1974.

72. Stevenson, J.G., Kawabori, I., Guntheroth, W.G.: Differentiation of ventricular septal defect from mitral regurgitation by pulsed Doppler echocardiography. Circulation *56*:14, 1977.

73. Yokoi, K., Kambe, T., Ichimiya, S., Toguchi, M., Hibi, N., Nishimura, K.: Pulsed Doppler echocardiographic evaluation of the shunt flow in ventricular septal defect. Jpn Heart J *24*:175, 1983.

74. Ludomirsky, A., Huhta, J.C., Vick, G.W., Murphy, D.J., Danford, D.A., Morrow, W.R.: Color Doppler detection of multiple ventricular septal defects. Circulation *74*:1317, 1986.

75. Barron, J.V., Sahn, D.J., Valdes-Cruz, L.M., Lima, C.O., Grenadier, E., Allen, H.D., Goldberg, S.J.: Quantification of the ratio of pulmonary: systemic blood flow in patients with ventricular septal defect by two-dimensional range gated Doppler echocardiography. (abstr) Circulation *66*(II):318, 1982.

76. Stevenson, J.G., Kawabori, I., Guntheroth, W.G.: Noninvasive detection of pulmonary hypertension in patent ductus arteriosus by pulsed Doppler echocardiography. Circulation *60*:355, 1979.

77. Daniels, O., Hopman, J.C.W., Stoelinga, G.B.A., Busch, H.J., Peer, P.G.M.: Doppler flow characteristics in the main pulmonary artery and the LA/Ao ratio before and after ductal closure in healthy newborns. Pediatric Cardiol *3*:99, 1982.

78. Gentile, R., Stevenson, J.G., Dooley, T., Franklin, D., Kawabori, I., Pearlman, A.: Pulsed Doppler echocardiographic determination of time of ductal closure in normal newborn infants. J Pediatr *98*:443, 1981.

79. Swensson, R.E., Valdes-Cruz, L.M., Sahn, D.J., Sherman, F.S., Chung, K.J., Scagnelli, S., Hagen-Ansert, S.: Real-time Doppler color flow mapping for detection of patent ductus arteriosus. J Am Coll Cardiol *8*:(5):1105, 1986.

80. Huhta, J.C., Cohen, M., Gutgesell, H.P.: Patency of the ductus arteriosus in normal neonates: Two-dimensional echocardiography versus Doppler assessment. J Am Coll Cardiol *4*:561, 1984.

81. Vick, G.W., 3rd, Huhta, J.C., Gutgesell, H.P.: Assessment of the ductus arteriosus in preterm infants utilizing suprasternal two-dimensional Doppler echocardiography. J Am Coll Cardiol *5*:973, 1985.

82. Wilcox, W.D., Carrigan, T.A., Dooley, T.J., Giddens, D.P., Dykes, F.D., Lazzara, A., Ray, J.L., Ahmann, P.A.: Range-gated pulsed Doppler ultrasonographic evaluation of carotid arterial blood flow in small preterm infants with patent ductus arteriosus. J Pediatr *102*:294, 1983.

83. Wilson, N., Dickinson, D.F., Goldberg, S.G., Scott, O.: Pulmonary artery velocity patterns in ductus arteriosus. Br Heart J *52*:462, 1984.

84. Allen, H.D., Sahn, D.J., Lange, L., Goldberg, S.J.: Noninvasive assessment of surgical systemic-to-pulmonary artery shunts by range-gated pulsed Doppler echocardiography. J Pediatr *94*:395, 1979.

85. Marx, G.R., Allen, H.D., Goldberg, S.J.: Doppler estimation of systolic pulmonary artery pressure in patients with aortic-pulmonary shunts. J Am Coll Cardiol *7*:880, 1986.

86. Sahn, D.J., Allen, H.D., Lange, L.W., Goldberg, S.J.: Cross-sectional echocardiographic diagnosis of the sites of total anomalous pulmonary venous drainage. Circulation *60*:1317, 1979.

87. Smallhorn, J.R., Sutherland, G.R., Tommasini, G., Hunter, S., Anderson, R.H., Macartney, F.J.: Assessment of total anomalous pulmonary venous connection by two-dimensional echocardiography. Br Heart J *46*:613, 1981.

88. Williams, R.G., Bierman, F.Z., Sanders, S.P.: Echocardiographic Diagnosis of Cardiac Malformations. Boston, Little Brown & Co, 1986.

89. Tajik, A.J., Seward, J.B., Hagler, D.J., Mair, D.D., Lie, J.D.: Two-dimensional real-time ultrasonic imaging of the heart and great vessels. Technique, image orientation, structure identification, and validation. Mayo Clin Proc *53*:271, 1978.

90. Del Torso, S., Goh, T., Venables, A.: Echocardiographic findings in the liver in total anomalous pulmonary venous connection. Am J Cardiol *57*:374, 1986.

91. Cooper, M.J., Teitel, D.F., Silverman, N.H., Enderlein, M.A.: Study of the infradiaphragmatic total anomalous pulmonary venous connection with cross-sectional and pulsed Doppler echocardiography. Circulation *70*:412, 1984.

92. Skovranek, J., Tuma, S., Urbancova, D., Samanek, M.: Range gated pulsed Doppler echocardiographic diagnosis of supracardiac total anomalous pulmonary venous drainage. Circulation *61*:841,1980.

93. Smallhorn, J.F., Freedom, R.M.: Pulsed Doppler echocardiography in the preoperative evaluation of total anomalous pulmonary venous connection. J Am Coll Cardiol *8*:1413, 1986.

94. Bass, J., Berry, J., Einzig, S.: Flow in the aorta and patent ductus arteriosus in infants with aortic atresia or aortic stenosis: a pulsed Doppler ultrasound study. Circulation *74*:315, 1986.

95. Barber, G., Helton, J.G., Aglira, B.A., Chin, A.J., Murphy, J.D., Pigott, J.D., Norwood, W.I.: The significance of preoperative regurgitation in hypoplastic left heart syndrome. (abstr) Circulation *74*(II):336, 1986.

96. Bierman, F.Z., Williams, R.G.: Prospective diagnosis of d-transposition of the great arteries in neonates by subxiphoid, two-dimensional echocardiography. Circulation *60*:1496, 1979.

97. Silverman, N.H., Snider, R.A.: Two-dimensional Echocardiography in Congenital Heart Disease. Norwalk, CT, Appleton-Century-Crofts, 1982.

98. Deal, B.J., Chin, A.J., Sanders, S.P., Norwood, W.I., Castaneda, A.R.: Subxiphoid two-dimensional echocardiographic identification of tricuspid valve abnormalities in transposition of the great arteries. Am J Cardiol *55*:1146, 1985.

99. Sanders, S.P.: Echocardiography and related techniques in the diagnosis of congenital heart defects. Part III. Conotruncus and great arteries. Echocardiography *1*:443, 1984.

100. Moro, E., ten Cate, F., Tirtaman, C., Leonard, J.J., Roelandt, J.: Doppler and two-dimensional echocardiographic observations of systolic anterior motion of the mitral valve in d-transposition of the great arteries: An explanation of the left ventricular outflow tract gradient. J Am Coll Cardiol *7*:889, 1986.

101. Areias, J.C., Goldberg, S.J., Spitaels, S.E.C., de Villeneuve, V.H.: An evaluation of range gated pulsed Doppler echocardiography for detecting pulmonary outflow tract obstruction in d-transposition of the great vessels. Am Heart J *96*:467, 1978.

102. Chin, A.J., Sanders, S.P., Williams, R.G., Lang, P., Norwood, W.I., Castaneda, A.R.: Two-

dimensional echocardiographic assessment of caval and pulmonary venous pathways after the Senning operation. Am J Cardiol *52*:118, 1983.

103. Smallhorn, J.F., Gow, R., Freedom, R.M., Trusler, G.A., Olley, P., Pacquet, M., Gibbons, J., Vlad, P.: Pulsed Doppler echocardiographic assessment of the pulmonary venous pathway after the Mustard or Senning procedure for transposition of the great arteries. Circulation *73*:765, 1986.

104. Stevenson, J.G., Kawabori, I., Guntheroth, W.G., Dooley, T.K., Dillard, D.H.: Pulsed Doppler echocardiographic detection of obstruction of systemic venous return following repair of transposition of the great arteries. Circulation *60*:1091, 1979.

105. Niederle, P., Stepanek, Z., Grospic, A., Ressl, J., Firt, P., Beranek, I., Dobovska, M.: Character of mitral valve flow in left atrial tumor. Eur J Cadiol *12*:357, 1981.

106. Panidis, I., Mintz, G., McAllister, M.: Hemodynamic consequences of left atrial myxomas as assessed by Doppler ultrasound. Am Heart J *111*:927, 1986.

107. Berman, W., Jr., Alverson, D.C.: Assessment of hemodynamic function with pulsed Doppler ultrasound. J Am Coll Cardiol *5*:104S, 1985.

108. Wallmeyer, K., Wann, S., Sagar, K.B., Kalbfleisch, J., Klopfenstein, H.S.: The influence of preload and heart rate on Doppler echocardiographic indexes of left ventricular performance: comparison with invasive indexes in an experimental preparation. Circulation *74*:181, 1986.

109. Sabbah, H., Khaja, F., Brymer, J., McFarland, T., Albert, D., Snyder, J.E., Goldstein, S., Stein, P.D.: Noninvasive evaluation of left ventricular performance based on peak aortic blood acceleration measured with a continuous-wave Doppler velocity meter. Circulation *74*:323, 1986.

110. Sabbah, H.N., Przybylski, J., Albert, D.E., Stein, P.D.: Peak aortic blood acceleration reflects the extent of left ventricular ischemic mass at risk. Am Heart J *113*:885, 1987.

111. Mehta, N., Bennett, D., Mannering, D., Dawkins, K., Ward, D.E.: Usefulness of noninvasive Doppler measurement of ascending aortic blood velocity and acceleration in detecting impairment of the left ventricular functional response to exercise three weeks after acute myocardial infarction. Am J Cardiol *58*:879, 1986.

112. Gardin, J.M., Iseri, L.T., Elkayam, U., Tobis, J., Childs, W., Burn, C.S., Henry, W.L.: Evaluation of dilated cardiomyopathy by pulsed Doppler echocardiography. Am Heart J *106*:1057, 1983.

113. Cogswell, T.L., Sagar K.B., Wann, L.S.: Left ventricular ejection dynamics in hypertrophic cardiomyopathy and aortic stenosis: Comparison with the use of Doppler echocardiography. Am Heart J *113*:110, 1987.

114. Gardin, J.M., Davidson, D.M., Rohan, M.K., Butman, S., Knoll, M., Garcia, R., Dubria, S., Gardin, S.K., Henry, W.L.: Relationship between age, body size, gender, and blood pressure and Doppler flow measurements in the aorta and pulmonary artery. Am Heart J *113*:101, 1987.

115. Mowat, D.H.R., Haites, N.E., Rawles, J.M.: Aortic blood velocity measurement in healthy adults using a simple ultrasound technique. Cardiovasc Res *17*:75, 1983.

116. Bennett, E.D., Barclay, S.A., Davis, A.L., Mannering, D., Mehta, N.: Ascending aortic blood velocity and acceleration using Doppler ultrasound in the assessment of left ventricular function. Cardiovasc Res *18*:632, 1984.

117. Bristow, J.D., Van Zee, B.E., Judkins, M.P.: Systolic and diastolic abnormalities of the left ventricle in coronary artery disease: Studies in patients with little or no enlargement of ventricular volume. Circulation *42*:219, 1970.

118. Hammermeister, K.E., Warbasse, J.R.: The rate of change of left ventricular volume in man: II. diastolic events in health and disease. Circulation *49*:739, 1974.

119. Brutsaert, D.L., Rademakers, F.E., Sys, S.U.: Triple control of relaxation: implications in cardiac disease. Circulation *69*:190, 1984.

120. Reduto, L.A., Wickemeyer, W.J., Young, J.B., Del Ventura, L.A., Reid, J.W., Glaeser, D.H., Quinones, M.A., Miller, R.R.: Left ventricular diastolic performance at rest and during exercise in patients with coronary artery disease: assessment with first-pass radionuclide angiography. Circulation *63*:1228, 1981.

121. Bonow, R.O., Bacharach, S.L., Green, M.V., Kent, K.M., Rosing, D.R., Lipson, L.C., Leon, M.B., Epstein, S.E.: Impaired left ventricular diastolic filling in patients with coronary artery disease: assessment with radionuclide angiography. Circulation *64*:315, 1981.

122. Danford, D.A., Huhta, J.C., Murphy, D.J., Jr.: Doppler echocardiographic approaches to ventricular diastolic function. Echocardiography *3*:33, 1986.

123. Fujii, J., Yazaki, Y., Sawada, H., Aizawa, T., Watanabe, H., Kato, K.: Noninvasive assessment of left and right ventricular filling in myocardial infarction with a two-dimensional Doppler echocardiographic method. J Am Coll Cardiol *5*:1155, 1985.

124. Kitabatake, A., Inoue, M., Asao, M., Tanouchi, J., Masuyama, T., Abe, H., Morita, H., Senda, S., Matsuo, H.: Transmitral blood flow reflecting diastolic behavior of the left ventricle in health and disease—a study by pulsed Doppler technique. Jpn Circ J *46*:92, 1982.

125. Snider, A.R., Gidding, S.S., Rocchini, A.P., Rosenthal, A., Dick, M., Crowley, D.C., Peters, J.:

Doppler evaluation of left ventricular diastolic filling in children with systemic hypertension. Am J Cardiol *56*:921, 1985.

126. Spirito, P., Maron, B.J., Bonow, R.O.: Noninvasive assessment of left ventricular diastolic function: comparative analysis of Doppler echocardiographic and radionuclide angiographic techniques. J Am Coll Cardiol *7*:518, 1986.
127. Tanouchi, J., Inoue, M., Kitabatake, A., Hori, M., Asao, M., Mishima, M., Shimazu, T., Morita, H., Masuyama, T., Abe, H., Matsuo, H.: Impaired early diastolic filling of left ventricle in hypertensive patients assessed by intracardial pulsed Doppler flowmetry. (abstr). Circulation *64*(IV):255, 1981.
128. Miyatake, K., Okamoto, M., Kinoshita, N., Owa, M., Nakasone, I., Sakakibara, H., Nimura, Y.: Augmentation of atrial contribution to left ventricular inflow with aging as assessed by intracardiac Doppler flowmetry. Am J Cardiol *53*:586, 1984.
129. Gidding, S., Snider, R., Rocchini, A., Peters, J., Farnsworth, R.: Left ventricular diastolic filling in children with hypertrophic cardiomyopathy: assessment with pulsed Doppler echocardiography. J Am Coll Cardiol *8*:310, 1986.
130. Takenaka, K., Dabestani, A., Gardin, J.M., Russell, D., Clark, S., Allfie, A., Henry, W.L.: Pulsed Doppler echocardiographic study of left ventricular filling in dilated cardiomyopathy. Am J Cardiol *58*:143, 1986.
131. Gardin, J.M., Rohan, M.K., Davidson, D.M., Dabestani, A., Slansky, M., Garcia, R., Knoll, M.L., White, D.B., Gardin, S.K., Henry, W.L.: Doppler transmitral flow velocity parameters: Relationship between age, body surface area, blood pressure and gender in normal subjects. Am J Noninvasive Cardiol *1*:3, 1987.
132. Pearson, A.C., Schiff, M., Mrosek, D., Labovitz, A.J., Williams, G.A.: Left ventricular diastolic function in weight lifters. Am J Cardiol *58*:1254, 1986.
133. Rokey, R., Kuo, L.C., Zoghbi, W.A., Limacher, M.C., Quinones, M.A.: Determination of parameters of left ventricular diastolic filling with pulsed Doppler echocardiography: Comparison with cineangiography. Circulation *71*:543, 1985.
134. Belkin, R.N., Mark, D.B., Svetkey, L.P., Daly, L., NeSmith, J.W., Kisslo, J.: Doppler-derived indices of diastolic filling in mild to moderate hypertension. Circulation (abstr) *74*:(II):47, 1986.
135. Ishida, Y., Meisner, J.S., Tsujioka, K., Gallo, J.I., Yoran, C., Frater, R.W.M., Yellin, E.L.: Left ventricular filling dynamics: influence of left ventricular relaxation and left atrial pressure. Circulation *74*:187, 1986.
136. Leeman, D.E., Feldman, M.D., Diver, D.J., Santinga, J.T., Come, P.C.: Effects of decreases in preload on pulsed Doppler indices of left ventricular filling: Circulation (abstr) *74*(II):46, 1986.
137. Drinkovic, N., Wisenbaugh, T., Nissen, S.E., Elion, J.L., Smith, M.D., Kwan, O.L., DeMaria, A.N.: Sensitivity and specificity of transmitral flow velocity measurements in detecting impaired left ventricular compliance. Circulation (abstr) *74*(II):46, 1986.
138. Appleton, C.P., Alderman, E.L., Popp, R.L., Hatle, L.K.: Can the mitral flow velocity curve be used to assess left ventricular diastolic function?: Circulation (abstr) *74*:(II):46, 1986.
139. Lin, S., Tak, T., Gamage, N., Kawanishi, D.T., McKay, C.R., Chandraratna, P.A.N.: Assessment of left ventricular diastolic function in coronary heart disease by Doppler ultrasound: (abstr) Circulation *74*(II):47, 1986.

CHAPTER *7*

VALVE AREA COMPUTATION FROM DOPPLER

THE GORLIN EQUATION

Gorlin and Gorlin[1] first introduced the concept of valve area to the cardiology community in 1951. All of their assumptions and computations are pertinent to Doppler methods for computing valve area. They found that standard fluid dynamic equations were generally applicable to humans. A cardiac valve was likened to a "rounded edge" orifice where:

$$\text{Flow} = C_c \times \text{Orifice Area} \times \text{Velocity through the orifice} \qquad \text{eq 1}$$

C_c is the coefficient of orifice contraction (also called coefficient of discharge). The value of this coefficient for a perfect orifice (one without viscous properties) is unity but since no perfect orifices exist, the jet that issues from a less than perfect orifice will have an area that is only a fraction of the area of orifice area. The difference between the orifice and jet area is expressed as a ratio, and that ratio is the coefficient of orifice contraction.

Gorlin and Gorlin next combined the above equation with a second equation, a form of the Bernoulli equation, which stated that:

$$\text{Velocity} = c_v \sqrt{2gh} \qquad \text{eq 2}$$

where c_v is a coefficient that defines the percentage of velocity converted to pressure drop at the orifice, g is gravitational acceleration (980 cm/sec/sec) and h is the height of a column of fluid above the orifice. The factor "gh" is pressure in a fluid column; the "2" comes from the $\frac{1}{2}MV^2$ term. The $\sqrt{2g}$ quantity is equal to $\sqrt{1960}$ which in turn is equal to 44.5, the familiar coefficient of the Gorlin equation.

Since the objective is to determine valve area, the two equations can be combined to demonstrate that:

$$\text{area} = \frac{F}{C_c \times c_v \sqrt{2gh}} \text{ or area} = \frac{F}{C \times 44.5 \sqrt{\text{mean pressure drop}}} \qquad \text{eq 3}$$

where C is a combined coefficient for c_v and C_c and pressure drop is in mm Hg. F is a value which also needs qualification. In the computation, flow is considered to be continuous but during the cardiac cycle, flow is intermittent. In cardiac work this intermittent nature of flow requires an adjustment to

293

represent cardiac flow as continuous. For example if cardiac output is 4500 ml/min and if the time of ejection is 30 sec/min, then valve flow rate would be 4500 (ml/min)/30(sec/min) to yield a value of 150 ml/sec. Finally, pressure drop refers to *mean* pressure drop during filling or ejection rather than the average of several peaks. The method for determining mean pressure drop from two simultaneous tracings on either side of a valve is shown, in pictorial form, in Figure 7–1.

The Gorlin equation computes actual valve area which is best defined as the area that the surgeon sees. Valve area also can be computed as effective area which is the product of actual area and the coefficient of contraction. Gorlin and Gorlin used coefficients of contraction of .7 for the mitral valve and .85 for the other valves. Numerous subsequent investigators have suggested modifications to the Gorlin equation, mainly in values for the coefficient of contraction, to better approximate area values found at surgery or autopsy. Nonetheless, principles of the original Gorlin equation have stood the test of time and Doppler methods have either been derived from the Gorlin equation or results have been compared to results of the Gorlin equation.

THE HOLEN EQUATION

Holen et al.[2] first approximated valve area by ultrasound using a variation of the equation of continuity but made no specific reference to that equation. The concept of the equation of continuity states that if flow enters a tube which has no leaks, the volume of flow exiting the tube will equal the volume of flow which entered it. Since flow is equal to the product of mean velocity (Vm) and flow area (A), the equation of continuity can be stated mathematically:

$$Vm_1 \times A_1 = Vm_2 \times A_2 \qquad\qquad \text{eq 4}$$

Subscripts 1 and 2 refer to pre-valve and post-valve respectively. In cardiac work the units of Vm are cm, but, in order to express flow in ml/minute, Vm is usually integrated over a minute and its true units become cm/min. Figure 7–2 shows the concept of the equation of continuity in a pictorial diagram. Note that A_2 and A_1, as shown in the lower panel, need not be similar in area.

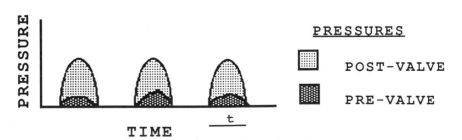

Fig. 7–1. Pictorial to explain computation of mean pressure drop across a valve from a pressure tracing. Pressure is shown on the vertical axis and time on the horizontal axis. Pictorial waveforms are depicted which consist of a pre-valve pressure (dark stipple) and a post-valve (light stipple) pressure. To compute mean pressure the area of the pre-valve and post-valve pressures are computed separately for each beat. The time "t" represents systolic ejection time. Mean pressure drop is computed for each beat as (post-valve area − pre-valve area)/t.

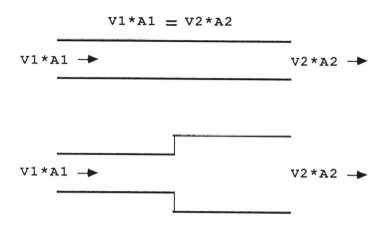

Fig. 7–2. Continuity equation. The product of velocity and area at the entrance of the tube equals the product of velocity and area at the exit of the tube. The lower panel shows that the same relationship holds even if the exit area is different from the entrance area.

Holen et al. began their reasoning by stating the familiar relationship that:

$$\text{pressure drop } (\Delta P) = \tfrac{1}{2}\rho V^2 \qquad \text{eq 5}$$

where ρ = density and V = velocity.

Next they restated the equation of continuity in a manner that is equivalent to that shown above as:

$$\frac{dQ}{dt} = A \times V \qquad \text{eq 6}$$

dQ/dt represents volume flow per unit time and is equivalent to the product of A and V. These two equations can be combined to show that:

$$\Delta P = \frac{r}{2A^2} \times (dQ/dt)^2 \qquad \text{eq 7}$$

Eq 6, the Holen equation, can be restated in a simpler form:

$$A = Q/(V_m \times T) \qquad \text{eq 8}$$

In this instance, T is ejection time or filling time depending upon the valve studied, and V_m is mean velocity. By substituting the value of r and taking into account the method for transforming a mean velocity difference into a pressure drop, the equation can be restated as:

$$A = \frac{Q}{51.7 \, T\sqrt{\Delta P}} \qquad \text{eq 9}$$

This equation bears a strong resemblance to the Gorlin equation since Q/T is equal to F, but the coefficient, 51.7, is different. This difference is due to the fact that the Holen et al. equation computes effective area and the Gorlin equation computes actual area. The area of the Holen et al. result can be transformed to the Gorlin area by dividing the area (Holen) by the coefficient of contraction. Holen et al. studied 10 patients by catheterization (using the Gorlin method) and by Doppler and found a correlation coefficient of .97 (Fig. 7–3) for mitral valve area. Flow in this study was computed by the Fick method and required invasive blood gas determinations. Accordingly, this method was not one that could be performed completely noninvasively. Flows, however, can be measured by Doppler, and a completely noninvasive method for valve area appeared possible.

PRESSURE HALF-TIME

Libanoff and Rodbard[3] reported a method for estimating mitral valve area by determining the time taken for the diastolic pressure difference between left atrium and left ventricle to fall to one half its original value. This time value was independent of heart rate and cardiac output. Hatle et al. first applied this method to Doppler tracings.[4] They reasoned that the pressure drop at any point in time could be approximated by $4V^2$. Since pressure drop rather than velocity had to be computed and since the pressure relationship is to the square of velocity, determining the time on the velocity curve at which pressure fell to half its original value required dividing the peak velocity by $\sqrt{2}$ (or its equivalent = 1.41). The methodology for determining pressure half-time is demonstrated in Figure 7–4 and correlation with the revised Gorlin method[5] is shown in Figure 7–5. Hatle et al. found that pressure half times in normals ranged from 20 to 60 msec, in patients with isolated mitral regurgitation from 35 to 80 msec and in patients with mitral stenosis from 90 to 383 msec. They also confirmed that pressure half-times were relatively unaffected by heart rate, cardiac output or presence of regurgitation. Further, they demonstrated that a reasonable estimate of pressure half time for a mitral valve area of 1 cm was 220 msec. Accordingly, dividing the measured pressure half time into 220 msec produces a result that approximates valve area. Limitations of the method include prolonged PR interval (because atrial contraction increases velocity early in diastole and precludes the measurement) and technical failure to align the beam with the jet. The pressure half time method has been reported to be effective for prosthetic valves, but the "normal" value is elevated over native

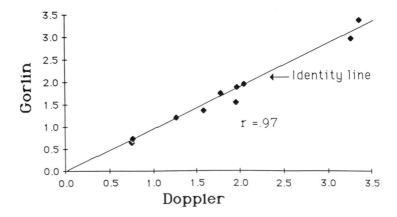

Fig. 7–3. Data of Holen et al.[2] are plotted to show the relationship of valve area by Doppler and catheterization.

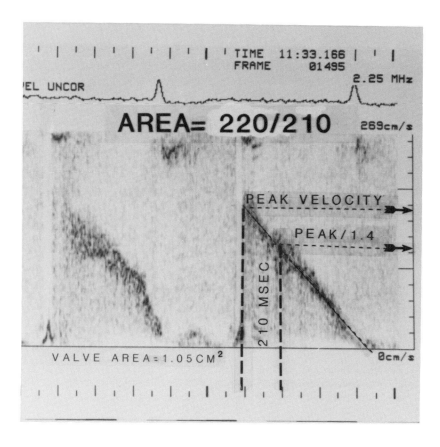

Fig. 7–4. Pressure half time calculation. Peak velocity is 175 cm/sec. This number is then divided by $\sqrt{2}$ (1.41) to determine the pressure half time. The time between these velocity markers is 210 msec. The area is computed by dividing 210 into 220 (the time for 1 cm²).

valves. The method is said to be useful in tricuspid stenosis, but does not seem appropriate for estimation of semilunar valve area.

THE KOSTURAKIS METHOD FOR SEMILUNAR VALVES

Kosturakis and co-workers[6] developed a Doppler method for determining semilunar valve area. They began with the standard Gorlin equation:

$$\text{area} = \frac{F}{C \times 44.5 \sqrt{\text{pressure drop}}} \qquad \text{eq 10}$$

and substituted the Doppler equivalent of pressure drop which is $4V^2$. The "V" in this equation is peak jet velocity. If pre-jet velocity exceeds 1 m/s, the value of pre-jet velocity² must be subtracted from jet velocity². Since the square root of $4V^2$ is $2V$, the latter quantity was substituted into the equation to give:

$$\text{area} = \frac{F}{C \times 44.5 \times (2V)} \text{ or } \frac{F}{89CV} \qquad \text{eq 11}$$

These authors utilized F in the same terms as Gorlin, C was set to unity and

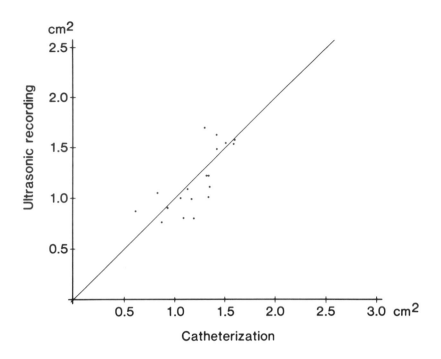

Fig. 7–5. Results in 20 patients with mitral stenosis. Correlation (r = 0.87) between Doppler predicted mitral valve area from pressure half-time and catheterization mitral valve area is shown. (From Hatle, L., Angelsen, B.: Doppler Ultrasound in Cardiology. Physical Principles and Clinical Applications. 2nd Ed., Philadelphia, Lea & Febiger, 1985.)

V could be expressed in m/s as above or cm/s by changing the denominator to .89CV as in the publication. V had one additional characteristic that separated it from the method of Gorlin and Gorlin: V, in the Kosturakis equation, was the peak velocity gradient and not the mean velocity gradient. Although the correlation of valve area by Gorlin equation and by Doppler was good, Doppler generally underestimated the result of the Gorlin equation (Fig. 7–6). This probably occurred because the denominator was excessively large as a result of substitution of peak gradient for mean and assumption of a coefficient of contraction of unity. Teirstein and co-workers used a variation of the Kosturakis method and had less underestimation.[7] The method of Kosturakis and co-workers is a time consuming one since a flow elsewhere in the heart must be measured, and has as the significant limitation that the measured flow can not be accompanied by a shunt or regurgitation. Further, the apparently simple measurement of systolic time proved to be a problem because time intervals were difficult to determine accurately from the relatively broad Doppler signal at the baseline. The lowest correlation between any measurement at catheterization and Doppler was for systolic ejection time (r = .65) even though studies were simultaneous. This is an important limitation because systolic ejection time is needed to compute the adjusted flow rate.

VALVE AREA ATTEMPT BY JET MAPPING

Veyrat and co-workers[8] reported that the post-valvular jet could be mapped in two planes by using a short sample volume and a nearly perpendicular angle

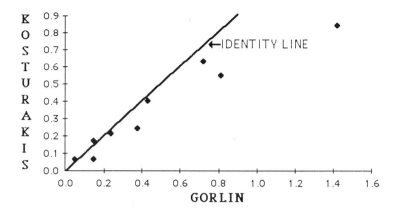

Fig. 7–6. Data of Kosturakis et al.[6] Valve area by the Kosturakis method (Y-axis) and by the Gorlin methods (X-axis) are compared. Units of both axes are cm² valve area. The line of identity is plotted. Note that the Kosturakis method generally underestimates results of the Gorlin method.

to the jet (Fig. 7–7). They reasoned that since the jet bears a definite relationship to valve area, as defined by the coefficient of contraction, measuring the jet in two dimensions should approximate the valve area. Although this concept has merit, an infinitely small sample volume is not possible, the jet may diverge after the orifice, and the mapping procedure is tedious. Color-coded Doppler does not improve matters since the beam width is sufficiently wide to make the jet appear wider than it really is. Further, some high energy eddies enter the parajet and the low Nyquist limit of color-coded Doppler systems images some of these eddies as though they were part of the jet.

CONTINUITY EQUATION STUDIES

Richards and co-workers[9] used the continuity equation to estimate aortic valve area in patients with aortic valvular stenosis. To simplify mechanics of making the computation, they showed that the ratio of mean mitral velocity (V_{mm}) and mean aortic velocity (V_{ma}) bore a close relationship to valve area determined by the Gorlin equation. Further they demonstrated that the ratio of mitral velocity-time integral (VT_m) and aortic time-velocity integral (VT_a) bore a close relationship to valve area determined by the Gorlin equation. Both relationships had a minimal standard error of the estimate. This relationship

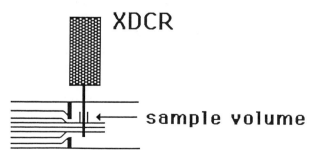

Fig. 7–7. A pictorial diagram for determining jet width after the method of Veyrat.[8] The beam must not be precisely perpendicular to the jet or no signal will be returned. The method assumes a small sample volume, no jet diversion, and no high energy eddies in the parajet.

is true probably because adult heart rates and valve areas are relatively constant across the population. As a result of this relatively constant empirical relationship they developed two equations from regression equations:

$$\text{Aortic valve area} = 9.35 \ (V_m)/(V_a) - .19 \qquad\qquad \text{eq 13}$$

$$\text{Aortic valve area} = 5.6 \ (VT_m)/VT_a) \qquad\qquad \text{eq 14}$$

Equation 13 produced results that correlated with results of the Gorlin equation with a coefficient of .90 (SEE = .23 cm^2). Equation 14 correlated with results of the Gorlin equation with a coefficient of .93 (SEE = .18 cm^2). The obvious advantage of these equations is that mitral valve area does not need to be determined. Two velocities, however, must be integrated.

All methods detailed thus far which compute semilunar valve area have required integration of at least two velocities, and integration requires an off-line computer. Zoghbi and co-workers[10] developed an adaptation of the equation of continuity that can be easily applied without off-line integration. The equation of continuity

$$V_{m1} \times A_1 = V_{m2} \times A_2 \qquad\qquad \text{eq 15}$$

requires that velocity terms MV$_1$ and MV$_2$ be integrated with respect to time. Zoghbi and co-workers hypothesized that the velocity proximal and distal to the aortic valve has the form of half an ellipse (Fig. 7–8). Since the formula for the area of an ellipse equals the product of the major axis length, minor axis length, and a constant ($\pi/4$), and since the minor axis (systolic time) is the same on either side of the valve, the only variables after cancellations become the amplitudes of the major axes. The major axes are merely the peak velocities proximal and distal to the aortic valve. Accordingly, the formula can be re-written as:

$$\text{Peak } V_1 \times A_1 = \text{Peak } V_2 \times A_2 \qquad\qquad \text{eq 16}$$

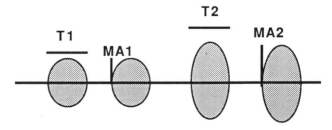

ELLIPSE AREA = T * MA * ∏/4

SINCE T1 = T2, AREA (f) MA1/MA2

Fig. 7–8. Simplified continuity valve area. A pictorial of the method of Zoghbi et al.[10] On the left are depicted two ellipses which represent pre-valve velocities, and on the right are depicted two other ellipses which represent post-valve velocities. The formula for area of an ellipse is the product of height or major axis (MA) and minor axis or time (T) and the constant $\pi/4$. Since T and $\pi/4$ are the same for both pre and post valve ellipses, area is a function (f) of the ratio of the amplitude of MA1 and MA2.

Zoghbi and co-workers measured A_1 as the diameter (d) of the left ventricular outflow tract just below the aortic valve in the annular area and converted the result to an area [area $= \pi(d/2)^2$]. They compared their result to the result of the Gorlin equation and found a correlation coefficient of .94 (SEE $= .16 cm^2$) and a slope near unity with no appreciable intercept. A small number of their patients had associated regurgitation and this addition did not appreciably affect the result. The major limitation of this technique is the requirement for detecting the maximal amplitude jet velocity.

Valve area is becoming a popular subject of abstracts and manuscripts at the present time. Whether the rather simple and easily applied method of Zoghbi and co-workers will become the standard or whether another variation will find more favor remains unclear at present. Whatever the eventual outcome, the ability to measure valve area noninvasively is a major forward step in application of Doppler to clinical cardiology.

REFERENCES

1. Gorlin, R., Gorlin, S.G.: Hydraulic formula for calculation of the area of the stenotic mitral valve, other cardiac valves, and central circulation shunts. Am Heart J *41*:1, 1951.
2. Holen, J., Aaslid, R., Landmark, K., Simonsen, S., Ostrem, T.: Determination of effective orifice area in mitral stenosis from noninvasive ultrasound Doppler data and mitral flow rate. Acta Med Scand *201*:83, 1977.
3. Libanoff, A.J., Rodbard, S.: Atrioventricular pressure half-time. Measure of mitral valve orifice area. Circulation *38*:144, 1968.
4. Hatle, L., Angelsen, B., Tromsdal, A.: Noninvasive assessment of atrioventricular pressure half-time by Doppler ultrasound. Circulation *60*:1096, 1979.
5. Cohen, M.V., Gorlin, R.: Modified orifice equation for the calculation of mitral valve area. Am Heart J *84*:839, 1972.
6. Kosturakis, D., Allen, H.D., Goldberg, S.J., Sahn, D.J., Valdes-Cruz, L.M.: Noninvasive quantification of stenotic semilunar valve areas by Doppler echocardiography. J Am Coll Cardiol *3*:1256, 1984.
7. Teirstein, P., Yeager, M., Yock, P.G., Popp, R.L.: Doppler echocardiographic measurement of aortic valve area in aortic stenosis: A noninvasive application of the Gorlin formula. J Am Coll Cardiol *8*:1059, 1986.
8. Veyrat, C, Lessana, A., Abitbol, G., Ameur, A., Benaim, R., Kalmanson, D.: New indexes for assessing aortic regurgitation with two-dimensional Doppler echocardiographic measurement of the regurgitant aortic valvular area. Circulation *83*:998, 1983.
9. Richards, K.L., Cannon, S.R., Miller, F.J., Crawford, M.H.: Calculation of aortic valve area by Doppler echocardiography: a direct application of the continuity equation. Circulation *73*:964, 1986.
10. Zoghbi, W.A., Farmer, K.L., Soto, J.G., Nelson, J.G., Quinones, M.A.: Accurate noninvasive quantification of stenotic aortic valve area by Doppler echocardiography. Circulation *73*:452, 1986.

INDEX

Page numbers followed by "f" indicate illustrations; numbers followed by "t" indicate tables.

303

flow area changes during cardiac cycle, 154-155

forward flow during opposite part of cardiac cycle, 156

mean velocity as description of velocity factor, 155

in cardiomyopathy, 187, 188f

descending aorta flow measurement for, 166

Doppler application to, 187-193

historical background of Doppler studies, 3-4

in mechanical alternans, 187

Cardiomyopathy

cardiac output measurement in, 187, 188f

E wave in, 284

Chirp Z analysis, 16

Coarctation of aorta, 123, 125f, 126. *See also* Aorta, coarctation

Coefficient of contraction, 73, 76

Color-coded Doppler

aliasing in, 71-72

in aligning with jet, 96-97

in aortic regurgitation, 210, 217, Plates 20, 21

apical five chamber plane, 58, Plate 11

right atrium, 52, Plate 8

tricuspid valve, 57, Plates 9-10

in atrioventricular valve regurgitation, 103, Plate 14

autocorrelation method for velocity, 33, 34-36f, 35-36

basic concepts, 30-36

in coarctation of aorta, 126

for correction of beam-flow intercept angle for ascending aorta, 165

for flow disturbance, 71

historical background, 2, 5

in jet mapping in valve area computation, 299

long axis parasternal plane in, 45, Plates 3-5

from long axis subcostal plane, 67, Plate 13

in mitral regurgitation, 194, Plate 16

in patent ductus arteriosus, 245, 249, Plate 30

pixels in, 32-33, 33f

prioritization in, 34

for pulmonary and systemic inflow velocities after Senning operation, Plate 31

in pulmonary regurgitation, 217, 225, Plates 22, 23

from suprasternal notch plane, 64, Plate 12

in tricuspid regurgitation, 201, Plate 17, Plate 18

mapping negative systolic velocities in right atrium, 205, Plate 19

after Senning operation, Plate 32

variance in, 34-36, 36f

in ventricular septal defect, 104, 136, 234, Plates 15, 28-29

Conduit

between systemic venous ventricle and pulmonary artery, 130

Continuity equation, 154-155, 154f, 294-295, 295f

in aortic stenosis, 299-301, 300f

Continuous wave Doppler

advantage over pulsed Doppler, 20-21

in aortic flow computation, 163

in aortic regurgitation, for diastolic retrograde velocities, 210, 214f

in aorticopulmonary shunts, 249, 252, 253f

for cardiac output, 3

for intracardiac masses, 271, 275f

in mitral regurgitation, 194, 197f

in patent ductus arteriosus, 245, 248f

physical concepts, 20-21

pressure drop determined by, 95, 96f

range ambiguity in, 20

in ventricular septal defect, 239f

small defect, 234, 241f

Contrast, Doppler studies using, 85, 85f

Coronary sinus

persistence of left superior vena cava to, 259, 261f

pulmonary venous drainage into, 252, 257f, 259

Cor triatriatum, apical four chamber plane for, 103

Crystal

phased array, 11-12, 13f

sector and aperture, 12, 14f

in transducer, 10-11, 10f, 11f

Deceleration half time for E wave, 281, 283f, 284

Deceleration instability, 80-81, 81f

Deceleration time, of E wave, 281, 283f, 284

Detector

quadrature, 27

zero crossing, 16, 17f

Diffuse reflectors, 13-14

Digitization, for mean velocity, 157f, 158-159

Doppler, J.C., 1, 2f

Doppler echocardiography

in aortic regurgitation, 210, 212-216f, 217, 218-221f

in atrial septal defect, 225, 229, 230-233f, 234, 235f

audio signal during pressure drop examination, 95-96

for cardiac function, 277-285

diastolic, 280-285

systolic, 277-280

in cardiac output measurement, 187-193

color-coded velocities, 30-36. *See also* Color-coded Doppler

continuous wave, 20-21, 20f. *See also* Continuous wave Doppler

conventional techniques, 16, 18-21. *See also* *under* normal examination *below*

differences between conventional modes, 21-22

effects causing interpretation difficulty, 79-84

deceleration instability, 80-81, 81f

induction, 82, 84f

masking, 83-84

series effect, 81

vortex shed distance, 82, 83f

examination technique for pressure drop, 95-97

frequency shift analysis in, 15-16, 17f

gray scale depiction of velocities, 28-30, 30f, 31f, 32f

high pulse repetition frequency, 20f, 21. *See also* Pulse repetition frequency, high

historical background, 1-6

in hypoplastic left heart syndrome, 262, 263f

in intracardiac masses, 271, 275-276f

in mitral regurgitation, 194, 195-200f, 201, 202f

normal examination, 39-67

Left atrium
  apical four chamber plane for, 52, 53f
  long axis plane for, 99-100
  mapping jet from mitral regurgitation in, 195-196f, 201
  shunting from right atrium with anomalous pulmonary venous drainage, 259
  suprasternal notch plane for, 106, 107f
Left heart, hypoplastic, 262, 263f
Left ventricle
  filling fraction as measure of function, 281, 283f
  function, 277-285
    diastolic, 280-285
    systolic, 277-280
  hypertrophy, E wave in, 284
  long axis plane for, 100
  outflow tract
    apical five chamber plane for, 58, 59f
    apical four chamber plane for, 104
    diastolic retrograde velocity in, 210, 212-213f
    flow measurement in, 177
    jets of regurgitant flow in aortic regurgitation in, 179f, 180
    long axis parasternal plane for, 45
    obstruction in transposition of great arteries, 266, 268f
    pressure drop at, 137-138
    truncal regurgitation in truncus arteriosus into, 252, 255f
    tumor occluding, 271, 275-276f
Left ventricular to right atrial shunt
  atrial septal defect distinguished from, 229
  tricuspid regurgitation jet distinguished from, 205
Long axis plane. *See under* Parasternal long axis plane; Subcostal plane
Lung disease, tricuspid regurgitation in, 205, 206f

Masking, 83-84
Mechanical alternans, cardiac output in, 187
Microbubbles, Doppler studies using, 84-85, 85f
Mitral regurgitation, 118-119, 119-121f, 194, 195-200f, 201, 202f
  aortic stenosis distinguished from, 110, 113f, 194
  apical four chamber plane for, 103, 194, 195-197f
  cardiac output measurement in assessing drug therapy, 190, 191f
  color-coded Doppler in, 194, Plate 16
  diagnostic Doppler findings, 194, 195-198f
  differentiation from other lesions by Doppler, 194, 201
  heart failure in, 119
  jet direction in, 194, 195-197f
  long axis imaging plane for, 99-100, 100f
  mapping regurgitant jet in left atrium in, 195-196f, 201
  in mitral valve prolapse, 119, 120-121f, 194, 198f
  mitral velocities in, 194, 199-200f, 201
  pressure half-time in, 296
  pulmonary hypertension in, 119
  quantitation of regurgitant flow, 181
  regurgitant velocities in, 201, 202f
  severity of disease estimation by Doppler, 201, 202f

subcostal four chamber plane for, 104, 104f
  suprasternal notch plane for, 106, 107f
  timing of, 194, 197f
  transducer placement in, 99-100, 100f, 103, 104, 104f, 106, 107f, 118, 194, 195-197f
  velocity waveform in jet in, 93, 93f
Mitral stenosis, 115-117
  aortic regurgitation distinguished from, 210, 216f
  long axis imaging plane for, 100, 100f
  parasternal short axis plane for, 101
  pressure drop in, 115-117, 117f
    historical background of Doppler studies, 4-5
  pressure half-time in, 296, 298f
  subcostal four chamber plane for, 104, 104f
  subcostal short axis plane for, 105, 106f
  transducer placement in, 100, 100f, 101, 105, 106f, 115
  tricuspid stenosis with, 117-118
  velocity waveform in jet in, 93
Mitral valve. *See also* Mitral regurgitation; Mitral stenosis
  A wave, 52, 53f, 54t
  apical four chamber plane for, 52, 53f, 55f
  atresia, hypoplastic left heart syndrome with, 262, 263f
  comparison of flow by indicator dilution and Doppler methods, 177
  E wave, 52, 53f, 54t. *See also* E wave
  flow area, 176-177
  flow measurement across, 4, 174f, 175-177
  pressure drop across, 4-5, 115-117, 117f
  pressure half-time method for area, 116-117, 296, 297f, 298f
  prolapse. *See* Mitral valve prolapse
  transducer placement for flow measurement, 175-176
  velocity findings, 52, 54t
    age related changes, 285
    ventricular function related to, 280-281, 282-283f, 284-285
Mitral valve prolapse
  mitral regurgitation in, 119, 120-121f
  systolic regurgitation jet in, 194, 198f
Motion, frequency related to, 9
Mustard operation
  pulmonary venous obstruction after, 266, 273f
  superior vena caval obstruction in, 271, 274f
  systemic venous inflow velocities after, 266, 271, 274f

Neoplasms, cardiac, 271, 275-276f
Nitroprusside, Doppler determination of cardiac output in assessing response, 190, 191f
Normal Doppler examination, 39-67. *See also* Doppler echocardiography, normal examination
Nyquist frequency limit, 23
Nyquist limit principle, 24

Obstruction
  flow disturbance at, 74-75, 76-78f
  jet distal to, 87
  jet flow at, 77